MENTAL HEALTH
Psycho-Social Perspectives

VOLUME FIVE: Adolescents & Childrens' Mental Health

The details of the volumes: Mental Health

Volume 1: Issues and Interventions

Volume 2: Multigroup Analysis

Volume 3: Strength of Human Resources

Volume 4: Therapeutic Applications

Volume 5: Adolescents & Children Mental Health

Volume 6: Women Mental Health

About the Editors

Aradhana Shukla (Ph.D.) is former Professor and Head, Department of Psychology and Dean (Arts) Kumaun University, Nainital. She is now Senior Fellow (ICSSR, New Delhi) at Department of Psychology, SSJ University, Almora. She has served here as a teacher for the last 35 years and before joining here she served as Research Associate (UGC,New Delhi), Gorakhpur University and Assistant Research Officer, at Department of Paediatrics, Banaras Hindu University. She guided 52 Ph.D. students and conducted five major research projects from NCERT, UGC, ICSSR and UNESCO. She served as a supportive supervisor in the GFATM Round 7 project. She has written 16 books and developed 15 psychological tests. She has published more than 200 research papers in national and international journals and edited volumes. Moreover, she has received 15 awards from the organisations of national and international repute. She has co-edited a series of mental health in 2015 (volume 1 & 2) and in 2017 (volume 3 & 4). She is an established motivational speaker and counselor. The major areas of her interest are Cross Cultural Psychology, Health Psychology, Positive Psychology and Mental Health Interventions. E-mail: aradhana.shukla5@gmail.com

Anubhuti Dubey is presently Professor and Head, Department of Psychology DDU Gorakhpur University, Gorakhpur and has been teaching here since 1998. Apart from publishing more than 60 research papers in journals, 10 chapters in edited volumes, she has written a book entitled 'Psychological Perspectives on Chronic Illness' (2012) and co-edited a series of mental health in 2015 (volume 1 & 2) and in 2017 (volume 3 & 4). Her research interests include Health Psychology, Positive Psychology, Gender issues, and Counselling. She is more interested in applying qualitative research methodology. She has carried out ICSSR research projects and 14 students have been awarded Ph.D. under her supervision and she has also guided 20 M.Phil. dissertation and more than 150 PG dissertations so for. She is also a Master Trainer and Supportive Supervisor for Training HIV/AIDS counsellors under GFATM-Round 7 Programme. E-mail: anubhutiddu@rediffmail.com

MENTAL HEALTH
Psycho-Social Perspectives

Volume Five

Adolescents & Children Mental Health

Edited by
Aradhana Shukla
Anubhuti Dubey

CONCEPT PUBLISHING COMPANY PVT. LTD.
NEW DELHI-110059

ISBN: 978-93-5125-173-6 (Series)
ISBN: 978-93-5439-017-3 (Vol. V)

First Published 2021

Published and Printed by

Concept
Since 1974

Concept Publishing Company Pvt. Ltd.
A/15-16, Commercial Block, Mohan Garden,
New Delhi-110059 (India)
T: 91 11 41101460, 91 11 25351460, 91 11 25351794
E: publishing@conceptpub.com, *W*: www.conceptpub.com

Cataloging in Publication Data--Courtesy: D.K. Agencies (P) Ltd. <docinfo@dkagencies.com>

Mental health : psycho-social perspectives / edited by Aradhana Shukla, Anubhuti Dubey.
volumes cm
Contributed articles.
Includes bibliographical references and index.
Contents: volume 5. Adolescents & childrens' mental health — volume 6. Women mental health
Volumes 5 6 received now
ISBN 9789351251736 (series)
ISBN 9789354390173 (vol. V)
ISBN 9789354390258 (vol. VI)

1. Teenagers—Mental health—India. 2. Child mental health—India. 3. Women—Mental health—India. I. Shukla, Aradhana, editor. II. Dubey, Anubhuti, editor.

LCC RA790.7.I5M46 2021 | DDC 362.20954 23

Preface

We desire to live a healthy and happy life. It is a common and well accepted fact that everyone desires to live a healthy life. The mind and bodily functions are closely embedded hence, the relative significance of mental health along with physical wellness cannot be denied. As mind and bodily functions are closely embedded we cannot deny the relative significances of mental health long with physical wellness. Mental health is an integral part of health, mental health is more than the absence of mental illness, and mental health is intimately connected with physical health and behaviour. Mental health is the foundation for well-being and effective functioning for an individual and for a community. Good mental health is a sense of wellbeing, confidence and self-esteem. It enables us to fully enjoy and appreciate other people, day-to-day life and our environment.

Mental health is the sheer responsibility of a person himself. The mental health field aims to deal with: (1) mentally ill people, (2) people at risk and, (3) promoting mental health of normal people so that their normality can be sustained.

If we go back into the history of mental health we can see that it was treated either as "boon of God "(good or positive mental health) or "curse of God "(bad or negative mental health). Both the eastern and western evidences support the notion. Not only in abroad but our ancient evidences also support this notion. The western literatures on mental health were seen hallucinations as communication of humans with bad souls, ghosts and witches. Moreover, in the ancient Indian literature of Ayurveda, Mental disorders are represented as various forms. The aetio-genesis of these disorders was thought to be endogenous because of provoked humours like vat, Pitta & Kalph. Exogenously the causes were attributed to sudden fear or association with ill influence of certain mythological gods or demon. Charak Samhita listed Psychiatry as 'Bhuta Vidya'. Psychotherapy was known as Ilaj-I-Nafsani in Unani Medicine. But time never remains stable.

Years and years were passed and the outlook of people towards mentally ill people become more and more aversive and they were treated like an undesirable social being for whom only such behaviour was required that was only meant for animals or criminals. Even with the advent of modern scientific methods and practical thoughts, the stigma and discrimination against mentally illnesses prevails the society. However, the advocates of Psychology started to cola soft touch and healing approach for the mentally ill people. Again it took decades to develop behaviour and psycho therapies against tying mentally ill people with iron chain, and treat them like prisoners. A complete soft and medico-human environment under single roof was constructed for them and it was termed as asylum or mental hospital. Psychologists attempted such patients to get out from the boundaries and from the trap of ojhas, neem-haquims and other such traditional healers and placed them at asylum. The patients were properly medicated along with different psychotherapies and many of them got complete recovery. At first the asylums were established in abroad but in India the first asylum was established in 1787 by Surgeon Kenderline in Calcutta and thereafter many asylums were made. This period was relatively longer but it opened the doors of a new era for the support and care of mental ill-health. Thcy not only paid attention to treat the mentally ill people but also concentrated on maintaining and nurturing public health, and trying to eradicate the stigma and discrimination faced by people with mental disorders. Psychologists and mental health care professionals are still trying to launch innovative programs for the same. The focal theme of these developmental programs is the utilization of community resources for mental health care. These programs have given new vision to the mental health care professionals to prevent mental disorders and promote mental health. This also needs a greater role for the non medical mental health care professionals and better utilization of cultural resources in terms of belief, practice and important social institutions like family and community groups. The contemporary world's realization about mental health and mental illness has come to a point where we find passionate discussions and caring mental health professionals to deal with mental disorder and promote well being.

Keeping these views into consideration the innovative thought of this series appeared in our mind and we decided to pool the thoughts of psychologists and health care professionals regarding various concerns of mental health. The basic aim of this series was: (i) to bring concepts, issues, strengths and treatment in a single jacket, (ii) bring a sense of mental health awareness in people so that they can make their health safe with additional attention on social health, (iii) to carve the research competence in young researchers, and (iv) to put forth the mental health policies before the readers, so that a better understanding of mental health can be developed.

About the Series Mental Health: Psycho Social Perspectives

It is a series on the psychology of mental health and we have tried to cover as many areas as possible and we could justify its name i.e. rethinking. Many traditional notions of mental health have been reconceptualised and many concepts in a new framework have been introduced. This series has four volumes:

1. **Mental health: Psychological Issues and Interventions:** In this volume we have covered various issues that foster or hamper mental health. Also, strategies to minimize negative mental health and improve positive mental health are discussed.
2. **Mental health: Multigroup Analysis:** This volume covers the conceptual background and psycho-social perspective of mental health in various social settings.
3. **Mental health: Strength of Human Resources:** In this volume we have tried to throw light on the promotional strategies of mental health following which a person can be relieved from negative mental health.
4. **Mental Health: Therapeutic Applications:** This volume covers a range of behavioural therapies which were found effective to minimize or overcome mental ill health.
5. **Mental Health of Adolescents and Children:** This volume presents a wide spectrum of the mental health of children and adolescents which are seen in them.
6. **Mental Health of Women:** This volume presents the mental health of women in different perspective

We have exercised our best attempt to seek out as many experiences as possible and we also anticipate that this will open new foresight for the researchers. However, we will be highly blessed to obtain the healthy and critical comments from our colleagues, seniors and friends and we will appreciate them from the bottom of our hearts.

Aradhana Shukla
Anubhuti Dubey

Acknowledgements

We, the editors, feel immense pleasure to present our series on mental health before the august readers. We hope that it will be admired by you all and the comments will be highly appreciated.

We fell our deep sense of gratitude and thankfulness to our respected contributors. If was their support that these volumes came in the shape. We are thankful to Mr. Abhishek and Mrs. Kavita Khawar for computer task.

Last but not least , we are thankful to Mr. Ashok Mittal, M/s. Concept Publishing Company Pvt. Ltd., New Delhi to shape our dreams in concrete form.

15 March, 2021

Aradhana Shukla
Anubhuti Dubey

Contents

Our Contributors

Adil Azeez is presently pursuing his Ph.D. from Department of Psychology, DDU Gorakhpur University, Gorakhpur, Uttar Pradesh. He has completed his Masters in Psychology (Gold Medalist, 2016) from Mahatma Gandhi Kashi Vidyapith, Varanasi, and one year Post Graduate Diploma in Counseling and Psychotherapy from Banaras Hindu University, Varanasi. His area of research includes social exclusion, socially excluded or marginalized children and adolescent groups like Orphans, Offspring of PLHA (People Living with HIV/AIDS) etc. **E-mail:** adilmgkvp.21.aa@gmail.com

Aishwarya Jaiswal is a research scholar at the Department of Psychology, Banaras Hindu University. She has strong interest in women and children mental health issues and rehabilitation approaches. In addition Ms. Jaiswal is working on exploring the dimensions and effectiveness of behavioural and psychological immune systems on human health and well-being. **E-mail**: aishj9000@gmail.com

Anubhuti Dubey is presently Professor of Psychology and has been teaching since 1998 at Department of Psychology, DDU Gorakhpur University, Gorakhpur (U.P.), India. Apart from publishing more than 45 research papers in journals, 33 chapters in edited volumes, she has written book entitled 'Psychological Perspectives on Chronic Illness' (2012) and also co-edited four volume series on Mental Health: Psycho-Social Perspectives: Issues and Intervention (Vol. 1, 2015); Multigroup Analysis (Vol. 2, 2015); Strength of Human Resources (Vol. 3, 2017); Therapeutic Applications (Vol. 4, 2017) and also 'Psyche of Asian Society' (2018). Her research interest includes Health Psychology, Positive Psychology, Gender issues, and Counselling. She is more interested in applying qualitative research methodology. She has carried out ICSSR research project and 11 students have been awarded Ph.D. under her supervision and she has also guided 4 M.Phil. dissertation and more than 100 PG dissertations so for. She is also a Master Trainer and Supportive Supervisor for Training HIV/AIDS counsellors under GFATM-Round 7 Programme. **E-mail:** anubhutiddu@rediffmail.com

Anushka Singh is school counselor, Sunbeam School, Lahartara, Varanasi.

Aradhana Shukla (Ph.D.) is former Professor and Head department of psychology and Dean (Arts) Kumaun University, Nainital. She is now Senior Fellow (ICSSR) at department of psychology, SSJ campus, Almora. She is serving here since last 35 years and before joining here she served as Research Associate (UGC), Gorakhpur University and Assistant Research Officer, at department of paediatrics, Banaras Hindu University. She guided 52 Ph.D. students and conducted four major research projects from NCERT, UGC and ICSSR. She served as supportive supervisor in GFATM Round 7 project. She has written 16 books and developed 15 psychological tests. She has come edited in a series of mental health. Its four volumes are appeared and two volumes are in progress. One edited volume on the Psyche of Asian Society is also co-edited by her. The major areas of her interest are cross cultural psychology, health psychology and mental health interventions. **E-mail:** aradhana.shukla5@gmail.com

Archana Shukla is Assistant Professor, Department of Psychology, and Coordinator of Institute of Women's Studies, University of Lucknow, Lucknow, Uttar Pradesh, India. Having more than 20 years of teaching experience, she has published 45 research papers in journals of national and international repute and contributed 15 chapters in edited books. Her research area of specialization includes gender, and LGBT community. **E-mail:** archana.kshitish@gmail.com

Dhananjay Kumar is Professor of Psychology in DDU Gorakhpur University, Gorakhpur, (U.P.), India, and has been teaching there for the past 21 years. His research interest includes cross cultural psychology, social cognition and intergroup relation, as well as health and counselling psychology. **E-mail:** dk_ddugu@yahoo.co.in

Garima Gupta is Assistant Professor in the Department of Psychology, Arya Mahila PG College, Varanasi. **E-mail:** grm.gupta2@gmail.com

Gunjan Joshi is pursuing her M.Phil. Clinical Psychology from King George Medical University, Lucknow, Uttar Pradesh, India. **E-mail:** gunjan051011@gmail.com

Kalpana Sahoo is an Assistant Professor in the area of Organizational Behavioural at Xavier School of Human Resource Management, Xavier University, Bhubaneswar, Odisha. She has published many papers in the areas of Learned Optimism, Positive Psychology, Competency Mapping, Employee Engagement, Emotional Intelligence and Personality in referred journals. Her teaching interests are in the areas of quality of work life, EQ & SQ, Psychological wellbeing, personality and leadership. **E-mail:** kalpana@xshrm.edu.in

Kanchan Verma is a Ph.D. Scholar in the Department of Psychology at Banaras Hindu University, Varanasi. Her present research focuses on correlates of body image dissatisfaction among adolescents and its association with their well being.

Lalawmpuia is M.Phil. Scholar, Department of Clinical Psychology, PGIBAMS, Raipur, Chhattisgarh. **E-mail**: oparalte6@gmail.com

Loisi Vanlalnguri is Research Scholar, Department of Psychology, Pachhunga University, Aizawl, Mizoram. **E-mail:** loisivlralte@gmail.com

Madhu G. Tapadia is Professor of Zoology at Banaras Hindu University, Varanasi, Uttar Pradesh. An expert of cell biology, she had completed major research projects from DBT, DST, SERB. She had written books on cell biology and published many research papers in journals. Her current researches are focused in the areas of Neurodegeneration, Innate Immune response, GENETic basis of depression in humans, and Development of Malpighian tubules.

Madhumita Roy is pursuing her doctoral research from Department of Zoology, Banaras Hindu University, Varanasi with a focus on molecular and genetic basis of depression. **E-mail:** madhubhu09@gmail.com

Madhurima Mukherjee is research scholar in the Department of Psychology, Banaras Hindu University, Varanasi, **E-mail:** madhurima.2323@gmail.com

Manish Kumar Jaisawal is Research Scholar in the Department of Psychology, Deen Dayal Upadhyaya Gorakhpur University, Gorakhpur. His area of interest is clinical psychology. He is a skilled Counsellor and Psychotherapist. Former Trainer at Bundl Tech. Pvt. Ltd. and at Prodigious Public School, Nema, Varanasi. He earned his Graduation and Post Graduation from Banaras Hindu University, Varanasi

Manoj Kr. Pandey is Assistant Professor, Department of Clinical Psychology, PGIBAMS, Raipur, Chhattisgarh. **E-mail:** manojpandey813@gmail.com

Mithilesh Kumar Tiwari is Assistant Professor in the Department of Psychology, SM College, TNB University, Bhagalpur, Bihar. His major area of interest is child rearing practices **E-mail:** mithilesh303318@gmail.com

Monika Shukla is pursuing B.Ed. at Kashi Vidyapith, Varanasi.

Neelam Verma is clinical psychologist, talk to cure online service.
E-mail: neelampsycho.86@gmail.com

Nishant Goyal, MD, DPM is Associate Professor of Psychiatry and In-charge Centre for Child and Adolescent Psychiatry, Central Institute of Psychiatry, Ranchi, Jharkhand. His research interest includes Child and Adolescent Psychiatry, Cognitive Neurosciences. He is working in the areas for more than 15 years. **E-mail:** psynishant@gmail.com

Purnima Awasthi is Associate Professor in the Department of Psychology, Banaras Hindu University, Varanasi. Her major area of expertise is cultural analysis of different social strata. **E-mail:** awasthip9@gmail.com

Rajbala Kumari is Research Scholar in Department of Psychology, Banaras Hindu University, Varanasi. Her area of research is clinical psychology. She is UGC NET & JRF. Gold Medalist in graduation from Women's College, Ranchi University, Ranchi and a Post-Graduate from Banaras Hindu University, Varanasi.

Rinpari Ralte is Associate Professor & Head, Department of Psychology, Pachhunga University, Aizawl, Mizoram. **E-mail:** mapari27@yahoo.co.in

Ruchi Tiwari is Academic Associate at Uttarakhand Open University, Haldwani. Her area of interest is cultural differentials in children. **E-mail:** rtewari@uou.ac.in

Saroj Verma is professor in the Department of Psychology at Banaras Hindu University, Varanasi. She has more than twenty years of teaching experiences. Her current research interests include parenting behaviours, adolescents' mental health, and personality.

Shakshi Priya Giri is presently a Research Scholar in the Department of Psychology, Deen Dayal Upadhyaya Gorakhpur University, Gorakhpur (U.P.). She had earlier worked as a Junior Research Fellow (JRF) in the Mental Health Division at Defence Institute of Psychological Research, DRDO, New Delhi. She has pursued her Masters in Psychology from DDU Gorakhpur University, Gorakhpur. As a research scholar she is working in the area of multidimensional loneliness and its relationship with emotional functionality and depressive symptomatology. **E-mail:** shakshipriyagiri@gmail.com

Shivangi Pandey is Research Scholar, Department of Psychology, DDU Gorakhpur University, Gorakhpur. She is doing research linking Triguna, Spirituality and identity with happiness and health in various age groups.

Shivani Pandey is Research Scholar, Department of Psychology, University of Lucknow, Lucknow, Uttar Pradesh, India.

Shobhna Joshi is a Professor of Psychology in the Faculty of Social Sciences, Banaras Hindu University. She has earned her Post Doctoral Fellowship from BHU. She had authored two books and has a teaching experience of twenty years. Her specialization is Developmental, Educational and Sports Psychology with special reference to adolescents. She is actively engaged in Haemophilia Society, Varanasi Chapter. She is also Co-ordinator and consultant of Career, Guidance and Counseling Cell, Student Welfare Centre, Banaras Hindu University. She has 47 research publications of national and International repute. **E-mail:** getshobhna@yahoo.com

Shubhra Sinha is Assistant Professor in the Department of Psychology, Vasant Kanya Mahavidyalaya, Varanasi, her major area of interest is cultural analysis of parent-child relationship. **E-mail:** usss_ss@rediffmail.com

Sweta Pathak is Assistant Professor in the Department of Psychology TNB College, TNB University Bhagalpur, Bihar, her major area of interest is parent-child relationship, **E-mail:** swetapsybhu@gmail.com

Tilottama Mukherjee is Associate Professor in the Department of Psychology, University of Calcutta, Kolkata. **E-mail:** tilottamamukherjee3@gmail.com

Turfa Ahmed is a Post-Graduate student in the Department of Psychology, University of Calcutta, Kolkata.

Tushar Singh: Dr. Tushar Singh is an Assistant Professor in the Department of Psychology, Banaras Hindu University. He is associated with various national and international research groups and is the recipient of several national and international awards. Presently Dr. Singh is serving as Treasurer of the National Academy of Psychology (NAOP), India and is the member of the

Board of Directors of the International Association of Applied Psychology. **E-mail**: tusharsinghalld@gmail.com

Usha Verma Srivastava is Clinical Psychologist and EDMR practitioner at Samvedana Centre of Neuropsychological Rehabilitation and Mental Well-being, Varanasi. **E-mail:** ushavermasri@gmail.com

Vandana Singh is presently a Research Scholar in the Department of Psychology, Deen Dayal Upadhyaya Gorakhpur University, Gorakhpur (U.P.). She is ICSSR Doctoral Fellow. She has pursued her Masters in Psychology from DDU Gorakhpur Univehrsity, Gorakhpur. As a research scholar she is working in the area of school psychology focusing on school climate and social skills in students. **E-Mail:** vandanasingh.9324@gmail.com

Vatsala Pathak is presently a Research Scholar in the Department of Psychology, Deen Dayal Upadhyaya Gorakhpur University, Gorakhpur (U.P.). She has completed her Masters in Psychology from DDU Gorakhpur University, Gorakhpur with gold medal. As a research scholar she is using qualitative research methods to understand psychology of visually challenged people. **E-mail**: vatsalapathak@ymail.com

Velprashanth Venkatesan, Senior Resident, Centre for Child and Adolescent Psychiatry, Central Institute of Psychiatry, Ranchi, Jharkhand. His areas of interest include Neurobiology of Mood Disorder and Child and Adolescent Psychiatry.

Vibha Kriti is Research Scholar, Department of Psychology, Banaras Hindu University, Varanasi, Uttar Pradesh, India.

Yogesh Kumar Arya is an Assistant Professor in the Department of Psychology, Banaras Hindu University, Varanasi. His major areas of Interest are cognition, health, and wellbeing. He has published several research papers in many reputed journals and is contributing as "Associate Editor" of Indian Journal of Social Sciences Researches. **E-mail**: yogeshatbhu@gmail.com

1

Introduction

Aradhana Shukla and *Anubhuti Dubey*

The concept of mental health can be thought as the absence of mental illness and presence of such psychological activities that come under the underpinnings of positive social behaviour, in general and personal growth and gratification in particular. It is the state of some one who is, "functioning at a satisfactory level of emotional and behavioural adjustment". From the perspective of positive psychology mental health may include an individual's ability to relish life and create a balance between life activities and efforts to achieve psychological resilience. In accordance with WHO (World Health Organization) mental health includes subjective wellbeing, perceived self-efficiency, autonomy, competence, intergenerational dependence and self-actualization of one's emotional and intellectual potential among others.

Mental health in childhood and adolescence means to achieve the required milestones of psychophysical, emotional and behavioural wellness that are the demand of that particular age group. It reflects the fact that mental health in adolescence and childhood is learning healthy social skills and the knowledge and application of better coping behaviour to meet and solve any problem. Mentally healthy children, at maximum have a positive and desirable quality of life in home, school and every domain of life.

Mental disorder in children is the outcome of the reformative behaviour produced by their parents, siblings, teachers and/or other members of the society. Although there are some features of childhood behaviour like shouting, running, quarreling, temper tantrums, pulling hair of each other, biting etc. are found more or less common in children but increase in these activities is a matter of problem. Mental disorders change the entire childhood and cause distress and problems getting through the day. Other conditions and concerns that affect children's learning, behaviour and emotions include learning and developmental disabilities, autism and risk factors like substance use and self-harm.

Moreover, children develop so many disruptive, impulse control and conduct disorders which in normal range becomes a part of life and with increase in magnitude it becomes "A problem" for the family and society. It is true that there is a need of understanding the psyche of children with proper care, handle them with full support for development and foster them by developing four H's (Hand, Head, Heart and Health) in them.

Keeping these views in consideration this volume is planned. Actually, this volume is the fifth appearance of a series on mental health entitled, "Mental health: Psychosocial Perspective" and it focuses on various issues and challenges pertaining to the mental health of adolescents and children.

This volume is consisted of twenty four research articles. They are review papers and/or empirical investigation reports. The first chapter "Introduction" written by the editors, Aradhana Shukla and Anubhuti Dubey have shared their views on the concept of mental health and briefed the papers incorporated here. The next paper is also written by Aradhana Shukla and Anubhuti Dubey and role of family and parenting is discussed in the realm of mental health promotion. Archana Shukla and Shivangi Pandey have shared their views on the mental health construct in many situations. They presented their views on the intellectually disabled children and related it with parental stress and their coping. In thc cra of globalization, children and adolescents' mental health is discussed widely by Nishant Goel and Velprashanatu Venkateshan. Neelam Verma explained the role of bullying in child development and the scenario of substance use in Mizorum is narrated by Manoj Kr. Pandey, Lalaumpuia, Rinpari Ralte and Loisi Vanlalnguri. Relative significance of peer group has discussed by Aradhana Shukla in her paper entitled, "Teenager Adolescents and Children in Schools: Peer Group Pressure and Mental Health. Shivangi Pandey and Anubhuti Dubey have shed light on the conjunction of spirituality and mental health and happiness in adolescents is discussed by Madhumita Roy, Shobhna Joshi and Madhu G. Tapadia. Also, they discussed stress and depression in adolescents as related with their genetic predispositions. Similarly, cognitive style and academic achievement is studied by Madhumita Mukherjee and Purnima Awasthi and Sakshi Priya Giri and Anubhuti Dubey have explained the concept of Parlous effect and academic anxiety as affected by cultural variation, gender and age is well narrated by Ruchi Tiwari and Aradhana Shukla.

Social anxiety as predicted with parenting style and perceived social support is thoroughly narrated by Turfa Ahmed and Tilottama Mukherjee and Manish Kumar, Raj Bala Kumari and Dhananjay Kumar have focused the burning issue of COVID-19 and discussed the issue of challenges and coping by the children during the time of COVID-19. Problems and challenges faced by adolescent orphans is described by Adil Azeez and Anubhuti Dubey and Sweta Pathak, Mithilesh Kumar Tiwari and Shubhra Sinha have shed light on the role of self-disclosure. Kalpana Sahoo described the role of empowerment in school-based community programme and Garima Gupta, Anushka Singh, Monika Shukla and Usha Verma Srivastava have explored the development of sustainable intervention programme for autistics in a case study perspective.

Vatsala Pathak and Anubhuti Dubey in a review paper shared their views on visually impaired children. A relationship between attachment and well-being is critically reviewed by Gunjan Joshi and Vandana Singh and Anubhuti Dubey discussed mental health promotion among students following school based approach. Further in the paper of Aradhana Shukla has sketched the role of counsellor in school settings to increase the strength of children and adolescents. Kanchan Verma, Saroj Verma and Purnima Awasthi have elaborately dealt with aggression among adolescents in relation to social intelligence and self-esteem.

Aishwarya Jaiswal, Tushar Singh and Yogesh Kumar Arya have brought to fore the ill-effects of the abuse or overuse of modern ICT tools on children whereas Sreeja Das, Rahul Varma, Tushar Singh and Yogesh Kumar Arya have addressed the issue of child sexual abuse in their chapter.

All the papers selected here are visionary and thought increasing. They present mental health of adolescents and children in a wide spectrum. We hope that they will satisfy the needs of mental health knowledge of researchers, teachers and mental health professionals and flourish new insight and vision in them.

2

Family and Parenting

Promotion of Mental Health in Adolescents and Children

Aradhana Shukla and *Anubhuti Dubey*

Health is a valuable asset for all and it is highly essential to maintain good quality of life. Good health provides optimism and better understanding of the world while a person being in poor health does not show good adjustment with the society and even with himself which results in terms of so many psychophysical disorders in him.

Mental health can be understood as a personal quality up to any extent or magnitude. Each person possess a set of mental health attributes and variation in the amount and magnitude of these attributes decide the presence/existence of positive and/or negative mental health in the concerned person. It is also felt or experienced as a mould of life and every situation is differently faced and experienced by different people due to their own experiences and explanation. Therefore, it can be said that mental health is- the state of someone anyone who is, "functioning a satisfactory level of emotional and behavioural adjustment (WHO, 2014). From the view of positive psychology mental health is the combined product of searching enjoyment in life and experiences it creating a positive balance between favourable and unfavourable events and having psychological resilience (Snyder, Lopez and Pedrotti, 2011). In accordance with World Health Organization mental health includes subjective well-being, perceived self-efficacy, autonomy, competence, intergenerational dependence and self-actualization of one's intellectual and emotional potential among others (WHO Report, 2001, 2014). A mentally healthy person is encompassed by the realization of his abilities, coping with normal stress in life, productive work and thus, contributes the overall community. Cultural setting, individual differences and circumstances decide the pattern and magnitude of mental health. It is not a state but it varies according to personal demands and external requirements.

Up to a large extent we cannot deny the fact that mental health is functioned by emotional maturity, positive conditions and favourable surroundings that are emerged at first from the family and cultivated by society and turns into emotional bonding. This emotional bonding, as the child grows up, increase with the help of positive and desirably favored social events. So, it can be claimed that positive family and social surroundings play an important and leading role in shaping the individual personality (Dwivedi, 2000; Lall, 2012; Ojha, 2005; Shukla, 2013; Pant, 2009; Thagunna, 2009). These determinants also, lay the foundation of mental health.

Home is the matrix of any individuals' mental health and parents, grandparents, siblings and other relatives perform a major role in the formation of life. A home atmosphere where mutual trust prevails, adds a sense of security, positive personality and increases mental hygiene. Theories and views of Baumrind (1991) have suggested that authoritative attitude of parents towards their children increases positivity in them (Srivastava, 1994). There are some and certain self-evident precautions to be observed in the way of not playing favourites by being more generous with one child than with another because there are so many psychological dangers of playing favourites.

The concept of mental health has found varied with more or less magnitude in different culture and it is determined by the cultural specificity and need of the time. Although self-esteem, tolerance, adjustment in a typical situation, feeling of security and self-confidence are commonly found in every culture yet, adequate self-knowledge and life goal, environmental mastery, growth, maturation and learning from experiences in life, integration and consistency of personality are also the other significant aspects of mental health.

Role of Family in Promoting Positive Mental Health Family is a unit of society which live under one roof, share the common kitchen and all sources of finance and most important is that they comprised with one male, one female and their children. Some time children are also nested with their grandparents. Also, most of the studies have shown that family at first responsible to observe the child's behaviour and notable differences have deficits found (Clark 1996; Goldman 1984; Dean & Hayat Baksh, 2014; Carli, Hoven and Wasserman et al. 2014; Hagequist 2009). As the parents are the pillars of the family and they bear a huge responsibility on their shoulders to upbring their children they should make a peaceful, encouraging and warm atmosphere of home to provide positive and nutritional cognitive and emotional diet to their children. McCloskey, Figuriolo and Ross (1995) and McClean, Sweating and Hunt (2010) have examined many families and the role of familial aggression in the resultant psycho-pathological behaviour of their children. They were aimed to find out the form of children's aggression that might take in violent home and whether close ties within the family (to the mother or a sibling) in buffered children. They found that different forms of abuse in the homes were highly interrelated and that children of battered women at risk for child abuse. Domestic violence predicted children's general pathology but specific forms of disorders was found absent. It was also noted that parental and sibling warmth was quite normal. Dubey and Srivastava (2013) studied the parental factors and achievement motivation and its relation to performance of adolescents. Amongst the four parental factors, parental approval emerged as the most significant predictor of achievement motivation and performance followed by resources made available by parents, parental engagement and parental pressure.

Children and adolescents were also studied in Kumaun Himalaya. In so many studies (Shukla & Joshi, 2017a, 2017b; Pandey & Shukla, 2018; Joshi & Shukla, 2018) it was noted that the development of children and adolescents and their behavioural mode is also determined by social support, stress and stress management, residential locale (Gailakoti & Shukla, 2012), emotional intelligence and many more affectors.

The role of family structure, its function and impact an children's mental health is very important and it has a lead role in shaping the child development. The interest in the area was started in the 1960 and 1970 and the impact of divorce and single parenting on the development of positive mental health was a matter to be studied (Avison, 2002; Oliver, Kuhns and Pomeranz, 2006; Holdon & Smock, 1991). It was also noted that most commonly, children coming from such families were suffered from ADHD, mood disorders, oppositional defiant disorder and physical abuse increasing the risk by more than twice.

Over a years, there has been a general concern that single parenting (whether mothering or fathering) lay its important on the child rearing. Such types of parenting is found less resilient, economically deprived/ financially insecured and hyper stressed. In case, such family possesses a well-of financial support it is found somewhere failed to provide acceptable and desirable rearing practices to their children. Further, economic disadvantage and cognitive insecurity in the parent (single) lead to high level of emotional and behaviour problem in children (Offord, Boyle and Jones, 1997).

Role of Parents in Promoting Mental Health in Children and Adolescents

Parenting is a complex activity that includes many specific behaviours that work individually and together to influence outcomes. Although specific parenting behaviours, such as speaking of reading aloud, may influence child development, looking at any specific behaviour in isolation may be misleading. Many writers have noted that specific parenting practices are less important in predicting child well-being than in the broad pattern of parenting. Most researchers who attempt to describe this broad parental milieu rely on Diana Baumrind's concept of parenting style. The construct of parenting style is used to capture normal variations in parents' attempts to control and socialize their children (Baumrind, 1991). Two views emerged after the classic explanation of Baumrind. First, parenting style is meant to describe normal variations in parenting. In other words, the parenting style typology Baumrind developed should not be understood to include deviant parenting such as might be observed in abusive of neglectful homes. Second, Baumrind assumes that normal parenting revolves around issues of control. Although parents may differ in how they try to control or socialize their children and the extent to which they do so, it is that the primary role of all parents is to influence, teach and control their children.

Parenting style captures two important elements of parenting: parental responsiveness and parental demandingness (Maccoby & Martin, 1983). Parental responsiveness (also referred to as parental warmth of supportiveness) refers to the extent to which parents intentionally foster individually, self-regulation, and self-assertion by being attuned, supportive and acquiescent to children's special needs and demands (Baumrind, 1991) while parental demandingness (also referred to as behavioural control) refers to the claims parents make on children to become integrated into the family whole, by their maturity demands, supervision, disciplinary efforts and willingness to confront the child who disobeys (Baumrind, 1991). Parents play a central, but not exclusive, role in shaping the lives of their children and teenagers. Extensive researches show that parents are more influential in their children's lives than anyone else, shaping their thoughts, feelings and behaviours. Yet parents are neither the only influences nor the only ones with responsibility. Peers, other adults, genetics the media, and various other sources also play important roles. Ideally, all these influences can work together with parents to promote young people's healthy development.

Parents Affect Children's Thoughts and Feelings

Researches and common sense state that emotional and cognitive developments are fostered through relationships with parents. The effects of parents on children begin at (or before) birth and last a lifetime. For example, parent's responsiveness to their infant children has long lasting effects on emotional adjustment and cognitive development. While it used to be a commonly held belief that responding to an infant's cries would spoil her or him. Researches now shows us the importance of creating a sense of security through comforting the baby on later emotional and cognitive development.

As infants turn into children and children become adolescents they begin to spent more unsupervised time with their friends and have increased exposure to sources of influence and information outside of their family such as media and school influences that parents often view as harmful to their children (Farkas et al., 2002). However, the importance of parents does not diminish as children age. While adolescents may go to their peers more often than their parents for advice for example, they still choose to go to their parents in time of real need or while making serious decisions (Freeman & Brown 2001) but choose to prefer school subject as their school friends do.

Parental Influence During Adolescence

Discussions about adolescent behaviour often focus on negative actions such as delinquency or early sexual behaviour. This focus treats successful adolescent and young adults as escape artists who manage to dodge the hazards of growing up rather than focusing on the ways that young people acquire and master skills construct positive identities and learn how to negotiate social roles simultaneously in the youth culture and adult world (Firstenberg, 2002).

There are several ways that parents and parenting affect adolescent's positive and negative behaviours. For example, family cohesion and having strong attachments to parents help kids make better decisions about which friends they choose (Warr, M., 1993). On side higher levels of supervision are associated with less delinquency and adolescents who feel close to their parents are more likely to having sex. Even among kids with deviant peers those with closer relationship to parents tended to get in less trouble than those with less close relationship (Ardelt et al., 2002).

Categorizing parents according to whether they are high or low on parental demandingness and responsiveness creates a typology of four parenting styles: indulgent, authoritarian authoritative, and uninvolved (Maccoby & Martin, 1983). Each of these parenting styles reflects different naturally occurring patterns of parental values, practices, and behaviours (Baumrind, 1991) and a distinct balance of responsiveness and demandingness.

Indulgent parents (also referred to as permissive or non-directive) are more responsive than they are demanding. They are non-traditional and lenient, do not require mature behaviour, allow considerable self-regulation, and avoid confrontation (Baumrind, 1991). Indulgent parents may be further divided into two types: democratic parents, who, though lenient, are more conscientious, engaged, and committed to the child, and non-directive parents.

Authoritarian parents are highly demanding and directive, but not responsive. They are obedience–and status-oriented, and expect their orders to be obeyed without explanation (Baumrind, 1991). These parents provide well-ordered and structured environments with clearly stated rules. Authoritarian parents can be divided into two types: non-authoritarian directive, who are directive, but not intrusive or autocratic in their use of power, and authoritarian-directive, who are highly intrusive.

Authoritative parents are both demanding and responsive. They monitor and impart clear standards for their children's conduct. They are assertive, but not intrusive and restrictive. Their disciplinary methods are supportive, rather than punitive. They want their children to be assertive as well as cooperative (Baumrind, 1991).

Modern Models of Parenting and Abroad

Parenting typically utilizes tools of reward and punishment method, but most child development experts now agree that corporal punishment is not an effective behaviour modification tool. In some jurisdictions corporal punishment (e.g., spanking or whipping) has been prohibited by law. Many parents have adopted non-physical approaches to child discipline, for example time-out. The other civilized forms of discipline behavioural control, structure, accountability, parental supervision, etc.

Other Modern Models of Parenting

Examples of other modern parenting models include:

- *Nurturant parent model*—a family model where children are expected to explore their surroundings with protection from their parents.
- *Strict father model*—places a strong value on discipline as a means to survive and thrive in a harsh world.
- Attachment parenting seeks to create strong emotional bonds, avoiding physical punishment and accomplishing discipline through interactions recognizing a child's emotional needs all while focusing on holistic understanding of the child.
- *Taking children seriously*—sees both praise and punishment as manipulative and harmful to children and advocates other methods to reach agreement with them.

Empirical Analysis of Parenting in India

The study of human development in general and of parenting, socialization and child rearing in particular has been a field neglected by the mainstream psychologists. It is only during the last three decades that some interest has been shown in this area. With the initiatives taken by D. Sinha (1988), Anandlakshmy (1980), Nandy and Kakar (1980), Krishnan (1998), Saraswathi (1987, 1997, 1999) and Saraswathi and Kaur (1979), work in this domain has been integrated and given further impetus. The studies published in this area have been of diverse kinds including theoretical analysis based on texts (e.g. Kakar, 1979) as well as empirical investigations. Commenting on the research scenario Saraswathi and Dutta (1987) observed that the study of child rearing practices and their consequences for personality development has continued to be an area of both theoretical and research interests. Researches have focused on social class and urban rural differences in child rearing and on the consequences of some child rearing practices for selected personality variables. Theorizing has remained essentially within the psychoanalytic framework". This trend still holds true for a large number of studies done in this field.

The studies in this area up to 1985 have been summarized by Saraswathi and Dutta (1987). Therefore, only a brief and selective account of relevant work is presented to indicate the trends in research. Some of these studies have focused on the customs and practices observed in birth and upbringing of children in specific groups. For instance Kaur, Sisodia and Mehra (1981) examined the positive and negative aspects of various practices observed during birth and upbringing the child of a village in Haryana and suggested some measures to improve the conditions of children. Swain (1978) studied the beliefs and customs associated with pregnancy and childbirth in rural Orissa and suggested to encourage the beneficial customs, ignore the neutral ones and try to change the harmful ones.

Some researchers have explored the reasons for having children like the one done by Singh, Bhargava and Kumar (1981). In this study the biological, cultural, political and economic motivations behind wanting children have been uncovered. Kakar (1979) has studied the traditional Indian ideas concerning the child' and how these ideas have influenced the contemporary reality of childhood. He has suggested the cultural proscriptions relating to childhood and how it informs the behaviour of adult caretakers. The values and behaviours in the context of child rearing as an aspect of individual modernity and traditionalism are also discussed. Raina, Kumar and Raina (1980) found a close agreement in a comparative study between 165 East Indian fathers and American parents concerning the characteristics to be encouraged or discouraged in children but found a poor correlation with the rankings of experts.

Seth and Saksena (1978) investigated the attitudes of literate and illiterate mothers towards child rearing with the help of Schaefer and Bells Parental Attitude Research Instrument (PARI). The literate mothers were found to encourage verbalisation in their children, believed more in seclusion of the mother, experienced greater marital conflict, were stricter, suppressed their aggression, rejected their home-making role, were more inconsiderate toward their husband and believed in the dependency of the mother. Illiterate mothers fostered dependency in there children, believed in approving the activities of their children, suppressed sexuality, and favoured the dependency of the mother. In an investigation by Seymour (1976) of child rearing practices among a upper, middle and low caste households in an Indian town revealed certain significant differences in parent-child behaviour between the lower socio-economic status households and the higher status ones.

Singh and Kaur (1981) found that the rural mothers interacted more with girls than with boys. They felt that girls needed more instruction and discipline than did boys. On the other hand mothers' interaction was related to her educational level mother-child interaction was greater when mothers were more educated. Both urban and rural mothers used tactics such as attention, diversion, discouragement, scolding and speaking to discipline their children.

The traditional Indian family has an authoritarian structure and it stresses conformity and deemphasizes autonomy and independence.

Gore (1978); Roland (1978), and Bisht and Sinha (1981), have reported significant influence of family structure on the interaction among family members. Sharma (1971), Mehra (1974), and Begum (1975) found positive influence of parents' educational level and SES on personality development of children.

Joshi and Tiwari (1977) studied personality development of children in relation to child rearing practices across different socioeconomic classes and that socio-economic status does affect child rearing practices. According to them, middle class mothers, who use praise and reward to inculcate obedience and desirable behaviours, are more punitive (spanking) and less consistent in their threatening and punitive behaviours than mothers of upper class. Extent of parental approval for disciplining techniques for children exists greater in middle class homes than in the upper class homes. Mostly fathers are considered as disciplinary agents for children in the middle class homes. Sharma, Saraswathi and Giri (1981) reported a positive relationship between parental warmth and affection, and sense of competence in their children.

Sinha (1984) has reported about pregnancy taboos of Bhil tribe of Madhya Pradesh, Gujarat and Rajasthan. The taboos were crossing a broom stick and the tying ropes of horse, ass and mare. They had a belief that the above said animals deliver their babies only in twelve months. Thus, a violation of the above taboo may lead to the same consequence to a pregnant woman and deliver a baby in twelfth month. Another taboo also observed that was seeing a dead body.

In a study done by Varinhva (1993) the beliefs and practices related to infant care among the Tangkhul Nagas of Manipur were investigated. These beliefs were related to pregnancy, childbirth, nutrition and physical care and health management. Also, the intergenerational differences were found out. In a sample of 20 families detailed interviews and observations of mothers were carried out. Traditional rituals and practices dominated all areas associated with the infant from prenatal period to birth process, diet pattern, routine care of the infants, methods of health care and interaction with the family.

Some of the researchers have studied the practices related to marriage and child birth among the non-tribals. Minturn and Hitchcock (1966) conducted a study on Rajputs of Khalapur as a part of famous six culture and found taboos during pregnancy. They included the avoiding of milk, cold rice, a pulse dish, food which combined either 'excessively hot' or 'cxccssively cold' and spicy foods such as pickles. It was noted that culture guides the food intake of the pregnant woman by providing suggestions for both the foods she should eat and the ones that are prohibited or at least undesirable. Different cultures and subcultures as well as the same culture in different historical periods and at different lends of economics development have idiosyncratic lists of permissible and prohibited foods. Particular foods become linked with beliefs about particular harms or benefits in the physiological, psychological and social realms of the child's and mother's lives (Valsiner, 1987).

As indicated earlier traditional child care attitudes and practices in India are guided by the principle of child-centredness. Children are considered as the gift of God. They are totally indulged, protected, and there is a belief in total gratification and minimum frustration for the child, permissiveness in training and little or no pressures to become autonomous and independent. Hence, in contrast to the Western conceptualizations, childhood in India is a golden period.

Carstairs' (1967) study has provided a psychoanalytic treatment of Hindu childhood. He has emphasized the physical closure between the Hindu mother and the child. In the first two years child and mother are seldom apart, commonly, the baby is seen astride the mother's hip. The mother held her child this way even as she does her chores. Past age too, when the child is somewhat less often by the mother's side it is common to see a relative, perhaps an older sister holding the child. The child sleeps with the mother, and the breast is kept accessible. No baby is allowed to cry for long since the breast is offered on demand. Citing a Hindu proverb Carstairs' compares the child to a king. What the baby wants. It gets. Its needs are indulged. Children, for example are rarely scolded for soiling in the home. Mothers uncomplainingly clean up a mess. Carstairs says, sucking is moderately prolonged, weaning taking place between the age of two and two-and-a half years. Weaning, Carstairs' informs, is difficult, provoking many days of crying and anger.

In Carstairs' (1967) account, one of the few frustrations in early childhood come in the presence of the father's mother i.e. the mother's mother-in-law. Carstairs' treatment of the mother-in-law's role illustrates the treatment of third-party caretakers in the traditional psychoanalytic model. In Hindu custom, if there is no cry for the breast, a mother ought not to pay attention to her child in her mother-in-law's presence. Often, if the mother-in-law is in attendance the child will be given over to her by the mother.

Kakar (1978) has observed that the psychosocial quality of infancy extends through the first four or five years of life. During this prolonged infancy, the Indian child is intensely and intimately attached to her mother.

The attachment is an exclusive one, not in the sense of being without older and younger siblings close in age who claim and compete for the mother's love and care, but in that the Indian child up to the age of four or five, exclusively directs his demands and affection towards his mother in spite of the customary presence in the extended household of many other customary caretakers and substitute' mothers.

Kakar's (1978) analysis has suggested that the intense relationship shared with the mother makes the child believe that the world is benign and that others can be counted on to act on his behalf. Social relationships built later are based on this belief in which suspicion and reserve are rare, trustworthiness and friendliness are in abundance. The spontaneous nuturance available to the child and the warm handling by several adults in the family contribute to vitality and intimacy in social relationship throughout one's life. Kakar states that unhurried and relaxed form to toilet training contributes to a relative feeling of timelessness and tolerance of contradictory impulses both within oneself and others.

Kurtz (1992) argues that the psychoanalytic work by Kakar and other in Hindu society is beholden to the dominance of concepts of individualism, individuation and primacy of single mother-child dyad. He has argued that in Hindu joint family a multiplicity of women, not a single natural mother, collectively rear children. This leads to an appreciation that the ineptness and goal of development in Hindu society is not individuation but an integration into the collective groups which structure the social order.

Neki (1976) has analysed the child rearing practices in the development of dependency by comparing the Indian and the Western cultures. He found that the western culture encourages independence whereas the Indian child rearing fosters dependence.

Srivastava, Banerjee and Tripathi (1995) studied parental views regarding the perceived values and costs in having a child. He identified two main value types—psychological and economical. The urban parents considered children to be more of psychological value such as children make life more meaningful and are a source of love and provide company. In contrast, rural parents value children for their economic values i.e. performance of domestic chores, followed by psychological value of children. Child rearing values also reflected family relations and changes in them. Regarding the costs of children the parental responses indicated the impact of urbanization and industrialization. Majority of the parents were worried about their children's future and wished their children to be successful in life. Parents' response indicated the change in the Indian setting from a collectivistic orientation in which greater emphasis was on societal functioning and family was the social unit to a personalized orientation due to the contemporary setup in the urban areas.

The context of childhood in the traditional Indian families involves a complex structure in which an interplay of personal and contextual factors takes place a dynamic fashion. Attention to balance the influences beyond one's control is always evident. It is believed that placement of stars at the time of birth of the child determines his/her fate. The horoscope or *janampatri* is often made and consulted on critical occasions (e.g. marriage, illness, job etc.). All this indicates a belief in some form of pre-determinism in parents (Misra, Srivastava and Gupta, 1999).

The traditional Indian view holds that each and every individual is endowed with certain competencies and ordered life course. Many people subscribe to the view that parents transfer merits and demerits to their children. A child is considered as an extension of her parents. The similarities between parents and children are often identified and emphasized during conversations in the family. Fathers and mothers also consider their children as self-objects, through which they are defined. As a result, for many Indian parents socialization happens to be an occasion for their own self-articulation. The locus of this articulation is often perceived to be lying within the psyche of parents themselves.

The description mentioned above denotes the fact that parenting is widely studied in India. Although the above mentioned review indicates that so many studies have done in Indian and Western setting and it is quite sure that they provide us a message and platform for child rearing and different models of parenting. They also provide a thought that the child reared up in a given cultural values and social norms reveals entirely different behaviour pattern. Even after rearing in a proper and well accepted mode children have a lot of problems. These problems may generate either by family or society or by themselves as they grow older and develop their peer group relation. It sometimes, causes disruption in them and they become the problem for the society and even for them also. Such disruption also destroys their mental health and they do not found well to adjust in the society. Moreover, they manifest many behavioural deficits like, inability to adopt change and use of coping behaviour, failure in maintaining the relationship with others, poor health conditions, mood disorder, irritability, temper tantrum, lying, back cheating etc. Such type of problems although arise due to stress, emotional insecurity, death of a loved one, suicidal thought, grief, addiction, ADHD, self-harm, mood swing or disorder or any other mental illness as well as learning disabilities

(Kitchner & Jorm, 2002; Shook 2012; Bertolote 2008), yet the role of parents in minimizing the problem with a deep concern to their children can not be avoided. Patternson and associates (1992) have found that the parents who are failed to:

(i) tell their children about accepted behaviour,
(ii) monitor their children's behaviour to ensure that it was desirable, and
(iii) enforce the rules promptly and unambiguously with appropriate rewards and penalties, proved them as failed parents of deficient children. So, there is a need to understand the behaviour, problem and individuality of the children following the rules of here, care and trust. Parents can understand the children and rear them in a way by which desirable and approved development could be possible. Here are some suggestions for parents to modify the behaviour of their children and promote good and positive mental health in them:

As the home environment is regarded the major determinant of human development (Alim, 2007) the parents should try to maintain a positive and supportive climate at home and minimize the level of stressful situation.

- They should be aware of the relative significance of psychophysical health which is highly based on good eating habits physical fitness, positive interaction with parents, siblings and other family members.
- They should also teach them socially adequate behaviour and act themselves accordingly.
- They should make a watch on the school related activities and peer group with their eye on the activities of children.

All these attempts are highly necessary for the parents and they should be strictly follow to make their children a good citizen.

References

Alim, F. (2007). Pattern of mental health in adolescents. In; S. Malhotra., P. Batra and A. Yadav (Eds.), *Health Psychology*, New Delhi, Globol.

Allen, J.P., Hauser, S.T., Bell K.L., and O. Conner, T.G. (1994). Longitudinal assessment of autonomy and relatedness in adolescent family interactions as predictors' adolescent ego development and self-esteem. *Child Development*. 65, 179-194.

Ardelt, M., and Day, L. (2002). Parents, siblings, and peers: close social relationships and adolescent deviance. *Journal of Early Adolescence*, 22, 310-349.

Avism. W.R. (2002). *Family structure and mental health London*. Ontario, Canada, The university of Western Onlano (Google, Scholar).

Bahn, A., Chandler, C.A., and Eisenherg, L. (1962). Diagnostic characteristics related to services in psychiatric clinics for children. *Kilbank Memorial Fund Quarterly,* 15, 289-318.

Barber, K., (1996). Parental psychology control. Revisiting a neglected construct. *Child Development*, 67(6), 3296-3319.

Bertolote, J. (2008). The sorts of the concept of mental health. *World Psychiatry*, 7, 2, 113-116.

Borr, W., Dean, A. Narman, J. and Hayat Baksh, R. (2014) Are Children and adolescents mental health problems increasing in the 21st century? A systematic Review. *Australian and New Zealand Journal of Psychiatry*, 48, 7, 606-616.

Carli, V., Hoven, C.W. and Wasserman, C. *et al.* (2014). A newly identified group of adolescents at invisible "risk for psychopathology and suicidal behaviour: findings from the STYLE study. *World Psychiatry*, 13, 78-86.

Clark, R.E. (1996). Family support for persons with dual disorders." In R.E. Drke and K.T. Mueser (Eds.) *Dual diagnosis of major mental illness and substance abuse* Volume 2 – Also in *Recent research and clinical implications*: (pp. 65-78). San Francisco: Lessey-Bass.

Dwidedi, V. (2000). Family Climate and achievement in children: A developmental analysis, *Unpublished Ph.D.* Thesis, Department of Psychology, Kumaun University, Nainital.

Dubey, A. and Srivastava, A. (2013). Parental factors, achievement motivation and performance of adolescents. *International Journal of Education and Management Studies*, 3,1, 66-70.

Farkas, S., Johnson, J., Duffett, A., and Collins, K. (2002). *Aggrevating circumstances: A status report on rudeness in America.* Washington D.C.: Public Agenda, accessed at http://www.publicagenda.org/specials/civility/civility.htm.

Freeman, H. and Brown, B.B. (2001). Primary attachment to parents and peers during adolescence: Differences by attachment style. *Journal of Youth and Adolescence*, 30, 653-674.

Furstenberg, F.F. (2000). The sociology of adolescence and youth in the 1990s: A critical commentary. *Journal of Marriage and Family*, 62, 896-926.

Gailakoti, Pooja, M. and Shukla, A (2012). Developmental impact of locale type and gender as environmental awareness. *Indian Journal of Social Science Research*. 9, 2. 50-57.

Goldman, H.H. (1984). "The chronically mentally ill: Who are they? Where are they ?" In M. Mirabi (Ed.) *The Chronically mentally ill: Research and services*. (pp. 31-44). Spectrum Publication.

Grotevent, H.D. and cooper, C.R. (1985). Patterns of interactions in family relationships and the development of identity exploration in adolescent, *Child Development,* 56, 415-428.

Hagguist, C. (2009) Psychosomatic health problems among adolescents in Sweden are the time trends gender related? *European Journal of Public Health*, 19, 331-336.

Holden, K.C. and Smock, P.J. (1991). The economic costs of marital dissolution: Why do women bear a Proportionate cost? *Annual Review of Sociology*, 17, 51-78.

Joshi, B. and Shukla, A. (2018). Life satisfaction of Kumauni women as affected by their cultural variation and age. *Recent Educational Psychological Research*. 6,4 22-29.

Joshi, S. (2011). A study of emotional disturbance and child rearing practices as affected by parenting type. Unpublished Ph.D. Thesis. Department of Psychology, Kumaun University, Nainital.

Kakar, S. (1978). *The inner world: A psychoanalytic study of childhood and society in Indian and cultural reshaping of psychoanalysis*, New York: Columbia University Press.

Kitchenes, B. B and Jorm, A. (2002). *Mental health first aid manual* (Ist ed). Canberra: Centre for mental Health Research, Australian National University.

Lall, A. (2012). A cross-cultural study of disruptive behaviour, academic motivation and academic anxiety, Unpublished Ph.D. Thesis, Department of Psychology, Kumaun University, Nainital.

Lavoie, J.C. (1994). Identity in adolescent: Issue of theory, Structure and Transition. *Journal of Adolescence*. 17-28.

Magnet, Myron (1992). "The American Family." *Fortune*, 10 Aug 1992; 42-47.

McClean, A., Sweeting, H. and Hunt, K. (2010). Rules for boys "guidance" for girls: gender difference in symptom reporting during childhood and adolescence. *Social Science and Medicine* 70, 597-604.

McCloskey, L.A., Figurido, A.J. and Koss, M.P. (1995). The effect of systematic family violence on children's mental health. *Child Development*, 66, 5, 1239-1261.

Ojha, N. (2005). A cross-cultural study of frustration tolerance and emotional disturbance in Kumauni tribal and non-tribals, *Unpublished Ph.D*. Thesis, department of Psychology, Kumaun University, Nainital.

O'Koon, J. (1997). Attachment to parents and peers in late adolescence and their relationship with self-image. *Adolescence*, 32,471-482.

Oliver, W.J., Kahns, L.R and Pomeranz, E.S. (2006). Family structure and child abuse. *Clinical Pediatrics*, 45, 111-8. (Google scholar).

Offord, D.R., Boyle, M.H and Jones, B.R. (1987). Psychiatric disorder and poor School performance among welfare children in Ontario. *Canadian Journal of Psychiatry,* 32, 518-525

Pandey, M.K. and Shukla, A. (2018). Effect of gender and internet use on interpersonal communication among the management students. *Pariplex.* 8,1,185-186.

Pant, B. (2009). Developmental patterns of mental health in children as affected by types and levels of calmative supportiveness: A cultural Analysis, *Unpublished Ph.D. Thesis,* Department of Psychology, Kumaun University, Nainital.

Patterson, G., Reid, B. and Dishion, T. (1992) A social International approach: Vol.4 *Antisocial Boys*. Eugene: Castila Publishing.

Shukla, A. (2013). Psychological patterns of children in Kumaun region of Uttarakhand: A cultural analysis. *Unpublished Project Report.* Department of Psychology, Kumaun University, Nainital.

Shukla, A. and Joshi, R. (2017). Social support and emotional intelligence as related to loneliness among college going first year students. *Indian Journal of Positive Psychology*. 8,3, 398-400.

Shukla, A. and Joshi, R. (2017). Academic stress among professional and non-professional students. *The International Journal of Indian Psychology*. 4, 4, 182-188.

Srivastava, P. (1994). Developmental impact perceived parental attitude and experiential deprivation an personality functioning. Unpublished Ph.D. Thesis. Department of Psychology, Kumaun University, Nainital.

Snyder, C.R., Lapez, S.J and Pedrotti, J.T. (2010). *Positive Psychology: The Scientific and Practical Explanation of Human Strength*. Sage. New Delhi.

Shook, J.R. (2012) (Ed.) *"Sweester William" Dictionary of Early American Philosophers,* Bloomsbury Publishing. U.S.A.

Steinberg, L; Dornbusch, S.M. and Brown, B.B. (1992). Ethnic differences in adolescent achievement: An ecological perspective. *American Psychologist,* 47 (6), 723-729.

Thagunna, N.S. (2010). Perceived Parenting, Emotional disturbance and supportiveness: A cross-cultural study, Unpublished Ph.D. Thesis. Department of Psychology, Kumaun University, Nainital.

Warr, M. (1993). Parents: Peers and delinquency. *Social Forces.* 72, 247-256.

Weiss, L.H., and Schwarz J.C. (1996). The relationship between parenting types and older adolescents personality, academic achievement, adjustment and substance use. *Child Development*, 67(5), 2101-2114.

WHO Report (2001). The world health report-2001- *Mental Health: New Understanding,* New Hope (PDF).

WHO Report (2014). *Mental Health: Strengthening Our Response*. World Health Organization.

3

Children with Intellectual Disability

Parents' Perceived Stress and Coping Strategies

Archana Shukla and *Shivani Pandey*

Introduction

From the time the child is born, parents' life start to change. Taking care of a child can turn parent's lives upside down. Parenting stress is a normative part of the parenting role. It becomes manifold difficult when it comes to that of a disabled child. Having an intellectually disabled child leads to variety of stresses related to the child's disability (Jaiswal, *et al.*, 2018). Research evidence suggests heightened amount of stress among parents of children with intellectual disability compared to parents of non-disabled children (Katkić *et al.*, 2018; Gupta & Kaur, 2010). Heightened stress among parents leads to inadequate care of children and have influence on the growth and development of children.

Parents struggle to cope with these stresses; the use of positive coping strategies has been shown to lower stress in parents of children with disabilities (Jones & Passey, 2004). In the absence of positive coping, parental stress is likely to have an effect on the child (Hadadian & Merbler, 1996). Thus, adequate coping could reduce the experience of stress and empower such parents. Thus, the present study aims to investigate perceived stress, and coping strategies of the parents of children with intellectual disability.

Moreover, managing stress in parents of children with intellectual disability is an important aspect of rehabilitation. In Indian context it is a neglected area so more studies are required in the area of intervention for parents of children with intellectual disability (Bhat, 2013). Hence, before providing the intervention to such parents it is essential that their current level of stress and coping strategies used by the parents should be assessed and understood to better plan intervention. Such Interventions hold promise for helping parents to deal with the stress of having a child with a disability. It can prove to be a big boon to parents and indirectly to these children.

Further, the incidence of intellectually disabled children is increasing year by year (Lakhan & Ekúndayò, 2017; NSSO, 2003). So empathetic understanding and adequate management is essential. A glance at the literature concerning these aspects is imperative at this juncture so as to get a clear picture of the current state of knowledge regarding stress and coping of parents of children with intellectual disability.

Studies focusing on the stress and coping strategies of parents of children with intellectual disability when reviewed it was observed that majority of studies in India and abroad have demonstrated that parents of children with intellectual disability are likely to experience significantly higher levels of stress than parents of non-disabled children (Katkić *et al.*, 2018, Thakuri, 2014, Gupta & Kaur, 2010, Roach *et al.,* 1999, Dyson, 1997). Moreover coping strategies of parents had been shown to be strong predictor of parental stress (Hsiao, 2018).

Further studies also report that mothers of intellectually disabled children experience more stress than fathers of intellectually disabled children. (Bonab *et al.*, 2017; Upadhyaya & Havalappanavar, 2008; Singer, 2006; Blacher, *et al.,* 2005; Saloviita, *et al.,* 2003).

The review of literature suggests that there is a paucity of systematic research focusing on the in-depth understanding and management of the stress experienced and coping used by the parents of intellectually disabled child especially in Indian scenario. This intrigued the researcher to take up the present research.

Therefore, the present research attempted to assess the level of perceived stress and coping strategies among parents of children with intellectual disability. To be specific, the objectives and hypotheses of the present study are given below.

Objectives of the Study

The objectives of the present study are as follows:

- To assess the level of perceived stress experienced by mothers and fathers of intellectually disabled children.
- To assess the level of coping strategies used by mothers and fathers of intellectually disabled children.

Hypotheses

On the basis of the available literature, following hypotheses were formulated:

- H1: Mothers of children with intellectual disability will have high level of Perceived Stress as compared to fathers of children with intellectual disability.
- H2: Fathers of intellectually disabled children will use more adequate coping strategies than Mothers of intellectually disabled children.

Methodology

The present study is an ex-post facto research that is exploratory in orientation and Descriptive in nature. Sample of the present study was 100 parents (50 mothers and 50 fathers) of intellectually disabled children who fulfil the selection criteria of the study. The method of sample selection was purposive sampling. The data was collected from the Out Patient Department of District Mental Health Programme Unit of District hospital Faizabad, Uttar Pradesh. Only those parents were included who were living together along with the child. Parents who have no psychiatric or chronic physical illness were included in the study. Further educational status and occupation of parents was also taken care of viz. those parents were included who had studied up to class 10th or above and mothers who were housewife. Moreover, parents who belong to urban class and nuclear family were included. Those parents were included who have children up to 12 years of age. The level of intellectual disability was taken care of, that is those parents were selected who have children with mild to moderate level of intellectual disability. Children with no severe physical disorder or condition requiring priority medical management or any co-morbid psychiatric disorder were included for the study. Those parents were excluded who were not staying with the child or were separated/divorced. Parents having any psychiatric or chronic physical illness were excluded from the present study. Those parents were excluded whose educational qualification was less than class 10th and mothers who were employed. Moreover, parents who belong to rural class and joint or extended family were excluded. Parents who have children more than 12 years of age were excluded. The level of intellectual disability was taken care of, that is those parents were excluded who have children with severe to profound level of intellectual disability. Parents of children with severe physical disorder or condition requiring priority medical management or any co-morbid psychiatric disorder were excluded.

Major characteristics of the sample of the study are depicted in Table 3.1:

Table 3.1: Characteristics of the Sample

Socio-Demographic Variable	*Fathers (N = 50)*	*Mothers (N = 50)*
Age		
Range	26 to 35 years	25 to 35 years
Mean	31.48	29.92
Standard Deviation	2.52	3.08
Education		
Intermediate	26%	56%
Graduate	50%	30%
Post-Graduate	24%	14%
Occupation		
Housewives	0%	100%
Self-Employed	38%	0%
Job	46%	0%
Unorganized sector Mechanic/Carpenter/ Labourer etc.	16%	0%
Religion		
Hindu	70%	
Muslim	30%	

Measures

- Informed consent form.
- Semi-structured Performa for socio-demographic details and clinical variables.
- Family Interview for stress and coping in mental Retardation (FISC-MR) (Girimaji *et al.* 1999)-Family Interview for stress and coping in mental Retardation (FISC-MR) developed by Satish Chandra Girimaji, Shobha Srinath, Shekhar Seshadri & D.K. Subba Krishna. (1999) was used to assess perceived stress and coping strategies among parents of children with intellectual disability. It is a standardized tool for Indian samples with a reasonable degree of reliability and validity; the coefficients of measures of reliability were between 0.36 to 0.9. The coefficients of validity measures were between 0.51 and 0.63. English version

of tool was available so it was translated into Hindi using back translation method.

Table 3.2: Structure of FISC-MR developed by Girimaji, *et al.*, (1999)

Sl. No.	*Sections*	*Areas*	*Sub-Scales*
I.	Perceived stress in family	Daily care stress (DCS)	Extra inputs for care
			Decreased leisure time
			Neglect of others
			Disturbed behaviour
		Family emotional stress (FES)	Personal distress
			Marital problems
			Other interpersonal problems
			Effects on sibs and other worries
		Social stress (SS)	Altered social life
			Social embarrassment
		Financial stress (FS)	Financial implications
II.	Coping strategies or mediators of stress	Awareness	General awareness
			Misconceptions
		Attitudes and expectations	Expectations from child
			General attitude towards child
			Attitude towards management
		Child rearing practices	General rearing practices
			Practices specific to training
		Social support	Social support
		Global	Global family adaptation

Procedure: Parents of intellectually disabled children who met the above mentioned inclusion criteria had been contacted. Rapport was established and a written consent was taken. Confidentiality was ensured. The data was collected by face to face structured interview. Parents were thanked for their cooperation. Analysis and interpretation of generated data was done using quantitative analysis.

Data were summarized and statistical analysis was done using MS Excel 2007 and SPSS version-20. To get inferences descriptive statistics and ANOVA were used. Significance was set at a standard of $p < 0.05$.

Results and Interpretation

The present study endeavours to explore the level of perceived stress and coping strategies used by mothers and fathers of intellectually disabled children. Stress was assessed on four areas i.e., daily care stress, family emotional stress, social stress and financial stress.

Descriptive statistics shows mean, standard deviation and standard error of mean of scores of perceived stress (overall and area-wise) of mothers and fathers. Further One way analysis of variance was done to assess the significance of difference in mean scores of perceived stress and coping strategies among mothers and fathers.

Perceived Stress: Data obtained on this section has been analyzed for both parents (mothers and fathers) separately on the four main areas (daily care stress, family emotional stress, social stress and financial stress) of this tool. The table below shows descriptive statistics of the scores of mothers and fathers on Perceived stress.

Table 3.3: Score of Mothers and Fathers on Perceived Stress

Perceived Stress Sub-scales	*Parents Groups*	*Mean*	*Std. Deviation*	*Std. Error of Mean*
Daily care	Father	7.40	4.72	.67
	Mother	11.62	4.07	.58
Family emotional stress	Father	6.82	4.22	.59
	Mother	8.80	3.93	.56
Social stress	Father	3.72	2.26	.32
	Mother	5.00	1.78	.25
Financial implications	Father	3.10	.79	.11
	Mother	2.70	1.01	.14
Total stress	Father	21.04	10.68	1.51
	Mother	28.12	9.63	1.36

The above table shows that the mean score of mothers is high for daily care stress, family emotional stress, social stress and total stress. However the mean score of fathers is high for financial stress.

Table 3.4 shows that F ratio was found significant for all the four subscales of perceived stress as well as for the total perceived stress. However, the mean values presented in Table 3.4 suggest that mothers perceive significantly more daily care, family emotional and social stress as well as overall perceived stress than fathers but fathers perceive significantly more financial stress than mothers of intellectually disabled children.

Now coming to the next section, of FISC-MR tool, it asses the coping strategies or which are likely to alter the perceived stress.

Table 3.4: One way ANOVA for Perceived Stress and its subscales

Subscales of Perceived Stress		*Sum of Squares*	*df*	*Mean Square*	*F*	*Sig.*
Daily care	Between Groups	445.21	1	445.21	22.87	.000
	Within Groups	1907.78	98	19.47		
	Total	2352.99	99			
Family emotional stress	Between Groups	98.01	1	98.01	5.89	.017
	Within Groups	1631.38	98	16.65		
	Total	1729.39	99			
Social life	Between Groups	40.96	1	40.96	9.88	.002
	Within Groups	406.08	98	4.14		
	Total	447.04	99			
Financial implica-tions	Between Groups	4.00	1	4.00	4.84	.030
	Within Groups	81.00	98	.83		
	Total	85.00	99			
Total stress	Between Groups	1253.16	1	1253.16	2.12	.001
	Within Groups	10131.20	98	103.38		
	Total	11384.36	99			

Coping Strategies

In the present study, to assess coping strategies of parents, FISC-MR Section-II (Girimaji *et al.*, 1999) had been used. The descriptive statistics of the scores of mothers and fathers on the subscales and overall coping strategies is presented in Table 3.5.

The Table 3.5 shows that the mean score of fathers is low in all the areas of coping *viz.*, awareness, expectation and attitude, child rearing practices, social support, global family adaptation and total coping.

Table 3.6 shows that F-ratio was found significant for coping strategies total, Expectations and attitude, Child rearing practices and Social support. However there is no significant difference in awareness and Global rating of family adaptation.

Discussion

In the present study stress experienced (perceived) by parents in caring for child with intellectual disability was assessed using FISC-MR Section-I (Girimaji *et al.,* 1999).

The obtained results indicate that there is statistically significant difference between mothers and fathers in total perceived stress (F (1, 98)

Table 3.5: Mean, S.D. and S.E.D. of perceived stress and its subscales for fathers and mothers groups

Coping Strategies Sub-scales	*Parents Group*	*N*	*Mean*	*SD*	*Std. Error Mean*
Awareness	Father	50	4.68	2.02	.29
	Mother	50	5.30	1.86	.26
Expectations and attitude	Father	50	6.92	2.69	.38
	Mother	50	8.02	2.58	.36
Child rearing practices	Father	50	4.70	1.57	.22
	Mother	50	5.60	1.52	.21
Social support	Father	50	2.50	1.03	.15
	Mother	50	2.98	1.02	.14
Global rating of family adaptation	Father	50	2.48	.97	.14
	Mother	50	2.84	.98	.14
Coping total	Father	50	21.28	7.51	1.06
	Mother	50	24.74	7.15	1.01

= 12.12, $p < .01$) and across all subscales of stress (Table 3.4). Further the analysis of mean score of total perceived stress (Table 3.3) shows that, the mean score of mothers (M = 28.12, SD = 9.63) is higher than mean score of fathers (M = 21.04, SD = 10.67).

Thereby, it can be concluded that mothers perceive more stress than fathers. Thus, the hypothesis is accepted viz. Mothers of children with intellectual disability will have high level of Perceived Stress as compared to fathers of children with intellectual disability. Similar findings had been reported by researchers from India and abroad (Chouhan *et al.*, 2016; Azeem *et al.*, 2013; Heller *et al.*, 1997).

Further, stress was assessed on four areas i.e., daily care stress, family emotional stress, social stress and financial stress (Girimaji, *et al.,* 1999). The analysis of each area is discussed below.

Daily Care Stress: Daily care stress is taken as that kind of parental stress which occurs during the caring task of their disabled child. Analysis of scores of daily care stress shows that the mean score of mothers (M = 11.62, SD = 4.07) is high for daily care stress than mean of fathers (M = 7.40, SD = 4.72) and there is statistically significant difference between mothers and fathers in daily care stress [$F(1,98) = 22.87$, $p < .01$]. Thus, it denotes that the mothers have high daily care stress. The present finding is also supported by (Upadhyaya & Havalappanavar, 2008) who reported that in the area of care mothers report higher stress in comparison to fathers.

Table 3.6: One way ANOVA for Coping Strategies and its Subscales

		Sum of Squares	*df*	*Mean Square*	*F*	*Sig.*
Awareness	Between Groups	9.61	1	9.61	2.54	.115
	Within Groups	371.38	98	3.79		
	Total	380.99	99			
Expectations and attitude	Between Groups	30.25	1	30.25	4.35	.039
	Within Groups	680.66	98	6.95		
	Total	710.91	99			
Child rearing practices	Between Groups	20.25	1	20.25	8.46	.004
	Within Groups	234.50	98	2.39		
	Total	254.75	99			
Social support	Between Groups	5.76	1	5.76	5.45	.022
	Within Groups	103.48	98	1.06		
	Total	109.24	99			
Global rating of family adaptation	Between Groups	3.24	1	3.24	3.41	.068
	Within Groups	93.20	98	.95		
	Total	96.44	99			
Coping total	Between Groups	299.29	1	299.29	5.56	.020
	Within Groups	5271.70	98	53.79		
	Total	5570.99	99			

A probable reason could be that women tend to spend more hours than men on family and household chores and in the present study all mothers were housewives.

Family Emotional Stress: This area of stress explores the feeling of parents that occurs after having a intellectually disabled children, for example, internal suffering, worries, and disappointments. It is also possible that birth of such a child might affect their family relationships. Analysis shows that the mean of fathers (M = 6.82, SD = 4.22) was found to be lower as compared to mothers (M = 8.80, SD = 3.93) and there is statistically significant difference between mothers and fathers in Family emotional Stress [$F(1,98) = 5.89$, $p < .05$]. Thus, it can be concluded that mothers perceived more family emotional stress than fathers.

Social Stress: The analysis of scores on social stress shows that, the mean score of fathers was (M = 3.72, SD = 2.26) lower than mean score of mothers (M = 5.00, SD = 1.78) and the difference is statistically significant [F(1,98) = 9.88, p < .05]. The results depict that mothers perceived more social stress as compared to fathers who have more supportive social network. This finding is corroborated by Upadhyaya and Havalappanavar (2008) and Orr, *et al.* (1993). A probable reason could be that fathers have more opportunity to maintain their social relationships.

Financial Stress: Financial stress is defined as the subjective, unpleasant feeling that one is unable to meet financial demands, afford the necessities of life, and have sufficient funds for the living. In this present study, it was taken as financial difficulties because of this child's condition.

On financial stress area the mean score of fathers was (M = 3.10, S.D. = 0.79) higher than mean scores of mothers (M = 2.70, SD = 1.01) and the difference is statistically significant [F(1,98) = 4.84, p < .05]. The results thus indicates that fathers had more financial stress than mothers, the picture that is emerged is in concordance with the traditional Indian setup where father is the bread-earner and looks after the financial responsibility of the family.

Now coming to analysis of Section II of FISC-MR, in the present study coping strategies used by parents in caring for child with intellectual disability was assessed using FISC-MR Section-II (Girimaji *et al.*, 1999).

Results obtained indicate that there is significant difference between mothers and fathers in Coping total (F (1, 98) = 5.56, p < .05]. The mean score of fathers (M = 21.28, SD = 7.51) is low in total coping as compared to mothers (M = 24.72, SD = 7.15). Thereby, denoting that fathers of intellectually disabled children use more adequate coping strategies than mothers. Thus, hypothesis 2, made in this regard had been accepted viz. "*Fathers of intellectually disabled children will use more adequate coping strategies than Mothers of intellectually disabled children*". Findings suggest significant gender differences in overall coping strategies, attitudes and expectations, child rearing practices and social support. And fathers are having more adequate coping strategies compared to mothers. Further Coping strategies were assessed on five areas. The analysis of each area is discussed below.

Awareness: In the present study, awareness is taken as having the knowledge about the child's condition among parents. The analysis of data of the area of awareness shows that there does not exist a statistically significant difference between mothers and fathers (F (1, 98 = 2.53), p >.05). However, the mean score of fathers is low (M = 4.68, SD = 2.02) compared to the mean score of mothers (M = 5.30, SD = 1.86). Studies have emphasized that awareness is an important coping strategy (Upadhyaya &

Havalappanavar, 2008). In the true sense, the awareness of the problem serves as a valuable resource of coping by which the individual cannot only understand the problem in fact, it can also increase the acceptance of the same.

Attitudes and Expectations: It is the second area of Coping Strategies, it explores the feeling and thoughts of parent's expectations and attitudes about the children with this kind of problem. Analysis of scores shows a statistically significant difference between mothers and fathers in Expectations and attitude [$F(1,98 = 4.35)$, $p < .05$] and the mean score of fathers is low ($M = 6.92$, $SD = 2.69$) compared to the mean score of mothers ($M = 8.02$, $SD = 2.58$), thus it can be concluded that fathers show more adequate attitudes and appropriate expectations towards child.

Child Rearing Practices: Child rearing practices involve ways which are related to the child's upbringing (Devi, 2013). In the present study, Child Rearing Practices explores how the child is treated by parents and family members. A statistically significant difference could be seen between mothers and fathers in Child rearing practice [$F(1,98 = 8.46)$, $p < .05$] and the mean score of fathers is low ($M = 4.70$, $SD = 1.57$) compared to the mean score of mothers ($M = 5.60$, $SD = 1.52$), thus it can be concluded that fathers used more adequate child rearing practices compared to mothers. A probable reason for obtained result could be that the mothers might feel stressed and exhausted due to high child caring demands so might employ inadequate child rearing practices out of exhaustion.

Social Support: In the present study, this area of coping strategies served as a "protective" factor to people's vulnerability on the effects of stress on health. (Cassel, 1976). Social Support is associated with how networking helps people cope with stressful events. Besides it can enhance psychological well-being. The analysis shows a statistically significant difference between mothers and fathers in social support. [$F(1,98 = 5.45]$, $p < .05$) and the mean score of fathers is low ($M = 2.50$, $SD = 1.03$) compared to the mean score of mothers ($M = 2.98$, $SD = 1.02$), thus, It is evident that fathers had better social support than mothers of children with intellectual disability.

Global Rating of Family Adaptation: This area of coping strategies which was taken in the present study in terms of overall global understanding of the degree to which the family has adapted to the predicament of having intellectually challenged child (Girimaji, *et al.*, 1999). The analysis of data of the area of Global rating of family adaptation shows that there does not exist a statistically significant differences between mothers and fathers [F ($F(1,98) = 3.41$, $p > .05$]. However the mean score of fathers is low (M = 2.48, SD = .97) compared to the mean score of mothers (M = 2.4, SD = . 98).

Conclusion

The present study highlights the gender differences in perceived stress and coping strategies among parents of children with intellectual disability. The obtained results highlight the gender differences in perceived stress and coping strategies used by parents of children with intellectual disability. It was found that mothers had high level of perceived stress than fathers. They had high level of daily care stress, family emotional stress and social stress than fathers. However, fathers had high financial stress than mothers. Furthermore, fathers used more adequate coping strategies than mothers. Fathers had more adequate expectations and attitude, child rearing practice and social support as compared to mothers. Hence, this study concluded that parents of intellectually disabled children and especially mothers require adequate intervention and support to reduce their stress and enhance their coping. Further it was also seen that mothers had high level of daily care stress, family emotional stress and social stress than fathers. However, fathers had high financial stress than mothers. Thus, interventions aimed at reducing daily care stress, enhancing emotional and social support would be beneficial in this regard.

Implications and Suggestions

The study is a step towards understanding the stress experienced by parents of children with intellectual disability. It could be suggested that professionals when diagnosing a child with intellectual disability must consider for the adequate assessment and management of stresses of parents, such steps would be beneficial not only for the parents but in long term also for the child with disability, as parents with adequately managed stress and coping strategies would be more able to take care of the child with disability.

References

Azeem, M.W., Dogar, I.A., Shah, S., Cheema, M.A., Asmat, A., Akbar, M., Kousar, S., Imran Ijaz Haider, I.I (2013). "Anxiety and Depression among Parents of Children with Intellectual Disability in Pakistan". *Journal of the Canadian Academy of Child and Adolescent*, *22*(4), 290–295.

Bhat, Abdul Majeed (2013). "Managing stress in parents of children with intellectual disabilities". *Indian Journal of Health and Wellbeing, 4*. 1794-1797.

Blacher, J., Neece, C., and Packowski, E. (2005). "Families and intellectual Disability". *Current Opinion in Psychiatry, 18*, 507-513.

Bonab, B.G., Motamedi, F. and Zare, F. (2017). "Effect of Coping Strategies on Stress of Parent with Intellectual Disabilities Children". *Asian Education Studies, 2*(3), 11-17.

Cassel, J. (1976). "The contribution of the Social Environment to Host Resistance". *American Journal of Epidemiology, 104*, 107-123.

Chouhan, S.C., Singh, P. and Kumar, S. (2016). "Assessment of Daily Parenting Stress and Depressive Symptoms among Parents of Children with Intellectual Disability". *International Multispecialty Journal of Health, 2* (4), 22-29.

Devi, N.B. (2013). "Child rearing practices in the Indian context". Department of Psychology, Mizoram University, *Retrieved from http://www.slideshare.net/naorembinitadevi/child-rearing-practices-inthe-indian-context.*

Dyson, L.L. (1997). "Fathers and mothers of school-age children with developmental disabilities: Parental stress, family functioning, and social support". *American Journal on Mental Retardation, 102*, 267-79.

Girimaji, S.C., Shobha, S., Sheshadri, S. and Krishna, S.D.K. (1999). "Family interview for stress and coping in mental retardation (FISC-MR): A tool to study stress and coping in families of children with mental retardation". *Indian Journal of Psychiatry, 41* (4), 341-349.

Gupta, R.K. and Kaur, H. (2010). "Stress among parents of children with intellectual disability". *Asia Pacific Disability Rehabilitation Journal, 21* (2), 118-126.

Hadadian, A., and Merbler, J. (1996). "Mother's stress: Implications for attachment relationships". *Early Child Development and Care, 125*, 59-66.

Hsiao, Y.J. (2018). "Parental Stress in Families of Children with Disabilities". *Intervention in School and Clinic, 53* (4), 201-205.

Heller, T., Hsieh, K. and Rowitz, L. (1997). "Maternal and paternal care giving of persons with mental retardation across the life span". *Family Relations, 46* (4), 407-115.

Jaiswal, S.V., Subramanyam, A.A., Shah, H.R. and Kamath, R.M. (2018). "Psychopathology and coping mechanisms in parents of children with intellectual disability". *Indian J. Psychiatry, 60*, 312-317.

Jones, J. and Passey, J. (2004). "Family adaptation, coping and resources: Parents of children with developmental disabilities and behaviour problems". *Journal on Developmental Disabilities, 11*, 31-46.

Katkić, L.O., Morović M.L. and Kovačić, E. (2018). "Parenting Stress and a Sense of Competence in Mothers of Children with and without developmental disabilities". *Hrvatska revija za rehabilitacijska istraživanja, 53*, 63-76.

Lakhan, R. and Ekúndayò, O.T. (2017). "Important Research Priorities in Intellectual Disability in India: A Public Health Perspective". *J Neurosci Rural Pract*, (Suppl 1), S150–S151. doi: [10.4103/jnrp.jnrp_102_17]

National Sample Survey Organisation (NSSO). (2003). *Disabled Persons in India. NSS 58th round* (July-December 2002), Report No. 485 (58/26/1), Ministry of Statistics and Programme Implementation: Government of India.

Orr, R.R., Cameron, S.J., Dobson, L.A., and Day, D.M. (1993). Age-related changes in stress experienced by families with a child who has a development delay. *Mental Retardation*, *31*(3), 171-176.

Oxford Dictionary.com. (2013). Definition of Awareness, Retrieved from http://www.oxforddictionaries.com/definition/english/awareness.

Roach, M.A., Orsmond G.I. and Barratt M.S. (1999). "Mothers and fathers of children with Down syndrome: Parental stress and involvement in childcare". *American Journal on Mental Retardation, 104*, 422-436.

Saloviita, T., Italinna, M., and Leinonen, E. (2003). "Explaining the parental stress of fathers and mothers caring for a child with intellectual disability: A double ABCX model". *Journal of Intellectual Disability Research*, *47*, 300–312.

Singer, G.H.S. (2006). "Meta-analysis of comparative studies of depression in mothers of children with and without developmental disabilities". *American Journal on Mental Retardation*, *111*(3), 155-169.

Thakuri, B.S. (2014). "Stress and Coping Mechanism among the parents of Intellectual Disable Children". *Journal of Advanced Academic Research*, *1*(I), 56-63.

Upadhyaya, G.R., and Havalappanavar, N.B. (2008). "Stress in Parents of the Mentally Challenged". *Journal of the Indian Academy of Applied Psychology*, *34*, 53-59.

4

Children and Adolescents Mental Health in the Era of Globalization

Nishant Goyal and *Velprashanth Venkateshan*

Globalization: Since Ancient Times

Human societies have always faced succession of empires bringing new trade and virtues that defied the normal accepted norms. Perhaps the Greek Imperialism under Alexander the Great (356-323 BCE) marks the first union of Mediterranean with Asia which was largely pushed by the great king's dream of cosmopolis, a world where all citizens lived harmoniously together. But this inevitably led to cultural imperialism, where a form of soft power enforced by one dominant culture over others, which changes the moral and cultural worldview of the subordinate country. The free trade of 16th century only marks the modern era where the colonial powers began to Orientalize the world into east and west resulting in a relentless intention of merging the two sides in form of economic liberalization. This isn't just summed up by a child listening to foreign music but the kid's expectation of own country to become like the dominant country (Rodrik, 2011).

Post-World War II, the new monetary system called Bretton Woods system which established rules for commercial and financial relations among the western countries of USA, Canada, Western European countries and Australia. Here each country had an obligation to adopt a standard exchange rate and a need to address lack of cooperation among other eastern countries to prevent competitive devaluation. This resulted in ambitious economic liberalization and hyperglobalisation eventually removing controls on international capital markets. Trade agreements extended to impingement on domestic policies and developing nations came under severe pressure to open their markets to foreign trades and investment. As Dani Rodrik puts it, Globalization became an end in itself (Rodrik, 2011).

Health Indices and Government Policies

Good health is crucial for human and economic welfare and positive effects of health play crucial roles in productivity and earnings. Child malnutrition and ill health during early childhood may result in irreversible damages to the child in later life. Globalization is a strong force that has improved health outcomes in rich and poor countries by improving national incomes and increased investment on health sector in order to be on par with international recommendations. But a more relevant indicator seems to be the regime type and quality of democracy which has a positive independent health impact. Thus, relation between globalization and child health is affected by a country's quality of its democratic institutions, thereby the poor are relatively empowered enough to be looked after by the policies. Overall there are likely and robust positive effects in terms of life expectancy in low income countries despite controlling for literacy, nutritional intake and income. But there are potential ill effects as well (Bergh & Nilsson, 2010). The same principles on the open trading front though, tend to create intense tax competitions in a race to bottom with eventual compromise of social services. This aspect is more relevant in developing countries. These factors along with incremental information flow across borders enables diffusion of medical technologies that enter the consumer markets, creating further unhealthy competition among health providers with no uniform standardization of resources. Poor countries will find themselves without means to buy patented drugs. The increased incentives in a more potent consumer markets would lead to educated experts preferring to migrate to places where wages are higher, all of which culminating in brain-drain, migration and urbanization related problems. Nissanke and Thorbecke (2007) point out that collective measure on economic, social and political integration have to be in place for developing countries to benefit from globalization. If not, this would only create opportunities for those that are best positioned to take advantage of them as seen in most capitalist promoting economies. Thus, democracy plays an important role in mediating negative effects of globalization (Welander *et al.*, 2014).

The efficiency of democratic powers are measured both as country's democratic status in a given period and as a country's historical experience with democratic administration. As globalization fosters growth, their effects over child health depends directly on quality of politico-economical institutions and whether the poor benefit from growth. According to Sen (1997) when democratic accountability is limited, resources made openly accessible may not reach a large share of population but rather imparts further discrepancy of services. But an open public sphere where at least the flow of information is free, it ensures political leaders do not disregard public welfare. Thus, the strength of the democracy rather than democracy per se will determine the success of globalized health provisions (Welander *et al.*, 2014).

Impact on Culture and Politics

Globalization affects culture through its effect on the forms of individual and collective identity. And also impacts the intermutual life that interacts with mental health through its impact over economic inequalities and through shaping and dissemination of knowledge of health and lifestyle itself. In essence, globalization contacts at first only a minority of people owing to poverty and lack of mobility. And the globalizing forces often meet their own counteraction in the tendency for communities to reassert their distinctive ethnic identity (Kirmayer & Minas, 2000). The ethno-cultural identity plays a role in individual's self-esteem and helps continue community role performance and can buffer the effects of racism and discrimination. The economic incapacitation of the state can directly influence an individual's self-role, self-esteem. Any economic impotence of state as well can influence how citizens see their role and their value in the larger scheme of things (Bhugra *et al.*, 2004). Hence the society is once again divided with respect to what the individual can identify oneself with respect to his perception of ethnicity and socio-economic status. This in addition only serves to accentuate the identity erosion of youth.

The time and space between cultures have been dramatically reduced by globalization. Societies are traversing through urbanization, acculturation, modernization and social and cultural change. There has indeed been economic disintegration, social disruption and unequal distribution of collective wealth and political repression causing increasingly surging gap between wealthy and poor in several under-integrated governments after globalization. There is a growing fear that this will soon turn individuals and spaces into more homogenous entities. The liberalized citizens begin to perceive their own traditional alter egos as backward and may curb their interaction with their own ethnic neighbourhoods. These behaviours manifest as private beaches and VIP inns with imported facilities where citizens try to escape the country within the country by living a more consumerist and individualistic lifestyles. This unavoidably creates further division within communities at an economic level. While the capitalist market tends to empower these citizens with superior purchasing capacity that fuels the market, power appears to have shifted from state to multinational corporations, some exceeding the market value of GDP of many countries (Bhugra *et al.*, 2004).

With the rampant free movement of capital, the economy is exempt from political control. Globalization has broken down natural boundaries with repeated exposures to news of violence and atrocities causing a perceptual numbness. Media has made citizens vicarious to disturbing atrocities in the fallen states. On the other hand, the media facilitated familiarity towards foreign cultures explains how several migrants experience no inhibitions in indulgence into a multinational culture. There is increasing bias in form of under appreciating minimalistic norms while appeasing the foreign consumerist experiences with a sense of emancipation associated with cultural hybridization. The global break down of boundaries make it possible today to enjoy Japanese anime games in India; enjoy Indian cuisine in Paris and visit the Eiffel tower in Vegas. The economic migrants if they are educated assimilate the experience with no barriers. But the economic refugees feel left behind and experience marginalization and acculturation stress due to loss of individuality. These unfortunate people who have difficulties assimilating these multi-cultural experiences have to experience cultural disempowerment and perhaps live life as vagabonds and not tourists (Bauman, 1998). The intense flow of capital, people and creed pulls the world into one tight net that can at times strangle the individuals it is supposed to liberate. Globalization has created dissonance between local practices and intercultural relations with daily circumstances causing an increased alienation of individuals from both localities and global space, especially children who are in their phase of identity crisis. The children may feel alienated if they do not change, making them feel backward or if they do change, it may still alienate them from their roots (Giddens, 1990).

The global economic system has resulted in a colossal increase in global wealth and also reduction in absolute poverty in several countries. But these have also lead to accentuated wealth inequalities, uneven cost distribution and privilege endearment. Globalization is a temporal phenomenon where there is speeding up of social interaction. The transformation isn't confined to economic spaces but also on socio-cultural and psychological aspects. The social determinants of globalization are more specifically on: (i) poverty and inequality, (ii) migration, (iii) socio-cultural values, and (iv) self and identity issues (Sharma, 2016). Friedman (2018) argues there is increased ascendancy of 'economic space' over 'life space', and that people's routine activities are marginalized by activities of rising global business class such as increased activities focusing on self-fulfillment, instant gratification and competitive manipulation. All these narcissistic goals create an environment of winners and losers—a kind of survival of the fittest, where there low incentive on social harmony (Timimi, 2010).

Globalization and Mental Health

In 2013, WHO published the Mental Health Action Plan, 2013-2020, in which the concepts of mental health promotion, mental illness prevention and treatment, and rehabilitation have been integrated into a protocol and has been refined for progress of global mental health (Saxena & Setoya, 2014). Schizophrenia, depression, epilepsy, dementia, alcohol dependence and neurological disorders encompass 13 per cent of global disease burden surpassing both cardiovascular disease and cancer. Depression is the third leading cause of disease burden. By 2020, an estimated 1.5 million people will die each year by suicide, and between 15 and 20 million will make the attempt (Collins *et al.*, 2011). The roots of psychosocial stressors are ingrained in the mold of a globalizing world.

Ethnic identity has direct influence on one's self-esteem and psychological well-being (Bhugra, *et al.*, 2004). Current processes threatened by multiple belongings, multi-ethnic communities, long distance networks and plastic identities (Bibeau, 1997). An essential process of progressive spatial segregation into local and modern combined with alienation can accumulate stress into vulnerable individuals. Thus, cultures may be denied of their psychologically protective qualities inherent in them. An important implication of globalization is increased 'existential uncertainty' with people being faced with rules from communities where individuals are obliged to participate as a member of a globalized society. This induces the person to seek affirmation from any localized group that can reduce their insecurity. Institutionalized religion and nationalism are used as identity markers in times of uncertainty (Hermans & Dimaggio, 2007). Individual's mental health is determined by positive self-concept and any insult to identity causes a mark of poor mental health. Any distortions of identity formation can be ascribed to combined effects of globalization and extreme forms of individualism. In the capitalistic society consumption and commodities are fast becoming important ways for youngsters to acquire and express their individuality. The contradictions of these expectations are reflected in problems of early depressive episodes, substance abuse and even suicide (Doku & Asante, 2011). According to Kirmayer and Minas (2000), globalization impacts mental health through its effect on economic inequalities on mental well-being and through shaping and dissemination of psychiatric principles itself. The original intent of Alexander's cosmopolis is quite unlikely, as experts argue homogenization of cultures is unlikely as this process of globalization affects only minority at the community level and is counteracted by the urge to assert one's own ethnic identity. But these economic pressures will eventually lead to capitalist pressures and urbanization resulting in rootlessness and reduced psychological protective factors. Urbanization has created a surge in behavioural disturbances—associated with broken families, abandonment and violence towards spouses, children and elderly as well as the increase in anxiety and depressive disorders.

Another emerging issue is immigration and second-class citizenships and lack of inclusion for non-westerners. They experience cultural differences and marginalization with respect to rights and responsibilities further worsened by lack of understanding of psychiatric symptoms in trans-cultural settings. Due to these pitfalls, globalization causes overwhelming shift of power to industry of pharmaceuticals which tend to be the essential guarantee for therapeutic benefit while undermining the absolute benefits of biopsychosocial model and the immense effectiveness of psychosocial and community treatments (Mezzina, 2001).

Effect on Children's Mental Health

50 per cent of all mental illnesses start by the age of 14 and 75 per cent by mid 20s (Kessler *et al.*, 2007). Predominantly anxiety and personality disorders have been presenting around 11 years age and in a survey across 10 countries, one fourth of youth had a diagnosis of mental disorder (Lievens, 2018). The oversight in addressing these disorders at their onset can culminate in affecting the entire life of the child with respect to development and contributing to poor educational outcomes (Choi, 2018).

Children's behaviour is influenced by child rearing attributes and social processes within a culture. The major effect of globalization is reflected in the tendency to regard western culture and its views in childcare practices as superior. People of any culture use an indigenous idea of childhood, its limitation, nature and duration based on their own network of ideologies and within their own context of social ecology. They may not categorically write about this, but instinctively conceive it and act according to these assumptions in all of their hopes and fears of their children. These practices nurture childhood with social practices that are legitimate within their local regime. But with globalization, there is dissemination of psychiatric knowledge itself that tends to publicize problems in a universalizing approach thereby with the western assumption of mental health dominating the ideology with its ready-made explicit solutions in black and white, eventually prevailing over local practices. The context behind these local rearing practices are often brushed aside (Harkness & Super, 1996).

Immaturity of children is a fact but the ways in which this is understood and made meaningful is a fact of culture (Prout & James, 2015). People from such diverse ecological framework have appreciation of the intentional person making sense from within broader social, political and cultural context. Thus, it's difficult to pass a scientific judgment that a child is better off in any particular society and hence the idea that all children can have universal rearing ideals can become unintelligible.

Since freedom is a dominant virtue of western market economy, it has also trickled into an appeal for ridding oneself from restrictions imposed by authority such as parents, community and governments. By application of this value system, it tends to encourage the idea of looking after the wants of the individual—narcissism. This leads to the idea of looking after oneself, who should be free of infringements and obligations other people demand (Richards, 1989). But the downfall is that the individual can end up being so insulated that they see harmony with wider community as an obstacle rather than objective. Globalization has helped to deliver this morale worldwide unfortunately. Children everyday coached in an environment that is born out of the free market economic ideology, that stresses oneself to be rid of any regulations that impedes the ability to compete with the idealization of success in forms of stories of individual conquest that is free of social responsibility (unless it helps increases your market share/fame). They are thus exposed through media and internet to a system that rejects authority and promotes competitiveness and individualism. In this level, the success stories in mass media reinforce the need to rid oneself of any authority (in fantasy) and become free to pursue own individual self-gratification, free from infringements other people represent. These lead to the isolation of the individual and any obligations to a wider community are seen as obstacles (Richards, 1989). Many non-western cultures welcome nurturing extended family structures where children are cared for despite their limitation and are appreciated for being an active part of the family irrespective of one's individual achievement, thereby the weak members aren't left behind to rot in the rat race. Anthropological studies also comment that family-centred cultures produce happier children who don't get exposed mental distress of a competitive free market society where each one fights for self (Timimi, 2005).

Attributes of Globalization

There are categorical phenomena of globalization that play a significant role in disrupting healthy childhood. The negative aspects of Individualism have been elaborated with respect to the narcissistic value system that applauds competitive manipulation and self-fulfillment, such that any development of deep interpersonal attachments from which a sense of social responsibility arises is thwarted. This perhaps explains the increasing trend of narcissistic disorders such as (Anti-social/Conduct behaviours, Substance abuse and eating disorders) (Timimi, 2012).

The other major attribute of free global trade is the encouragement of ever-increasing acquisition of goods and services called Consumerism. This aspect of consumer culture is driven into the social arrangement of buying and selling services including health services. Childhood distress which was the onus of parents has increasingly shifted into categorized states of behavioural deviance that enter the market with professionals selling treatments in a consumer world of parents. These tend to further relegate individual differences and promote a standardized package that Roberston (2000) called as the 'functional abstraction' where individual cases are considered as 'instances' of the generic category, which stands over and above them.

But perhaps the most robust evidences point to the effect of Urbanization, which is perhaps the unprecedented and the most sinister of all the after effects of globalization. The ever-increasing exacerbation of relative poverty and inequalities created by the consumerist markets cause an rural-urban divide in infrastructure resulting is internal migration and people moving to cities with dreams of a life promised by globalization. They affect mental health by increased stressors of pollution, overcrowding, changing family dynamics, violence and unemployment. Here it is apt observation that reduced social capital is a significant mediator of the connection between mental health and urbanization (Mckenzie, 2008).

Family disruption in form of increased nuclear families has been major aftermath of increased neo-liberal free markets with reduced continuity of family trade among members in pursuit of more profitable businesses and also as a direct result of urbanization (McMunn *et al.*, 2001).

On the contrary, third world countries that lack efficient democratic governments amidst a capitalist world economy tend to offer another level of problems for children such as regional wars, ecological catastrophe, lack of state resources, migration, fragmentation of communities and malnutrition (Timimi, 2012).

Newer Challenges for Children

The way we conceptualize children and their problems has been impacted by cultural pressures and practices around families and community. Current globalization policies promote a narcissistic value system. Especially within the western and the globalized cultures where the first impacts of the free market were felt shows certain important concerns. Some of them include:

1. Family structure has seen the demise of the extended family, an increase in separation and divorce, an increase in the working hours of parents, and a decrease in the amount of time parents spend with their children; Family disruption in form of increased nuclear families has been major aftermath of increased neo-liberal free markets with reduced continuity of family trade among members in pursuit of more profitable businesses and also as a direct result of urbanization (McMunn *et al.*, 2001).
2. Family lifestyles have been transformed by an increase in mobility, a decrease in 'rooted' communities, and more time spent in pursuit of individual gratification; An adolescent is meant to lead a life finding his own path and a lack ties with his native is encouraged and a path leading him to an urbanised surplus life is desired and seen as progress (Timimi, 2010).
3. Children's lifestyles have been changed by a decrease in exercise and the 'domestication' of childhood due to fears about the risks for children, resulting in more indoor pursuits such as computers and TV; Parents who aren't themselves largely present to ensure safety of child during outdoor play or be able to spend enough time in physical play, in turn encourage children to stay indoors or play online/video games for entertainment and learning. The urban overcrowding leading to increased condominium/apartment

living that disables optimal outdoor play and interaction. Thus, there is increased promotion of virtual socialization through 'Facebook', 'WhatsApp', 'Instagram', 'Snapchat' personalized TV in form of Android/iOS devices discouraging joint family entertainment watching and augmenting alienation.

4. The commercialization/commodification of childhood has emerged with an increase in consumer goods targeted at children and the creation of new commercial opportunities in childhood, such as the 'parenting' industry (Timimi, 2010). A child who enters a supermarket is instantly drawn towards a plethora of stuffed dolls/action figures and an ever growing list of digital toys that are constantly commercialised and the competition in the toy market ensures there is always something new, thereby the child's expectations are instant gratified by default. Parents are equally drawn towards a whole list of educational/interactional devices marketed as the state of the art and the possession of these are also an indication of social status.
5. There are changes in education system as well with decreasing role and influence of the nation-state in unilaterally determining domestic policies, and given the fiscal crisis of public revenues in most societies, there will be a corresponding decline in the state's commitment to educational opportunity and equality. There is a greater turn toward the market, privatization, and choice models that regard the public as consumers who will only obtain the education they can afford, turning education into an industry. These changes produce an overall decline in the civic commitment to public education itself. Children are encouraged in a more result-oriented education that puts less emphasis on each ones' uniqueness and the pursuit of creative thinking (Burbules & Torres, 2013).
6. Children's diets have been modified to fit a fast paced life style that reduces the active participation of parents in active preparation and feeding. Markets are brimming with globalised food that are attractive in colours and branded with toys and gifts that draw children towards them. These foods are mass produced in a cut-throat food industry that demands constant renovation of food items thus leading to increase in sugar, saturated fats, salt, chemical additives that increase cravings in children and decreased in certain essential fatty acids and fresh fruit and vegetables. In a Canadian study, 19.8 per cent of all

breakfast cereals were child-targeted, and these were significantly lower in total and saturated fat. Child-targeted cereals were significantly higher in sodium and sugar and lower in fibre and protein, and were three times more likely to be classified as "less healthy" compared to not child-targeted cereals. No child-targeted cereals were sugar-free, and sugar was the second most common ingredient in 75 per cent of cereals. Six breakfast cereal companies had child-targeted product lines that consisted entirely of "less healthy" cereals (Potvin Kent *et al.*, 2017).

Medicalization of Childhood and Adolescent Behavioural Patterns

The diagnosis and prescription of medications for childhood disorders has steeply increased in that last 3 decades across all Industrialized nations (Northern America, Northern Europe and Australasia) (Timimi & Leo, 2009). Perhaps due to increasing awareness and scientific understanding, the under-diagnosed conditions are now more easily recognized. Other possibility being a significant change in perception and our own conceptualization of "Normal Child" has changed, therefore a child who would have been brushed off as a normal, 'boisterous' kid may now likely get a diagnosis of ADHD. The possibility is perhaps, both the above phenomena are playing a role and Globalisation has significantly contributed to the latter.

As Timimi (2009) puts it, "It's now harder than ever to be a 'normal' child or parent. Our standards of what are considered to be acceptable behaviour and child rearing in young is constricting. There is increased tendency to intellectualize common issues and avoid responsibility by 'blame culture'. Instead of introspecting our specific roles, the guilt averting narcissism plays into the idea of tagging them to biological diseases that require medical attention as explanation (Blaming the genes). This sets into motion a rampant tendency to categorize all behaviours into an illness or abnormal developmental trajectory, by widening diagnostic boundaries. This causes their aggressive promotion in public awareness campaigns in order to expand their markets for treatment. This criticism has even received a very reproachful term called 'disease mongering'.

This dynamic eventually causes excessive surveillance of children's normal behavioural variants and undue anxiety in parenting where people will leave essential social and problem-solving life skills to be discharged by professional and experts as they lose confidence in own abilities. The increased medical explanation sold across the world is changing our ideas of free will, choice and personal responsibility for behaviour. As an eventuality, the progressive application of techniques of medicine and psychiatry to manage children's behaviour, particularly using drugs sums up the consumer culture where parents brand the problem behaviour and demand a service provider for drugs in a form of quick fix. This consumer culture of expecting immediate readymade solutions for behaviour problems branded into an illness category and channelized into a prompt prescription is what we can term as 'McDonaldisation' of children's mental health (Timimi, 2012).

The medical model of the West has always served evidence-based system of identifying and treating distinct pathological entities but as often in psychiatry and behavioural medicine, the syndrome approach can deliberately pathologize certain normal cultural variants that appear to be problematic under the medical model. The root of the issue lies in its overwhelming cultural power of pharmaceutical industries and a movement towards more uniform diagnostic systems. This further contradicts the need to address distress with a social meaning so that support systems can be made more efficient in treating the condition with cultural appropriation.

In children's mental health the globalized medical model has resulted in creation of new diagnostic categories, using western cultural ideas of normal childhood. These are further viewed as having genetic causes, with the broader environmental context being only a disease modifier. Individualization of children's suffering runs the risk of undermining local ways of solving problems and masking real life circumstances of poverty and exploitation that the children might have faced. This sets motion a system vulnerable to institutional racism in the dominant societies and foreign standards of normality may come to be viewed as primitive and their populations will be viewed as needing to be psychoeducated.

The direct impact is marginalizing family and diverting attention from real social injustice. Further research is needed to identify and label culture's role in development and long term course of emotional distress and cultural deviance among children. Another major setback was stigma, that arose from public acceptance of biomedical explanations of psychotic disorders resulting in further distance from patients. Certain cultural beliefs aided in keeping the diseased persons bound to the family and their socially accepted ministration served a better prognosis (Mezzina, 2001). Globalization on the contrary may promote the indulgence into non-Western collectivist cultures for a more cohesive parenting and child rearing. The cultures where value systems are oriented towards the importance of group as opposed to individual, helps people to be integrated into strong cohesive groups from birth onwards and continue to offer them protection and emotional shock absorption in exchange for loyalty throughout person's life (Hofstede, 1994).

There are several examples of the drawbacks of extensive promotion of biomedical model, such as the over-inclusive diagnostic criteria in DSM-5 for ADHD, Disruptive Mood Dysregulation Disorder, Intermittent Explosive Disorders, Oppositional Defiant Disorder and Conduct, all of which tend to describe variations of impulsivity and aggression by a child as being solely caused by a brain disorder such that parents may not be able to consciously control them and transfer of onus towards the medical experts and pharmaceuticals. The anxiety loaded, narcissistically primed vision of childhood also encourages the conditions of childhood depression, Autism Spectrum Disorders to eventually lead to viewing these disorders as purely the fault of one's biology thus sparing all from scrutiny. And fast forwarding to readymade solutions, particularly the use of second-generation antipsychotics and stimulants extensively right from toddlerhood, summing up the process of McDonaldisation of Child Psychiatry as well (Tait, 2006).

Impact of Virtual World on Child and Adolescent Mental Health

One of the several consequences of a narcissistic-consumerist society interconnected by popular media and Internet are the rise of newer behavioural addictions that deviate distinctly from traditional psychotropic substance abuse. And the propensity of these behaviours to affect the millennial children, largely encompassing child and adolescent population throw emphasis on the role of globalization in mediating this phenomenon. Every behavioural disorders appear too based on an impairment of three functional systems of motivation-reward, regulation of affect and behavioural inhibition. In an increasingly competitive win-lose interactions in this globalized society, the adolescent often becomes impaired in emotional regulation, further exacerbated by poor family support. This is worsened by increased anxiety levels due to constant comparison and need to be socially approved resulting in impulsivity and poor curbing of the need for immediate gratification.

The mass availability and usage of digital technology is a relatively recent phenomenon, there is such that a paucity of hard information. But there are increasing associations between internet usage and mental health. While not directly contributory, excessive use of social media is associated with mental illnesses (McCrae, *et al.*, 2017) and poorer sleep and sleep deprivation, especially with video games usage (Billari, *et al.*, 2018).

More recent data, in a world where children and adolescent are growing up in an era of digitalization with effortless familiarity with mobile phones and computers, studies show on an average across OECD countries, a typical 15 year old adolescent had been using internet since the age of 10 and spent on an average 29 hours/week on internet which is a striking increase from the average 21 hours spent by an average 15 year old in 2012. One fourth of students report themselves to be excessive internet users during weekends, more than 6 hours/day and with 16 per cent spending a similar amount of time even during weekdays (OECD, 2017).

One of the more recent upsurges in internet addictions has been the 'Internet Gaming Disorders' which has been included in DSM-5 as conditions for further study. It has found its way into both western and non-western societies at alarming rates largely contributed by the "Massively Multiplayer Online Role Playing Games' (MMORPGs) which clearly target children with easy access to smart phones and internet. Most of these children show clear disruption in family environment and their own self-esteem thereby these addictions serve to gratify their need for dominance and power as seen in the types of games that gain popularity such as 'PUBG' (Player Unknown Battle Ground). There are distinct gender differences: playing online games is more popular with boys (56% vs. 13%) while girls are more likely to participate in social networks by uploading personally created content (78% vs. 69%) (OECD, 2017). In USA, girls are more likely than boys to say Snapchat is the site they prefer (42% vs. 29%) while boys are more in the mood to use YouTube as their preferred social media app (39% vs. 25%) (Pew Research Centre, 2018).

Digital platforms provide tools for cyber-bullying with evidence of a rise in cyber-bullying is several countries. Perpetrators of cyber-bullying are found equally in among boys and girls and across adolescence whereas younger children preferentially commit bullying in-person (Livingstone *et al.*, 2016). Cyber bullying is associated with rapid creation and sharing of offensive comments and contents, spreading rumours, excluding someone from an online groups and other similar harassments that has been showing to lead up to several negative outcomes such as depressive symptoms, substance use, suicidal attempts and ideations (Bottino *et al.*, 2015).

With the rise of online merchandise and the materialistic norms of an individualist society, there appears to be an increase in 'Compulsive Buying' or in Kraepelinian terms, 'Oniomania'. The capitalist surge and the rise of startups and online shopping-delivery models along with massive social networking of brands enhance these maladaptive behaviours with never ending cues and consequences to ensure the subject continues buying. The industrialization of glamour/sex in form of porn industry and fashion industry creates unrealistic expectation to be in shape and constant exposure to sexual cues that invariably escalate the prevalence of sex addiction and exercise addiction syndromes (Pinna *et al.*, 2015). In these scenarios, there is rising evidences pointing towards association between social media and body image concerns/disordered eating (Holland & Tiggemann, 2016). Social media is exclusively conducive to allow individuals to present themselves in the most attractive images in front of peers to play persuasive impact on an individual's body image (Fardouly & Vartanian, 2016).

The constant idealization of a hard working corporate and the romanticization of the materialistic success lead to excessive goal-setting in terms of monetary achievement at the expense of personal life and transcendence as seen by the increase in Work Addictions. The evolution of internet services into a human-machine interface promotes further addictive tendencies in using Technologies and internet. Recent reports identify materialism and impulsiveness both drive a dependence of cell phone and instant messaging. The personality trait most consistently associated with these problematic addictions is low self-esteem, quite evidently contributed by an individualistic culture.

Most of these above entities are yet to get a separate diagnostic criterion as perhaps the whole venture would be a tautological exercise where in further blaming of biology and relinquishing of responsibilities would ensue in this already consumerist society (Pinna *et al.*, 2015). In view of the above newer challenges, the OECD Recommendation on the Protection of Children Online (OECD, 2012) requests remedial steps in the form of 4 Es namely:

1. Empowering children and youth to be responsible online participants.
2. Educate families about appropriate digital usage.
3. Encourage industry to develop appropriate content.
4. Ensure children and young people who show signs of mental illness get help early.

Current Treatment Issues and Future Directions

In caring for children and adolescents with mental disorders the importance of 'contextual understanding and context of disorder' in terms of family, community and nation plays an essential role. Disorders cannot be seen as static diagnostic labels, but rather a dynamic response to environmental stressors along with genes. The epigenetic principle has perhaps laid rest the age-old debate of nature vs. nurture such that both play an interdependent role in determining outcome.

It is essential to emphasize the degree of impairment with a diagnosis in developing countries. The degree varies with circumstances and demands of the society and the government. Thus, specific diagnosis may be less important than degree of impairment and the ability of the individual to participate in society. The main barriers to treatment include lack of resources (financial, human resources, facilities) and stigma. Some of the World Health Organization (2003) recommended interventions to reduce the barriers include:

1. Improving family communication and cohesiveness.
2. Increasing awareness of psychosocial development.
3. Educating religious personnel about disorders and establishment of treatment alliance.
4. Encouraging the development of national child and adolescent mental health policy.
5. Utilizing scarce resources.

Globalization can always create discrepancies in social norms, but it also opens door for reverse cultural flow and thus new emergence of fusion of identities, beliefs and practices and even rediscovery of importance of certain aspects of traditional culture. Increased legislative attention is needed in strengthening social cohesion and reducing inequality to improve child protection. With regard to policy, support for more pro-social and minimalist systems will eventually bring forth stronger families and healthier children. A wider debate is needed to engage public with politicians, where knowledge about children's development, mental health and their relation to culture should be included.

References

Bauman, Z. (1998). *Globalization: The Human Consequences*. Columbia University Press.

Bergh, A., and Nilsson, T. (2010). "Good for living? On the relationship between globalization and life expectancy", *World Development*, *38*(9), 1191-1203.

Bhugra, D., and Mastrogianni, A. (2004). "Globalisation and mental disorders:

overview with elation to depression", *The British Journal of Psychiatry*, *184*(1), 10-20.

Bibeau, G. (1997). "Cultural psychiatry in a creolizing world: Questions for a new research agenda", *Transcultural Psychiatry*, *34*(1), 9-41.

Billari, F.C., Giuntella, O., and Stella, L. (2018). "Broadband internet, digital temptations, and sleep", *Journal of Economic Behaviour and Organization*, *153*, 58-76.

Bottino, S.M. B., Bottino, C., Regina, C.G., Correia, A.V. L., and Ribeiro, W.S. (2015). "Cyberbullying and adolescent mental health: Systematic review", *Cadernos de saude publica*, *1*, 463-475.

Burbules, N.C., and Torres, C.A. (2013). *Globalization and Education: Critical Perspectives*. Routledge.

Choi, A. (2018). Emotional well-being of children and adolescents. OECD Education Working Papers, No. 169, OECD Publishing, Paris. http://dx.doi.org/10.1787/41576fb2-en.

Collins, P.Y., Patel, V., Joestl, S.S., March, D., Insel, T.R. Daar, A.S., ... and Glass, R.I. (2011). "Grand challenges in global mental health". *Nature*, *475*(7354), 27.

Doku, P.N., and Asante, K.O. (2011). "Identity: Globalization, culture and psychological functioning". *Journal of Human Sciences*, *8*(2), 294-301.

Fardouly, J., and Vartanian, L.R. (2016). "Social media and body image concerns: Current Research and future directions". *Current Opinion in Psychology*, *9*, 1-5.

Fisher, J., Cabral, D.M. M., Izutsu, T., Vijayakumar, L., Belfer, M., and Omigbodun, O. (2011). "Adolescent Mental Health in Resource-Constrained Settings: A review of the evidence of the nature, prevalence and determinants of common mental health problems and their management in primary health care". *The International Journal of Social Psychiatry*, *57*(1 Suppl), v.

Friedmann, J. (2018). *Life Space and Economic Space: Third World Planning in Perspective*. Routledge.

Giddens, A. (2007). *The Consequences of Modernity*. Cambridge: Polity.

Harkness, S., and Super, C.M. (Eds.). (1996). "*Parents' Cultural Belief Systems: Their Origins, Expressions, and Consequences*". Guilford Press.

Hermans, H.J., and Dimaggio, G. (2007). Self, Identity, and Globalization in Times of Uncertainty: A Dialogical Analysis. *Review of general psychology*, *11*(1), 31-61.

Hofstede, G., Hofstede, G.J., and Hofstede, G.J. (1994). *Cultures and Organisations: Software of the Mind*—The Successful Strategist Series.

Holland, G., and Tiggemann, M. (2016). "A systematic review of the impact of the use of social networking sites on body image and disordered eating outcomes". *Body Image*, *17*, 100-110.

Kessler, R.C., Amminger, G.P., Aguilar-Gaxiola, S., Alonso, J., Lee, S., and Ustun, T.B. (2007). "Age of onset of mental disorders: a review of recent literature", *Current Opinion in Psychiatry*, *20*(4), 359.

Kirmayer, L.J. and Minas, H. (2000). "The future of cultural psychiatry: an international perspective", *The Canadian Journal of Psychiatry*, *45*(5), 438-446.

Lievens, E. (2018). Is self-regulation failing children? or Realising children's rights in the digital environment through self-and co-regulation: challenges and opportunities. In *OECD expert Workshop on the Protection of Children in a Connected World.*

Livingstone, S., Stoilova, M., and Kelly, A. (2016). Cyber-bullying: incidence, trends and consequences. In: Ending the Torment: Tackling Bullying from the Schoolyard to Cyberspace. United Nations Office of the Special Representative of the Secretary-General on Violence against Children, New York, USA, pp. 115-120.

McCrae, N., Gettings, S., and Purssell, E. (2017). Social media and depressive symptoms in childhood and adolescence: A systematic review. *Adolescent Research Review*, *2*(4), 315-330.

McKenzie, K. (2008). "Urbanization, social capital and mental health", *Global Social Policy*, (*3*), 359-377.

McMunn, A.M., Nazroo, J.Y., Marmot, M.G., Boreham, R., and Goodman, R. (2001). "Children's emotional and behavioural well-being and the family environment: Findings from The Health Survey for England", *Social Science and Medicine*, *53*(4), 423-440.

Mezzina, R. (2001). "Globalisation and the challenge for mental health services", In Nissanke, M., and Thorbecke, E. (Eds.). (2007). *The Impact of Globalization on the World's Poor: Transmission Mechanisms*. Springer.

OECD (2012), Recommendation of the Council on the Protection of Children Online, https://legalinstruments.oecd.org/en/instruments/OECD-LEGAL-0389 (acccssed on 24 July 2018).

OECD, P. (2017). Results (Volume III): Students' Well-Being.

Pew Research Centre (2018), How Teens and Parents Navigate Screen Time and Devise Distractions.

Pinna, F., Dell'Osso, B., Di Nicola, M., Janiri, L., Altamura, A.C., Carpiniello, B., and Hollander, E. (2015). Behavioural addictions and the transition from DSM-IV-TR to DSM-5. *Journal of Psychopathology*, *21*(4), 380-9.

Potvin Kent, M., Cameron, C., and Philippe, S. (2017). The healthfulness and prominence of sugar in child-targeted breakfast cereals in Canada. Les bienfaits pour la santé et la prédominance du sucre dans les céréales pour déjeuner destinées aux enfants au Canada. *Health promotion and chronic disease prevention in Canada: research, policy and practice*, *37*(9), 266–273. doi: 10.24095/hpcdp.37.9.02.

Prout, A., and James, A. (2015). "A new paradigm for the sociology of childhood?: Provenance, promise and problems". In *Constructing and Reconstructing Childhood* (pp. 6-28). Routledge.

Richards, B. (1989). "Visions of freedom: The subject in market relations". *Free Associations*, *1*(16), 31-42.

Robertson, M.M. (2000). "No net loss: wetland restoration and the incomplete capitalization of nature". *Antipode*, *32*(4), 463-493.

Rodrik, D. (2011). "The globalization paradox: Democracy and the future of the world economy". WW Norton & Company.

Saxena, S., and Setoya, Y. (2014). World Health Organization's Comprehensive Mental Health Action Plan: 2013–2020.

Sen, A.K. (1997). "From income inequality to economic inequality", *Southern Economic Journal*, *64*(2), 384-401.

Sharma, S. (2016). "Impact of globalisation on mental health in low-and middle-income countries". *Psychology and Developing Societies*, *28*(2), 251-279.

Tait, G. (2006). "A brief philosophical examination of ADHD". In *Critical New Perspectives on ADHD,* pp. 95-107, Routledge.

Timimi, S. (2005). "Effect of globalisation on children's mental health", *BMJ*, *331*(7507), 37-39.

Timimi, S. (2009). *A Straight-talking Introduction to Children's Mental Health Problems*. Pccs Books.

Timimi, S. (2010). "The McDonaldization of childhood: Children's mental health in neo-liberal market cultures", *Transcultural Psychiatry*, *47*(5), 686-706.

Timimi, S. (2012). "Children's mental health in the era of globalisation: Neo-liberalism, commodification, McDonaldisation, and the new challenges they pose". *Essential Notes in Psychiatry*, 413-438.

Timimi, S., and Leo, J. (Eds.). (2009). *Rethinking ADHD: From Brain to Culture*. Palgrave.

Welander, A., Lyttkens, C.H., and Nilsson, T. (2014). *Globalization and Child Health in Developing Countries: The Role of Democracy*.

World Health Organization (2003). Caring for children and adolescents with mental disorders: Setting WHO Directions.

Young, M., Wolfheim, C., Marsh, D.R., and Hammamy, D. (2012). World Health Organization/United Nations Children's Fund joint statement on integrated community case management: An equity-focused strategy to improve access to essential treatment services for children. *The American Journal of Tropical Medicine and Hygiene*, 87(5_Suppl), 6-10.

5

Bullying and Budding Minds

The Psychological Bearings

Neelam Verma

Introduction

Bullying is a behaviour that consists of power, aggression, domination and intimidation on or with a person who is perceived less powerful. According to American Psychological Association (APA), bullying is a form of aggressive behaviour in which someone intentionally and repeatedly causes another person injury or discomfort. World Health Organization (WHO) suggests that bullying is a multifaceted form of mistreatment, mostly seen in schools and workplace. It is characterized by the repeated exposure of one person to physical and/or emotional aggression including teasing, name calling, mockery, threats, harassment, and taunting, hazing, social exclusion or rumours (WHO, 2010). Commonly the issue is encountered during early years of life; however, its impact may have long-lasting effects which may continue to harm one's psychological health and wellbeing till adulthood or even later.

Schools or academic institutions are a place where child begins to learn in a formal setting. Here, children come from different backgrounds to gain knowledge and they undergo different experiences which may be positive and negative. It is suggested that the major experiences of bullying take place in a school environment as it is a place where the child interacts with most people of his/her age or above. School bullying is described as victimization and intimidation of students by their fellow classmates or peers in a school environment. Threatening repeatedly, verbal cursing, teasing, physical attacks and exclusion from the group are some common forms of school bullying and they can happen anytime within the school (Mayer-Adams & Conner, 2008). Many times childhood bullying is neglected as it seems to be a common issue amongst peers. Around 35 per cent to 40 per cent people are estimated to face bullying at least once in their life time. According to American Psychological Association (APA), approximately 40 per cent to 80 per cent of school going children experience bullying at some point during their school careers (Graham & Sandra, 2012).

Ways to Target the Victim: Various Forms of Bullying

Bullying may take place in different ways and affect differently individuals being bullied. Children and adolescents are the most targeted population for such behaviours and sometimes it is misunderstood with normal teasing behaviours amongst peers. Bullying is something which needs to be identified and intervened as it may cause serious mental health issues later. Following are the major types of bullying amongst which some may be obvious to spot while others could be a little subtle.

Physical Bullying: Physical bullying includes use of physical power to bully the other such as pushing, pinching, hitting or damaging the property of the one being bullied.

Verbal Bullying: Verbal bullying includes use of abusive words and language against the person being bullied such as name calling in an abusive way, insults, teasing, intimidating, racial comments or remarks etc.

Social Bullying: Social bullying sometimes is difficult to identify as it is performed behind the back of the person being bullied. It is used to harm someone's reputation and put them in a humiliating situation. It is done by spreading false rumours about them, contemptuous looks, saying nasty things, unkind or teasing mimicry, encouraging others to socially exclude or boycott them and damaging their social acceptance.

Cyber Bullying: Cyber bullying involves use of digital technologies to bully someone through instant messaging or texts on social media, websites or other online platforms. It can be done in a private space or publically through sending abusive or unwanted text messages, emails, images and videos. It also includes deliberately excluding someone online, spreading nasty rumours, using their log-in IDs and damaging their social image.

Sexual Bullying: Sexual bullying includes passing sexual comments, touching someone inappropriately, sending nude photos or any similar pictures or videos without their permission, objecting their sense of humour when they are not taking part in such activities etc.

It is assumed that the frequency and incidents of bullying must decrease with time. They may decrease actually, but their scars on the young minds may persist throughout and their impact may be as dangerous as of any type of child abuse. Data suggests that approximately 20 per cent people who experienced bullying in childhood suffered from some kind of mental illness in their later lives. Some of the conditions are easy to diagnose, whereas some are difficult. Some of the conditions may not even fit in particular diagnostic criteria, but there may be evident signs of adjustment, anxiety and inferiority issues during adulthood. They may exhibit signs of somatic symptoms such as sleep disturbances, headaches, stomach aches, fatigue, bed-wetting, etc. They may also experience low self-esteem, suicidal ideations, social rejection and isolation. Bullying can also lead to various health issues, alcohol or drug abuse, and major trust issues amongst the peer group when no support is received from them during their victimization period and this mistrust may persist life-long.

Recognizing the Signs of Bullying

Since the impacts of bullying are critical to mental health of young minds, it is important to know the warning signs of bullying. Following are some signs identified by organizations catering help to children and their parents in this regard. According to these, parents must speak to their children if they start to notice following signs or behavioural changes in them:

1. **Reluctant Behaviour towards Attending School:** Since school is one of the major spot for bullying, mostly children start to avoid waking up and getting ready for school. If they don't show reluctance at home they may exhibit frequent medical complaints at school so that they are picked up early by their parents from school. Children of a little higher age may start skipping the school altogether which increases school absenteeism.
2. **Frequent Somatic Complaints:** The most common manifestation of stress and anxiety is headaches, stomach aches and other pain related complaints. Usually, children who are being bullied at school regularly start giving frequent complaints similar to these. They may always have an excuse to avoid school and stay at home.
3. **Developing Aloofness within the Family:** Children being bullied may exhibit signs of aloofness at home. If there is a difference in pattern of interacting with other family members, staying alone mostly in the personal room, not showing interest

in family interactions, and acting out against siblings are the major things to observe.

4. **Disturbed Sleep or Major Change in Sleep Pattern:** Bullying episodes are so traumatic that they keep rolling in the mind always. Children may find difficult to fall asleep due to anxiety of going to the school next day and facing it all again. Thoughts of going through that everyday makes them anxious and it disturbs the quality of sleep. If the child is tensed specially during night time, or finds it difficult to fall asleep, it must be taken cautiously by parents.
5. **Extreme Emotional Responses:** Bullying may result in extreme emotional reactions such as crying spells, aggression and agitation when there is a conversation related to school or other social activities. This should be a matter of concern for the parents and other family members if the child reacts in an intense manner whenever talked about such activities. Also, evading the discussion is an additional point to be kept in mind and explored further.
6. **Change in the Friend Circle:** Sometimes, when bullying takes place children prefer to change their friends or evade the social gatherings with their group. It is more likely to happen in the adolescent group as this age group is more vulnerable emotionally and have a better understanding of other's behaviours as compared to younger kids. Parents must observe if their kids are denying for social gatherings, outings, picnics etc.
7. **Withdrawal or Excessive Use of Electronic Devices:** In cases of cyber bullying the child might be seen withdrawing or excessively using the electronic devices. Children fear to share about it as they think that their devices might be withdrawn by the parents and they may not get them back. In both the conditions, parents should take their children in confidence and assure them that they wish to help them and solve their problem and withdrawing the devices will not help.
8. **Injury Marks and Stained Clothes:** These signs are most visible in bullying which include torn, stained and ruined clothes along with bruises or physical scrapes. This mainly happens during recess where there is no one to watch the kids. The one who bullies avails the opportunity to target the victim mostly while playing as it's the safest way to do that. If anything happens, it would be well explained. If it happens once in a while, it's fine. But,.if it's a routine, it's high time to speak with the child.

Often, bullying involves Bully (the one who targets other person to show power on), the Bully Victim (the one who is the target of bully or is being bullied), and the Bystanders (those who are present during the bullying episode regardless of their level of participation). Barbara Coloroso, in her book *"The Bully, The Bullied and the Bystander"* divided bullies into several types:

- *The Confident Bully:* The one who feels a sense of superiority over other students.
- *The Social Bully:* The one who uses rumours, gossips and verbal taunts to insult others. Mostly, females with low self-esteem are categorized in this type.
- *The Fully Armored Bully:* The one who shows little emotions and usually bullies others when no one can watch or stop them.
- *The Hyperactive Bully:* The one who has issues with academics and social skills. They usually bully others and put the blame on someone else.
- *A Bullied Bully:* The one who has been bullied in past or is currently being bullied by an older one.
- *A Bunch of Bullies:* Those who gang up for fun to show desired power on others.

Bullying has a negative impact on the scholastic performance and academic achievement on all involved in the bullying process regardless of their category (whether it's a bully, bully victim or the bystander).

Why Bullies Bully?: A Background Analysis

According to *Ditch and Label* (An International Anti-Bullying Charity, UK and USA) there are some reasons behind bullying. They conducted a study over 8,850 participants and explained why people bully others. Around 14 per cent of their participants agreed and accepted that they bullied someone in past years and following were the reasons obtained from the study outcome:

1. **Past Traumatic Experiences and Stress:** Their study results showed that those who bullied others had some events in the past such as separation of parents, arrival of a young sibling at home, death of a loved one etc. These events were stressful for those individuals and resulted in bullying behaviour. We all

react to stressful situations differently, such as some believe in relaxation, meditation, seeking help from others to relieve stress, whereas, some react negatively such as bullying others, violence, alcohol or drug abuse etc. The study indicated that some people do not know how to respond in a stressful condition so they use bullying as a coping mechanism.

2. **Cultural Influence:** In every culture, there is a difference in the way girls and boys are brought up. Though, there is enough talked about equality and rights of males and females but one thing which persists common in all cultures is one's response to the emotional reactions of their kids. When a boy starts crying he is told to stop behaving like a girl and stay strong. Whereas a girl is asked to speak up for the things which affect them. Their study revealed that amongst those 14 per cent bullies of their sample were males. It was suggested that since they were not allowed to broke, they started to respond aggressively. Bullying was the way to cope with a situation which was affecting them. This is the reason why boys attack or bully others more often as compared to girls because they are not born with this; it's a kind of learned behaviour.
3. **Issues with Self-Esteem:** People who bully mostly suffer from low self-esteem. Since they do not want others to pay attention on them they try everything to shift that attention on others. Hurting and bullying others make them feel good and powerful which helps to boost up their self-esteem and feel confident.
4. **Previous Experiences of Being Bullied:** The study suggested that those who had a past experience of being bullied were most likely to bully others. They either had a bullying experience in past or being bullied currently, and they used bullying as a defence mechanism. It works like a vicious cycle of negative behaviours because they start to believe that by bullying others they will develop immunity to get bullied themselves.
5. **Difficult Family Life:** It was found that 1 in 3 of those who bully others was not happy with their family life. They responded that their family had no time for them and listen to their problems. Most of them belonged to large families and often faced rejection and lacked unconditional love. They also faced violent atmosphere within the family with lots of hostility and arguments.
6. **Lack of Access to Quality Education:** education is an institution and a mean to learn to behave in a desirable and socially

appropriate manner. It is not true that those who are uneducated are not socially good with people, but education does play an important role. The study suggested that lack of access to education was an important factor to speak in derogatory way with people and bully them.

7. **Insecure Relationships:** The study also revealed that those who bully others are most likely to feel insecure about their relationships, be it family or friends. They may have a feeling that their close members make them do things they are not comfortable in doing and also, they are not supportive and loving enough.

Since there are episodes of such events in everyone's life at least once in a lifetime, it is important to understand that if any of the mentioned things have happened by chance or once in a while it should not be labelled as bullying. '*Any single episode of social rejection, nasty comment, random intimidation and fights due to mutual arguments and disagreement are not considered as bullying, because bullying is always 'deliberate and repeated*'.

A Database of Psychological Conditions Associated with Bullying

As the earlier discussion suggested that bullying is critical to the emergence of psychological disturbance and may have long lasting effects which could last forever, it is important to review some literature and address the most prominent conditions associated with childhood bullying.

Researches often correlate bullying victimization and depressive disorders. The onset of the symptoms could occur due to mediated losses, abuse, frustration and ongoing conflicts (Birmaher, *et. al.*, 2007). Also, victimization to violence acts as a traumatic event and predisposes children and adolescents to depressive disorder (Laugharne, Lillee, & Janca, 2010). During adolescent years, when peer relationships are of utmost importance, victimization from bullying is most likely to represent abuse, frustration and conflict (Larson, & Richards, 1991). The data suggests that being bullied could cause emotional dysregulation, low self-esteem and psychological trauma which may further lead to depression (Turner, Finkelhor, & Ormrod, 2010). Children and adolescents being bullied have been characterized as submissive as they exhibit signs of helplessness. They are usually said to be less popular amongst peer group and suffer from low self-esteem (Sweeting, *et al.* 2006; Scholte, *et al.*, 2007). Many cross-sectional studies conducted over different phases of adolescence, across the countries have demonstrated a strong correlation between being bullied and developing signs of depression and suicidality (Brunstein Klomek, et al., 2007; Fitzpatrick, Dulin & Piko, 2010). Case histories of adult clients diagnosed with depression also showed a correlation between depressive symptoms and being bullied in childhood and adolescence (Gladstone, Parker, & Malhi, 2006). A similar research also reported that being a victim of school bullying increases the risk of depression in adulthood (Lund, *et al.* 2009; Jordanova, *et al.* 2007). Another research result showed that school bullying could result not only in clinical depression but also in social anxiety and functional impairment (McCabe, *et al.*, 2003). A study conducted by Roeger *et al.* (2010), suggested an association between being bullied at school and suicidal ideations after completing school. Follow-up studies suggested that being a victim of bullying could be an antecedent of emotional, behavioural and psychosocial issues in both long term and short term (Hanish & Guerra, 2002; Sourander, *et al.,* 2007). One study examined association between subtypes of bullying victimization, social connectedness and suicidal risk. Obtained results highlighted a continuum in severity of bullying involvement, social connectedness and suicidal risk (Alejandra *et al.*, 2016). A study conducted by Dorte (2012) showed an association between bullying and social exclusion anxiety in schools. The results were based on the empirical data generated over a five years period of studying bullying. In another study a history of being victimized and having poor social relationship with peers was found to be a predictor of emotional problems in adolescence (Lyndal *et al.*, 2001). Salmon and associates (1998) found a positive correlation between bullying self-reported anxiety, depression and low self-esteem in secondary school children.

The UN World Report on Violence Against Children (2006) showed that victims of corporal punishment may lead to increased aggressive behaviour and predictor of anti-social and criminal acts in adulthood. A link between being bullied and increased risk of eating disorders and social relationship difficulties was also noted in some of the studies (UNICEF, 2014; UNESCO, 2017).

Bullying has a strong relation with a child's academic performance especially if the child is being bullied in school environment. According to Stopbullying.gov (An Anti-Bullying Website Managed by Department of Health and Human Services, United States) approximately 50 per cent students of grades 4th to 12th experience bullying and around 70 per cent students admitted bullying taking place in their schools. The data suggested that nearly 160,000 students miss school or absent due to the fear of being bullied by other students. Every single day, around 280,000 students are physically attacked in schools and one out of ten of them drop school due to repeatedly being bullied. Dropouts, absenteeism and escapism cannot be taken lightly as it could have a serious impact on a child's educational experience. Violence and bullying at school makes children and adolescents afraid to attend school and interfere with their ability to concentrate and participate in school activities (UNESCO, 2017). Children who face consistent bullying at school are likely to have lower academic performance and less likely to opt for higher education. Analysis of international learning assessment highlighted the impact of bullying on learning outcomes suggesting reduced performance in key subjects like mathematics (Devries *et al.,* 2014). Researches also suggested that bullying and violence at school reduces the amount of trust students have in teachers and create an insecure environment in school which further reduces the quality of education for all (UNESCO, 2017). There is ample literature available that supports bullying has a negative impact on a child's academic performance. According to a study conducted by UCLA Centre for Health Policy Research, there was a link identified between bullying at school and low academic achievement. The author of the study quoted that "students who are repeatedly bullied in school receive poorer grades and participate less in classroom discussions. They may get mislabelled as low achievers because they fear from bullying and do not speak up in the class. Once they are labelled as low achievers they are bullied by calling 'dumb' and it make their performance even worse (Juvonen, Wang & Espinoza, 2011). A study conducted by Chandran, Krishnan & Madhavan (2018) found that academic performance of a student is negatively influenced by bullying victimization and those who were bullied were found to be more aggressive as compared to those who did not face bullying. It was also suggested that their academic performance could be improved by 20 per cent with their involvement in extracurricular activities.

A review article which included longitudinal studies analyzed through quantitative methods published between the years 1960 and 2015, indicated result of childhood bullying in adulthood in three major areas of mental health i.e. psychopathology, suicidality and criminality. The results showed that those involved in bullying in different ways i.e. bully victims and bullies are at most risk of developing psychological issues in later life. Victims were found to be more prone to develop internalizing disorders; whereas, bullies seem to be at risk of externalizing disorders, criminality and illicit drug misuse. Frequent exposure to bullying in childhood was strongly associated to adult adversities (Anat, Andre, & Henrik, 2015). Another study aimed at investigating bullying as predictor of later violence, heavy drinking and marijuana use in adulthood. Results of the study indicated that childhood bullying was significantly associated with violence and substance use among young adults (Kim, *et al.*, 2011). Niemela, *et al.* (2011) studied childhood bullying behaviours, as risk factors for substance use. The data regarding childhood bullying and psychopathology at the age of eight were collected from teachers, parents and students themselves. At the age of eighteen, data regarding frequent drinking behaviour, heavy smoking and illicit drug use was collected using self-reports from the remaining sample, i.e. 78 per cent (subjects who participated in the study at the age of eight years). Results indicated that bullying others predicted illicit drug use and being a victim of bullying predisposes subsequent smoking.

Researches based on the gender differences suggested that boys are more likely to bully others as compared to girls. This finding was consistent across countries and cultural groups (Gruber & Fineran, 2007; Peterson & Ray, 2006). The prevalence rate of bullying was higher amongst boys than girls across 40 countries (Currie, *et al.,* 2008). Boys were found to get engaged more in physical and sexual forms of bullying as compared to girls (DeSouza & Ribeiro, 2005). Boys reported being victims of physical bullying whereas girls reported being victimized by sexual means and emotional aggression (Delfabbro, *et al.,* 2006; Dao, *et al.,* 2006). A study conducted by Abdul Kareem (2017) revealed that common forms of bullying amongst males involved hitting and pushing whereas amongst females it was done through calling bad names. Males preferred bullying others on the way back to home from school, while females preferred bullying in classroom. Boys tend to bully others on the basis of their physical weakness, short temper, and friend circle and clothing status; whereas, girls tend to bully others on the basis of facial appearance, emotional factors, being overweight and academic status (Beaty & Alexeyev, 2008).

Studies on bullying based on socio-economic backgrounds suggested that students from lower socioeconomic backgrounds and students with disabilities are more likely to experience bullying as compared to other students (Agirdag, *et al.*, 2011; Jackson *et al.*, 2018). Students with emotional and behavioural disorders, autism spectrum disorder, specific learning disabilities, and speech and language impairments suffer from more victimization as compared to their peers without disabilities (Rose & Gage, 2017).

National Centre for Education Statistics (2016) suggests that the most cases of bullying take place at hallway and stairway at school which was reported around 42 per cent, inside the classroom the reported rate was 34 per cent, in cafeteria it was reported 22 per cent, outside on school grounds the reported bullying rate was 10 per cent, and in bathrooms and locker rooms it was reported around 9 per cent.

The Gay Bullying Statistics (2015), suggested that individuals who were homosexual, bisexual or transgender, they were likely to experience bullying five times higher than others. They also felt unsafe to attend school because of their sexual orientation and being bullied. According to the U.S. Centre for Disease Control and Prevention, approximately 11 per cent to 30 per cent of gay and lesbian students and 12 per cent to 25 per cent of bisexual students did not go to school at least one day during the 30 days preceding the survey due to safety concerns.

Bullying Prevention in Schools

Bullying prevention in schools involves interference of authorities to stop bullying in school premises. According to a report published in *The Telegraph*, 19th March (2015), the Central Board of Secondary Education (CBSE) has recommended that schools must mediate to step forward about anti-bullying programmes and conduct them successfully with the help of teachers, staff, parents and involvement of students. The board also recommended few methods to intervene bullying and made them a part of curricular. The circular states that anti-bullying committee should include vice-principal, a senior teacher, school doctor, counsellor, school management representative, and legal representative. Along with these there must be a peer educator who is usually the head student or house captain of the school. The curricular emphasizes that the committee must work on developing anti-bullying programmes for employees, parents and students so that they are aware about bullying and know how to deal with it. As a preventive act, CBSE suggested to form an anti-bullying committee with various stakeholders and developing training programmes for staff, students and parents. As an intervention their policy suggested to give oral and written warning, suspension from attending classes or school for a specific time period, withholding or cancelling the results, and expulsion or rustication from school in extreme cases of bullying.

It is important for the school authorities to involve students in activities which provide information regarding bullying. These activities may include internet or library search to read and understand about bullying, its types, prevention and how to respond in a situation when someone is being bullied. Conducting workshops, presentations, group discussions to spread awareness about bullying can be really helpful. Students could be encouraged to role play about bullying situations and share knowledge about how to stop it. As an intervention mean, students who have been bullied could be encouraged to engage in creative writing, public speaking against bullying and spreading awareness about how to cope with such situations. Teachers and parents can play an important role in educating students about respect giving behaviour. It is a duty of every parent and teacher to discuss with children why everybody needs to be given respect and why no one deserves bullying. They should be told about healthy peer relationships and why its importance to maintain a healthy psychological space (U.S. Department of Health and Human Services, 2018).

Since students with disabilities need special attention there has to be a special plan for taking care of their safety at school. Rose and Monda-Amaya (2012) suggested few successful strategies to prevent bullying among students with disabilities such as: (1) involvement of teachers and peers in more meaningful and appropriate interactions, (2) creating ample opportunities for disabled students to increase social competence and positive interactions, and (3) active involvement of school authorities to encourage social awareness and provide individualized interventions for disabled students.

The effectiveness of anti-bullying programmes is critical to the extent they are followed properly and strictly. There has to be a clear and strict action plan in order to identify, manage and stop bullying in school environment. According to U.S. Department of Justice (2004), teachers, staff members, and other administrative authorities apart from canteen workers, bus drivers, and playground monitors could be given training to recognize and respond to bullying. It has been studied that when consistent anti-bullying policies are made and implemented in schools, bullying incidents and rate of violence is significantly decreased (Cohn & Canter, 2003). To make these programmes even more effective, it is important to work with students on one to one basis. They must be assured that their problems would be intervened with utmost care (Harris & Willoughby, 2003). Schools can provide increased adult supervision especially in those areas where bullying takes place more often (Shellard & Turner, 2004). Also, in order to make the anti-bullying programmes more effective, school staff must educate and involve parents so that they observe early signs of bullying and interfere accordingly (U.S. Department of Justice, 2004). Day and Snapp (2016) suggested that, to intervene bullying it is important for the schools to adopt more supportive practices such as: (1) providing adequate counseling and services for students, (2) considering sanctions for violation of rules on the basis of individual cases with a range of options, (3) ensuring confidentiality of information disclosed and referral services if required, (4) helping students to deal with their emotional and behavioural problems caused by bullying, and (5) fostering resilience, youth development and promotion of assets.

The efficacy of school-based intervention programmes to stop bullying behaviour in school was analyzed in a meta-analytical review done by Hannah, David and Maria (2019). Major highlights of the review suggested that anti-bullying programmes effectively reduce school bullying perpetration by approximately 19-20 per cent and school bullying victimization by approximately 15-16 per cent. The review also suggested need for consistent researches to explore about specific components of school bullying which are most effective. Bullying programmes set up in schools with the engagement of faculty and other staff showed significantly reduced victimization and bullying in schools (O'Brennan, Waasdrop, Bradshaw, 2014). Incidents of victimization were also found to be reduced when students themselves disapproved bullying (Guerra, Nancy, *et al.*, 2010). Success of any intervention is highly associated with early detection and early intervention, their constant evaluation to assess effectiveness and student volunteers to spread and share awareness about dealing with bullying (Berger & Kathleen Staseen, 2007). According to McCallion and Feder (2013), school-based bullying prevention programmes significantly decrease bullying up to 25 per cent.

In order to stop bullying, Government of India had circulated a regulation called "UGC regulations on curbing the menace of ragging in higher education institutions (2009)". In higher education institutions, India's anti-ragging laws lead to immediate arrests of individuals caught ragging other students. The victim of ragging or bullying has the right to file FIR under thirteen different Indian penal codes in the police station under the area where incident had taken place. Former HRD minister formed a committee of academic and mental health experts to look and interfere in such incidents taking place in schools. Regarding cyber bullying there is a provision for victim to file complaint under IT Act 2000 where two kinds of offences could be taken, one is publishing information which is obscene and breach of confidentiality.

In current era, cyber bullying has become extremely prevalent. Approximately 95 per cent teens reported being bullied or witnessed someone being bullied on social media. Children and adolescents of current time have easy access to electronic means and it is now considered common also to be on a social media platform. Now, it is a call of parents to guide their children to be safe while using and handling social media accounts. All social media platforms come with pros and cons and they have to be considered seriously. Teenagers need to be informed about safe usage of their account IDs and passwords and not sharing that with anyone at any cost. Researchers have indicated that many times cyber bullying is left unreported due to mistrust of teens in their adults around. Study conducted by Nixon and Charisse (2014), identified four major reasons of cyber bullying not being reported: 1. The bully victims do not feel connected to the adults around them, 2. The students do not see cyber bullying as an issue worth discussing with others, 3. Students don't see the adults around capable enough of dealing with such issues, 4. Teenagers have increased feelings of shame and humiliation regarding cyber bullying.

There is plenty of literature available exploring and discussing outcomes of bullying, its impact on child and adolescent mental health and interventions to deal with such situations; however, there is still scope for improvement to conduct researches with more fruitful outcomes. Issue of bullying may not appear much important to many, but in reality it needs attention of parents, authorities, and most importantly the victims. Many times individuals who are being bullied do not know what is happening. They keep suffering from the anxious feelings and cope with it in maladaptive ways. Though there is fair awareness about bullying nowadays amongst school authorities, but it takes strength to resolve any problem. So, there is a need that teachers, students, parents, and mental health professionals come forward together to prevent and stop bullying, and save the budding minds to suffer from its outcomes.

References

Abdul-Kareem, J. (2017). "Gender differences in bullying and victimization among early adolescents in Jordan people", *International Journal of Social Sciences, 3,* 440-451.

Agirdag, O., Demanet, J., Van Houtte, M., Van Avermaet, P., Bettelheim, K.A. (2011). "Ethnic school composition and peer victimization: A focus on the interethnic school climate", *International Journal of Intercultural Relations, 35*(4), 465-473.

Aljendra, A., Kiel, J., Opperman., Polly, Y., Gipson., Cheryl, A. King. (2016). "Suicidal ideation and suicide attempts among youth who report bully victimization, bully perpetration and/or low social connectedness", *Journal of Adolescence. 51,* 19-29.

Anat B.K., Andre, S., Henrick, E. (2015). "Bullying by peers in childhood and effects on psychopathology, suicidality, and criminality in adulthood", *The LANCET Psychiatry. 2*(10), 930-941.

Beaty, L.A., Alexeyev, E.B. (2008). "The problem of school bullies", *Adolescence. 43*(169), 1-11.

Berger, Kathleen, S. (2007). "Update on bullying at school: science forgotten?" *Developmental Review. 27,* 90-126.

Birmaher, B., Brent, D., Bernet, W., Bukstein, O., Walter, H., Benson, R.S., Chrisman, A., Farchoine, T., Greenhill, L., Hamilton, J., Kaeble, H., Kinlal, J., Schoettle, U., Stock, S., Ptakowski, K.K., Medicus, J. (2007). "Practice parameter for the assessment and treatment of children and adolescents with depressive disorders", *Journal of American Academy of Child and Adolescent Psychiatry. 46*(11), 1503-26.

Brunstein Klomek, A., Marrocco, F., Kleinman, M., Schonfeld, I.S., Gould, M.S. (2013). "*Bully Facts and Statistics",* Achieved from the original on 25 December (2013).

Centres for Disease Control and Prevention. HIV Surveillance Report, 2014; Vol. 26. Published November (2015).

Chandran, R., Krishnan Namboodiripad, P.C., Madhavan, V. (2018). "Bullying and academic performance among school children", *International Journal of Pure and Applied Mathematics. 118*(5), 587-602.

Cohn, A., and Canter, A. (2003). "Bullying facts for school and parents", *National Association of School Psychologists.* Retrieved from http://www.naspcenter.org.

Coloroso, B. (2004). "The bully, the bullied, and the bystander: From preschool to high school: how parents and teachers can help break the cycle of violence: New York: Quill.

Currie, C. Nic Gabhainn, S., Godeau, E. (eds.) (2008). "Inequalities in young people's health: HBSC international report from the 2005-2006 survey. Copenhagen, WHO Regional Office for Europe. (Health Policy for Children and Adolescents, No. 5).

Dao, T.K., Kerbs, J.J., Rollin, S.A., Potts, I., Gutierrez, R., Choi, K., Creason, A.H., Wolf, A., Prevatt, F. (2006). "The association between bullying dynamics and psychological distress", *Journal of Adolescent Health. 3* (2), 277-282.

Day, J.K., and Snapp, S.D. (2016). "Supportive, not punitive, practices reduce homophobic bullying and improve school connectedness", *Psychology of Sexual Orientation and Gender Diversity, 3,* 416-425. Retrieved from http://psynet.apa.org.ezp3.lib.umn.edu/fülltext/2016-41520-001.pdf.

Delfabbro, P., Winefield, T., Trainor, S., Dollard, M., Anderson, S., Metzer, J. (2006). "Peer and teacher bullying/victimization of South Australian secondary school students: Prevalence and psychosocial profiles", *British Journal of Educational Psychology. 76,* 71-90.

DeSouza, E.R, and Ribeiro, J., (2005). "bullying and sexual harassment among

Brazilian high school students", *Journal of Interpersonal Violence. 20*(9), 1018-1038.

Devries, K.M., Child, J.C., Allen, E., Walakira, E., Parkes, J., Naker, D. (2014). "School violence, mental health and educational performance in Uganda", *Pediatrics. 133*(1), 129-37.

Dorte, M.S. (2012). "Bullying and social exclusion anxiety in schools", *British Journal of Sociology of Education. 33*(3), 355-372.

Fitzpatrick, K.M., Dulin, A., Piko, B.J. (2010). "Bullying and depressive symptomatology among low-income, African-American youth", *Journal of Youth and Adolescence. 39*(6), 634-45.

Gladstone, G.L., Parker, G.B., Malhi, G.S. (2006). "Do bullied children become anxious and depressed adults?: a cross-sectional investigation of the correlates of bullying and anxious depression", *Journal of Nervous Mental Disorders. 194*(3), 201-8.

Graham and Sandra (2012). "Bullying: A module for teachers. Retrieved from American Psychological Association on 30 December 2012.

Gruber, J.E., and Fineran, S., (2007). "The impact of bullying and sexual harassment on middle school and high school girls", *Violence against Women. 13,* 627-643.

Hanish, L.D., Guerra, N.G. (2002). "A longitudinal analysis of patterns of adjustment following peer victimization", *Developmental Psychopathology. 14*(1), 69-89.

Hannah G., David P.F., and Maria, M.T. (2019). "Examining the effectiveness of school bullying intervention programmes globally: A metal analysis", *International Journal of Bullying Prevention. 1*(1), 14-31.

Harris, S., and Willoughby, W. (2003). "Teacher perceptions of student bullying behaviours", *ERS Spectrum, 21*(3), 11-18.

Jordanova, V., Stewart, R., Goldberg, D. (2007). "Age variation in life events and their relationship with common mental disorders in a national survey population", *Social Psychiatry Epidemiology. 42,* 611-16.

Jorge, C.S. and Bennett, L.L. (2010). "Prevention of bullying-related morbidity and mortality: A call for public health policies", *Bulletin of the World Health Organization* 2010. *88,* 403-403.

Juvonen, J., Wang, Y., and Espinoza, G. (2011). "Bullying experiences and compromised academic performance across middle school grades", *The Journal of Early Adolescence. 31*(1), 152-173.

Kim, M., J., Catalano, R., Abbott, R. (2011). "Bullying at elementary school and problem/behaviour in young adulthood: A study of bullying, violence and substance use from age 11 to age 21." *Criminal Behaviour and Mental Health: CBMH. 21,* 136-144.

Larson R., and Richards M.H. (1991). "Daily companionship in late childhood and early adolescence: Changing developmental contexts", *Child Development. 62,* 284-300

Laugharne, J., Lillee, A., Janca, A. (2010). "Role of psychological trauma in the cause and treatment of anxiety and depressive disorders", *Current Opinion Psychiatry. 23*(1), 25-29.

Lund, R., Nielsen, K.K., Hansen, D.H. Kriegbaum, M., Molbo, D., Due, P., and Christensen, U. (2009). "Exposure to bullying at school and depression in adulthood: a study of Danish men born in 1953", *European Journal of Public Health. 19*(1), 111-116.

Lyndal, B., John, B.C., Lyndal, T., Kerryn, R., and George, P. (2001). "Does bullying cause emotional problems? A prospective study of young teenagers", *The BMJ. 323*, 480.

Mayer-Adams, Nancy and Conner, B. (2008). "School violence: Bullying behaviours and the psychosocial school environment in middle schools", *Children and Schools. 30,* 211-221.

McCabe, R.E., Antony, M.M., Summerfeldt, L.J., Liss, A., and Swinson, R.P. (2003). "Preliminary examination of the relationship between anxiety disorders in adults and self-reported history of teasing or bullying experiences", *Cognitive Behaviour Therapy. 32,* 187-93.

McCallion, G., and Feder, J. (2013). "Student bullying: Overview of research, federal initiatives, and legal issues", *Congressional Research Services.* Retrieved from http://www.fas.org/sgp/crs/misc/r43254.pdf.

National Centre for Education Statistics. (2016). "Indicators of school crime and safety." U.S. Department of Education. Retrieved from https://nces.ed.gov/pubs2017/2017064.pdf.

Niemela, S., Brunstein-Klomek, A., Sillanmaki, L., Helenius, H., Piha, J., Kumpulainen, K., Moilanen, I., Tamminen, T., Almqvist, F., Sourander, A. (2011). "Childhood bullying behaviours at the age eight and substance use at age 18 among males. A nationwide prospective study", *Addiction Behaviour 36*(3), 256-260.

Nixon, C.L. (2014). "Current perspectives: The impact of cyber bullying on adolescent health", *Adolescent Health, Medicine and Therapeutics. 5,* 143-158.

O'Brennam, L.M., Waasdrop, T.E., and Bradshaw, C.P. (2014). "Strengthening bullying prevention through school staff connectedness", *Journal of Educational Psychology. 106*(3), 870-880.

Peterson, J.S., and Ray, K.E. (2006). "Bullying and the gifted: victims, perpetrators, prevalence, and effects." *Gifted Child Quarterly, Sage Journals. 50*(2), 148-168.

Prevention at School. U.S Department of Health and Human Services. 29 February 2012. Retrieved 26 April 2018.

Roeger, L., Allison, S., Rebecca, Eckert, K.A., and Goldney, R. (2010). "Is a history of school bullying victimization associated with adult suicidal ideation?: a south Australian population-based observational study", *The Journal of Nervous and Mental Disease. 198*(10), 728-733.

Rose, C.A., and Gage, N.A. (2017). "Exploring the involvement of bullying among students with disabilities over time", *Exceptional Children. 83,* 298-314.

Rose, C.A., and Monda-Amaya, L.E. (2012). "Bullying and victimization among students with disabilities: effective strategies for classroom teachers", *Intervention in School and Clinic, 48.* 99-107. Retrieved from http://journals.sagepub.com.ezp3.lib.umn.edu/doi/abs/10.1177/1053451211430119.

Salmon, G., James, A., and Smith, D.M. (1998). "Bullying in schools: self-reported anxiety, depression, and self-esteem in secondary school children", *BMJ (Clinical Research ed.) 317*(7163), 924-925.

Scholte, R., Engels, R., Overbeek, G., de Kemp, R., and Haselager, G. (2007). "Stability in bullying and victimization and its association", *Journal of Abnormal Child Psychology. 35,* 217-228.

Shellard, E., and Turner, J.R. (2004). "Safe and secure schools. ERS Focus on... Arlington, V.A.: Educational Research Service.

Sourander, A., Jensen, P., Ronning, J.A., Niemela, S., Helenius, H., Sillanmaki, L., Kumpulainen, K., Piha, J., Tamminen, T., Moilanen, I., Almqvist, F. (2007). "What is the early adulthood outcome of boys who bully or are bullied in childhood? The Finnish "From a Bou to a Man", *Paediatrics, 120*(2), 397-404.

Statistics from the Annual Bullying Survey (2017). Ditch and Label. England, U.K., California, U.S.A. retrieved from https://www.ditchthelabel.org.

Stopbullying.gov. A federal government website managed by the U.S. Department of Health and Human Services, Washington, D.C. 20201.

Sweeting, H., Young, R., West, P., Der, G. (2006). "Peer victimization and depression in early-mid adolescence: A longitudinal study", *British Journal of Educational Psychology. 7,* 577-594.

The Gay Bullying Statistics—*Bullying Statistics*. 7 July 2015. Retrieved 19 February (2016).

Turner, H.A., Finkelhor, D., Ormrod, R. (2010). "The effects of adolescent victimization on self-concept and depressive symptoms", *Child Maltreat. 15*(1), 76-90.

U.S. Department of Justice (2004). "Bullying in schools." *Community-oriented policing services' problem oriented guides for police. Problem specific guides series, No. 12.* Retrieved from http://www.cops.usdoj.gov.

UGC regulations on curbing the menace of ragging in higher education institutions, (2009). http:/www.iitr.ac.innewsuploadsfileacademic/updatedraggingnotification.pdf.

UNESCO (2017). "School violence and bullying: Global Status Report (PDF). Paris, UNESCO. Pp. 17, 29, 31.

UNICEF (2014). "Hidden in plain sight: A statistical analysis of violence against children.

Wolpret, S. (2010). "Victims of bullying suffer academically as well, UCLA psychologists report." UCLA Centre for Health Policy Research.

6

Adolescents' Attitude towards Substance Use in Mizoram

Manoj Kr. Pandey, Lalawmpuia, Rinpari Ralte and *Loisi Vanlalnguri*

Introduction

Alcohol and Drug Abuse

National Institute on Drug Abuse (2009) defines drug addiction as a condition of intense and, at times, uncontrollable drug craving, along with compulsive drug seeking and use that persists even in the face of devastating consequences.

It further clarifies that addiction is something beyond an impulsive drug taking, which can likewise deliver enduring adverse outcomes. For instance, drug abuse and addiction can lead into a risk of mental and physical illnesses. Furthermore, a wide scope of dysfunctional behaviours due to abuse interferes with typical working in family, the occupation, and the more extensive network such as community.

Drugs appear to play a crucial role in "group culture" of children and adolescents. They create their "group identity" which brings them proximate to the group, where such activities are normal and it feels them a sense of adulthood. In addition it decreases their anxiety, inhibition, promotes enjoyment and results in an enhanced shared experience among the group. Unfortunately, when these drugs are taken in small amount, damage health and adversely affect socio-occupational functioning. But when these drugs are taken into large amount they can cause remarkable physical and/or social impairment and sometimes can causes death (Turk, Graham, & Verhulst, 2007).

Keane, Reaper-Reynolds, Williams and Wolfe (2005) define the drug is any substance which changes the way the body functions mentally, physically or emotionally. They further added that these substances are also known as psychoactive drugs because they affect central nervous system and bring changes in mood, thinking, perception and behaviour of an individual.

Jiloha (2009) cited Kastner and Silbereisen (1984) and reported that as per them, drug abuse/dependence is closely associated with the developmental pressures. The drug abuse can develop in as many as 6 ways:

1. A deliberate violation of social norms.
2. Testing whether the adolescent is able to behave like an adult.
3. Excessive and ritualized behaviour in the sense of testing one's limits.
4. A lack of self-control.
5. An age related life-style, aimed at peer-group integration.
6. An emergency reaction to age-related every day stress, thus developmentally irrelevant coping strategy.

American Psychiatric Association (2013) entailed that essential feature of a substance use disorder is a cluster of cognitive, behavioural, and physiological symptoms indicating that the individual continues using substance despite significant substance-related problems. An important feature of substance use disorders is an underlying change in brain circuits that may persist beyond detoxification, particularly in individuals with severe disorders. The behavioural effects of these brain changes may be exposed to drug-related stimuli. These persistent drug effects may benefit from long-term approaches to treatment. Substance used disorders are often associated with other disorders of mental illness. These disorders vary with the use of substances (abuse and dependence). The common mental disorders associated with substance use are psychotic, bipolar, depressive, anxiety, obsessive-compulsive, sleep, sexual dysfunction, delirium, and neuro-cognitive disorders.

American Psychiatric Association (2000) have given comprehensive definition and criteria for substance abuse and dependence, which often have more devastating impact on all spheres of abusers' life than other forms of substance use.

(A) Abuse: Substance abuse is described as a 'maladaptive' pattern of substance use leading to clinically significant impairment or distress, as manifested by one (or more) of the following within a 12 month period:

- Recurrent use leading to failure to fulfill major role obligations (work, home, school, etc.).
- Recurrent use in situations where it is physically hazardous (e.g., drunk driving).
- Repeated substance-related legal problems (repeated disorderly conduct while drunk).
- Persistent use despite recurrent social/interpersonal problems caused or exacerbated by the effects of a substance (e.g., arguments with spouse or physical fights).

(B) Dependence: Substance dependence is described as a 'maladaptive' pattern of substance use leading to clinically significant impairment or distress, as manifested by three (or more) of the following within a 12 month period:

- Tolerance: a need for increased amounts of a substance to achieve the desired effect or a diminished effect with ongoing use of the same amount of substance.
- Withdrawal.
- The substance taken in larger amounts over longer periods than was intended.
- Persistent desire or unsuccessful efforts to cut down or control use.
- A great deal of time spent in activities relating to obtaining the substance, using the substance or recovering from use.
- Significant social, occupational or recreational activities are given up or reduced because of use.
- Use continued despite knowledge of having a persistent or recurrent physical or psychological problem that is likely to have been caused or exacerbated by the substance.

Types of Drugs

Centre for Mental Health in Schools (CMHS) (2003) has classified drugs, their major roots of administration and their origins. In the following sections authors have listed these drugs with their characteristics and their impact on mental and physical health of an individual as per description by CMHS.

1. **Crack or Cocaine:** Crack is common name of cocaine in public domain. Cocaine is a powerful addictive drug of abuse and dependence. Once an individual try it, cannot control its use. It is processed through cocaine hydrochloride. It is taken by abuser through sniffing or snorting, injecting, and smoking. It stimulates the nervous system so strongly that it inhibits the re-absorption of dopamine, a neurotransmitter that is highly associated with the pleasure and movement. As a result of dopamine's excessive amount it produces immense sense of pleasure to individuals. Abusers/dependants reports irritability, anxiety, restlessness, and depression and many other physical symptoms, when they do not take, which provokes them to take is again. Its use in high dose is associated with paranoia or suspicion. It is also associated with depression. Prolonged cocaine snorting can result in ulceration of mucous membrane of the nose and can damage the nasal septum and can cause deaths as result of cardiac arrest or seizures followed by respiratory arrest.
2. **Heroin:** Heroin is a highly addictive drug. It is a processed form of morphine, extracted from the seedpod of the Asian poppy plant. It appears as white or a brown powder. Often is named as brown sugar. It is taken through injection, snorting or smoking. After intake of it, user feels a high of euphoria ("rush") accompanied by warm flushing of the skin, a dry mouth, and heavy extremities. Following initial euphoria, the user goes "on the node," an alternatively wakeful and drowsy state. Mental functioning becomes clouded due to depression of central nervous system. Chronic users often develop collapsed veins, infection of the heart lining and valves, abscesses, cellulites, liver disease, pneumonia.
3. **Inhalants:** Inhalants are breathable chemical vapours that produce psychoactive (mind-altering) effects. Adolescents are more likely to abuse inhalants, because are easily available and inexpensive. These are administered through nose or mouth, which provides feeling of stimulated. Excessive consumption may lead to sense of inhibition and less control and finally may result in a loss of consciousness. Physical adverse impacts of their use include liver and kidney damage, blood oxygen depletion etc. Inhalants fall into three categories:
   a) Solvents:

- Industrial or household solvents such as paint thinners, cleaning fluids, gasoline, and glues.
- Art or office supply solvents such as correction fluids, felt-tip-marker fluid, and electronic contact cleaners.

b) Gases

- Gases used in household or commercial products, including butane lighters and propane tanks, whipping creams or disappears (whippets), and refrigerant gases.
- Household aerosol propellants such as spray paints, hair spray and fabric protector spray.

c) Nitrites

- Aliphatic nitrites such as cyclohexyl nitrite, amyl nitrite and butyl nitrite.

4. **Lysergic acid diethylamide (LSD):** LSD is one of the drugs in hallucinogen class and one of the most potential mood-changing chemicals. It is derived from lysergic acid, which is found in ergot, a fungus that grows on rye and other grains. It is sold in form of tablets, capsules, and, occasionally, in liquid form. Its administration route is mouth with variety of forms.
Immediate physical effects include dilated pupil, higher body temperature, increased heart rate and blood pressure, sweating, loss of appetite, sleeplessness, dry mouth, and tremors. Other longer effects include for users rapid mood swing. If taken in large amount, it produces delusions and visual hallucination, sense of time and self is often found altered. Along with other symptoms, heavy users may have long lasting psychoses, schizophrenia and severe depression.
5. **Marijuana:** It is the most commonly used illicit drug worldwide. It is a product from a dry, shredded green/brown mix of flowers, stems, seeds, and leaves of hemp plant, *Cannabis sativa*. It is usually smoked in cigarette (join nail), or in a pipe (bong or hukka). It is also taken by mouth in form of cannabis round tablet. The main active chemical in it is THC (delta-9-tetrahydrocannabinol). The membranes of certain nerve cells in the brain contain protein receptors that bind to THC. Once reaches there, THC kicks off a series of cellular reactions that ultimately lead to high that users experience when they smoke it. It has serious health impacts. It impairs the immune system of the body that fight against cancer. Depression, anxiety, and personality changes are all associated with the longer use of

it. It impairs the cognitive abilities of the individuals such as attention, memory and learning ability, which affect the person's functioning in different areas of life.

6. **Methamphetamine:** It is an addictive stimulant drug that strongly activates the certain nervous system. It is a chemical related to amphetamine group, but its effects in central nervous systems are stronger. Its street names are such as speed, meth, and chalk. It is usually administered through inhalation (smoking), orally, or by intravenous injection. It releases high levels of dopamine, which stimulate brain cell resulting in enhancement of mood and body movement. Longer use of it appears to reduce the levels of dopamine, which can result in symptoms like those of Parkinson's disease, a severe movement disorder.
   In its small amounts it produces increased wakefulness, increased physical activity, decreased appetite, increased respiration, hyperthermia, and euphoria. Other CNS effects include irritability, insomnia, confusion, tremors, convulsions, anxiety, paranoid ideas, and aggressiveness. Increased heart rate and blood pressure can cause irreversible damage to vessels in brain, producing strokes. It can also result in cardiovascular collapse and death in high doses.
7. **Phencyclidine (PCP):** PCP was manufactured in the 1950s as an intravenous anaesthetic. It is produced illegally and in some parts of world legally in laboratories and is sold in by the names of "angel dust", "ozone", "wack" and "rocket fuel" in western countries. It is a white crystalline powder that is easily soluble in water or alcohol. It is usually administered in three ways i.e., snorted, smoked, or eaten.
   There are many adverse effects of it on physiology. At low to moderate doses it produces increase in breathing rate, blood pressure and pulse rate. Respiration becomes slow and flushing and profuse sweating occurs. Generalized numbness in extremities and muscular incardination also seen. At high doses, it drops the blood pressure, pulse rate, and respiration. Often may be accompanied by vomiting, blurred vision, flicking up and down of the eyes, drooling, loss of balance and dizziness. It may cause seizure, coma, and death. Psychological effects of it include illusions, hallucination, disordered thinking, and often catatonia.
8. **Methylphenidate:** It is a medication prescribed for individuals

who have an abnormally high level of activity known as attention-deficit hyperactivity disorder. It is a central nervous system stimulant. It has effects similar to, but more prominent than, caffeine and less prominent than amphetamines. There are reports worldwide that it is misused by the individuals because of its stimulant properties. It has several effects if not taken under proper prescriptions such as appetite suppression, wakefulness, increased focus/attentiveness, and euphoria. It is usually orally taken in form of tablets. Some abusers crush it and dissolve the tablets in water and inject. The mixture-complication can arise from this because insoluble fillers in the tablets can block the small blood vessels that may be dangerous to health of the individuals.

9. **Steroids (Anabolic-Androgenic):** Anabolic refers to muscle-building and androgenic refers to increased masculine characteristics. Steroid is a class of drugs. This drug is prescribed for low amount of testosterone. It is also prescribed in controlling pain in different medical conditions (Vyey, 2010). It is misused by athletes to enhance performance and to improve physical appearance. Major side effects of improper use of it lead to liver tumour, cancer, jaundice, high blood pressure, increase in LDL (bad cholesterol) and decrease HDL (good cholesterol).

Risk and Protective Factors

Hawkins, Catalano, and Miller (1992) proposed common risk and protective factors in context of substance abuse prevention. Commonly risk factors are understood to increase the vulnerability to particular clinical condition and protective factors work as buffer against those clinical conditions. The risk factors and protective factors for drug abuse described in this chapter are adapted from the findings, which were derived from the research and discussion conducted on substance abuse and its treatment (Hawkins, Catalano, and Miller, 1992). They categorized these risk factors into two broad categories. First category includes environmental variables and second includes personal factors.

A. Risk Factors

a) **Environmental variables:** Environmental risk factors/variables refer to those that have been present in the socio-cultural context of the individual.

- Community/school/family factors where there is an favourable attitude towards drug use
- Availability of drugs
- Extreme economic deprivation
- High levels of mobility
- Low neighbourhood/family attachment
- Community organization and friends who engage in the problem behaviour
- Academic failures
- Family history of alcohol/drug abuse/problem behaviours
- Family conflict.

b) **Personal variables:** Personal risk factors/variables refer to those that have been present in individuals before starting of drug use/abuse, which is usually called pre-morbid features of an individual. The following factors are categorized into personal risk factors:

- Elevated degrees of withdrawal
- Alienation
- Impulsiveness
- Defiance
- Aggression
- Poor school performance.

B. Protective Factors

National Institute of Drug (1999) laid down a list of protective factors that can buffer against the involvement of children and adolescent in alcohol/ drug abuse. These factors are following:

- Stable temperament
- A high degree of motivation
- A strong parent-child/adolescence bond
- Consistent parental supervision and discipline
- Bonding to pro-social institutions
- Association with peers who hold conventional attitudes.

Keane, Reaper-Reynolds, Williams, & Wolfe (2005) provided a comprchensive model to explain why people use drug. As per them there are basically two factors. First, risk factors that increase the likelihood of use/abuse of drug and second, protective factors that decrease the likelihood of drug use/abuse. The model is given below.

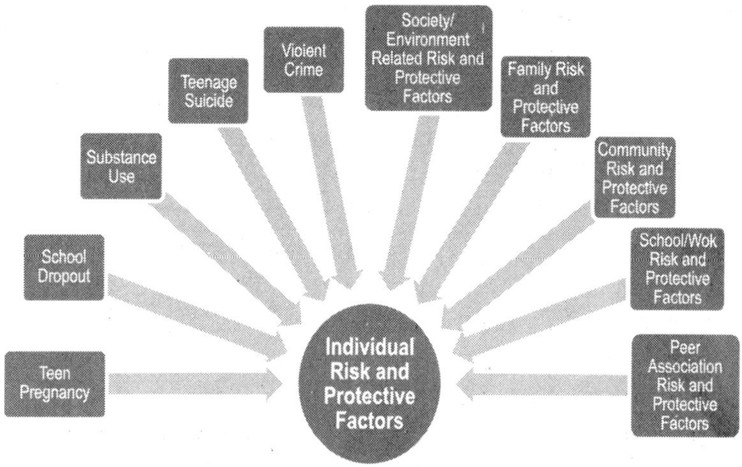

Source: Based on Keane, Reaper-Reynolds, Williams, & Wolfe (2005).

The above model explains different factors (risk and protective) which are usually found in the adolescents or individuals with various sorts of drug/alcohol abuse or dependence. These factors are either responsible for or are associated in some ways with the drug abuse problems. This information is quite worthwhile for the clinicians or policy-makers look after how to control or prevent such problems in youths.

Screening or Assessment Measures

CMHS (2003) has given a list of brief, paper and pencil, self-report questionnaires which can be helpful in screening the presence of drugs/ alcohol abuse/dependence and will be helpful for either management of cases or further detailed psych-physiological assessment. This chapter has limited scope to provide the details about these tools. However, these tools are provided here for readers to be aware of and so that they can search about these in details at the time of need.

- Adolescent Drinking Index (Psychological Assessment Resources; Harrell & Wirtz, 1989).
- Adolescent Drug Involvement Scale (Moberg, 1983).

- Client Substance Index (Olympic Counseling Services; Moore, 1983).
- Drug Abuse Screening Test—Adolescent version (Skinner, 1982).
- Drug and Alcohol Problem Quick Screen (Schwartz & Wirtz, 1990).
- Drug Use Screening Inventory (Tarter, 1990, Tarter & Hegedus, 1991).
- Perceived Benefit of Drinking & Drug Use Scales (Petchers & Singer, 1987; Petchers, Singer, Angelotta, & Chow, 1988).
- Personal Experience Screen Questionnaire (Western Psychological Services; Winters, 1992).

Prevalence of Alcohol and Drug Abuse in India and North-Eastern Regions

Ambekar *et al.* (2019) stated that this was first time in the history of India that a survey was conducted, in which all states and UTs have been covered and more than 1500 personnel were involved in data collection, which took place from December 2017 to October 2018 in representative population of aged 10 to 75. It included two kinds of surveys. Household Sample Survey (HSS) and Respondent Driven Sampling (RDS). HSS covered 200,111 households and 186 districts of the country with a total of 473,569 individuals were interviewed. RDS was conducted in 135 districts and covered 72,642 people suffering from dependence on illicit drugs. As a result from this extensive countrywide survey eight categories of psychoactive substance (including alcohol and drugs); Alcohol, Cannabis, Opioids, Cocaine, Amphetamine type stimulants, Sedatives, Inhalants and hallucinogens were found to be prevalent in the country.

They further found that alcohol was the most common (14.6%) psychoactive substance used in country. In terms of absolute numbers 16 crore persons consume alcohol in the country and men overpower women in this context. After alcohol, cannabis and opioids are next commonly used substances. About 2.8 per cent (3.1 crore persons) reported having used any product of cannabis in previous year. About 2.1 per cent of country's population (2.26 crore) were found using opioid in different forms. Opioids includes Opium (or its variants like poppy husk from smack or brown sugar) and variety of pharmaceutical Opiods. The most common opioid used was Heroin (1.14%). Survey further reported that sufficient number of people used sedatives and inhalants (1.08%). Other categories of drugs such as Cocaine (0.10%), Amphetamine Type Stimulants (0.18%), and

Hallucinogens (0.12%) were used by a small proportion of country's population.

The above national survey reported that highest prevalent drug in Mizoram state are Opioids, Sedatives, Inhalants and followed by alcohol and cannabis. These drugs are also most prevalent in other north-east states (Nagaland, Arunachal Pradesh, Sikkim and Manipur) along with Mizoram at almost top.

The scope of present study is to explore the attitude of adolescent population towards alcohol/drug abuse in Aizawl district of Mizoram.

Impetus Behind Current Study

In a same geographical or community or family environment why few people are more vulnerable to any sort of substance abuse than others. This is the milestone question. Keane, Reaper-Reynolds, Williams and Wolfe (2005) suggested attitude and values are important individual factors which may or may not lead the individual towards the alcohol/drug abuse/dependence. Positive attitude towards consumption of alcohol and other drugs is a worldwide scenario among youth about their attitude towards drug abuse/dependence (UNDCP, 2003). Taremian *et al.* (2018) found in their study that among other factors such as low religiosity, anxiety, depression, and anger, *attitude of individuals towards substance abuse was one of the key factors in determining their likelihood of substance abuse*. Similarly, Gray and Squeglia (2018) suggested that adolescent's attitudes are crucial in development of substance use disorders. This is not an entity which develops in a single day. It develops gradually and many factors that have major roles in its development such as peer pressure, media, availability of substance and public policy.

In addition, Hohman. Carno, Siegel, and Alvaro (2015) explained that theory of planned behaviour is responsible for one's attitude to intentions and resulting behaviour. In the context of substance abuse, they further proposed that behavioural intentions (inclination towards any behaviour, here particularly substance use) are best determinants of action, attitude and other personal constructs that are related to social norms of adolescents, which are directed by peer belief that adolescents hold. As per the authors this theory include attitudinal belief as one of the important components, which directs the multipurpose behaviours of adolescent's including the action for taking substance abuse.

Another influential theory related to attitude and beliefs, particularly about substance use and/or in form of experimental substance use, is one of the major components of Peer Cluster Theory by Oetting & Beauvais (1987). This theory further posited that even those adolescents with Not to Use attitude if involve in experimental substance use, many times causes substance abuse or dependence. Therefore, attitude is such an important individual internal factor along with other factors must be assessed and so that it can be an integral part of a multimodal management programme for adolescent's with substance abuse.

The above mentioned national survey reported that highest prevalent drugs in Mizoram state are Opioids, Sedatives Inhalants and followed by alcohol and cannabis. These drugs are most prevalent in other north-east states (Nagland, Arunachal Pradesh, Sikkim and Manipur) along with Mizoram at almost top. The present study is focused in studying the attitude of adolescent population and its associated factors in Aizawl district of Mizoram.

Aim of the Current Study

This study was intended to explore the attitude towards substance use (alcohol and drugs) and determinants of this attitude in the adolescents living in Aizawl District of Mizoram.

Objectives

1. To find out the variation in adolescents' attitude towards alcohol and other drugs.
2. To explore the effect of gender on attitudes towards alcohol and other drugs use among adolescents.
3. To explore the effect of settlements (rural and urban) on attitude towards alcohol and other drugs use.
4. To find out the combined effect of gender and settlements on attitude towards alcohol and other drugs use among adolescents.

Hypotheses

1. There will be a variation in adolescents' attitude towards alcohol and other drugs use.
2. There will be a significant effect of gender on attitudes towards alcohol and other drugs use among adolescents.
3. There will be a significant effect of settlements (rural and urban) on attitudes towards alcohol and other drugs use.

4. It is assumed that there will be a significant combined effect of gender and settlement on attitude towards alcohol and other drugs use among adolescents.

Method

Design of the Study: The current study employed 2×2 factorial design (2 settlement groups × 2 genders) to carry out the research.

Size of sample: The sample consists of 260 subjects (130 male and 130 females selected in equal numbers from rural and urban settlements) studying in higher secondary schools in Aizawl district. Stratified random sampling was used to identify and select the certain schools from all higher secondary schools in Aizawl and then students were randomly selected from each identified school for both genders and settlement in equal numbers. Age of the participants ranged from 15 to 18 years. The mean age of male was $M = 17.29$, $SD = 0.91$ and of female was $M = 17.09$, $SD = 0.76$.

Table 6.1: Schematic Presentation of Quasi-Experimental Design

Urban *n = 130*		*Rural* *n = 130*		
Male	n = 65	Male	n = 65	130
Female	n = 65	Female	n = 65	130
				N = 260

Tools

1. **Demographic data sheet:** It was a semi-structured self-prepared sheet to collect information about age, gender, monthly family income etc., although demographic variables (expected age, gender, and settlements) were not included in main analysis of the study.
2. **Alcohol and Drug Attitude Scale (Saini & Singh, 2010):** Alcohol and Drug Attitude Scale is a uni-dimensional scale which gives estimates of attitudes towards alcohol and drug use of an individual. It is a 5-point Likert scale. Five response categories, i.e., Strongly Disagree (5), Disagree (4), Can't Say (3), Agree (2), Strongly Agree (1). The minimum and maximum score range is 28-140. High score is interpreted as positive attitude towards use of alcohol and drug use and low score is indicated negative attitude towards alcohol and drug use. This scale has adequate psychometric properties (Saini & Singh, 2010).

Procedure

In the initial phase of the study, certain schools in Aizwal district were randomly selected using random table and permission from the identified schools authority to conduct the study was retained. Then from each identified school, as per the criteria of the study, male and female participants from both forms of settlements were randomly selected in the sample of the study. Their willingness to participate in the study was checked and from those who were found willing to participate in the study formal consent was taken. They were assured about the confidentiality of the data. The test was administered in different schools. Thereafter, study tools were administered and obtained data were analyzed using IBM Statistical Package for Social Sciences (SPSS 20 version).

Statistical Analysis

The obtained data were analyzed by descriptive statistics such as mean, standard deviation, percentage, Shapiro-Wilk test for normality, Levin's test for homogeneity and thereafter, when the data were found to be appropriate for parametric statistics; Two Ways Analysis of Variance and t-test were used to derive meaningful outcomes from the data.

Results

Table 6.1: Percentage of participants for three levels of attitude towards substance use

Levels of Attitude	*f (N = 260)*	*%*
Low Favourable Attitude	67	25.80
Favourable	66	25.40
High Favourable Attitude	127	48.80

It was found (Table 6.1) after the analysis that around fifty per cent (48.80%) of the adolescents living in Aizawl district of Mizoram found to have high favourable attitude towards substance use. Rest of the fifty per cent of adolescents found to have either favourable (25.40%) or low favourable attitude (25.80%). This result is suggestive that around fifty per cent of school going adolescents had highly favourable attitude towards the use of substances.

Table 6.2: Age difference between male and female adolescents

Gender	*Mean age*	*SD*	*Df*	*T*	*Sig.*
Male (n = 130)	17.29	0.91	258	1.91	.057
Female (n = 130)	17.09	0.76			

Results in Table 6.2 is suggestive that there is no significant difference $t(258) = 1.91, p > 0.05$ between the age of the male and female participants. Therefore, age of male and female is not going to have any confounding impact on the interactions of our main study variables. Chi-square test was run to check the income variation between male and female participants to rule out the impact of income on attitude towards substance use through its variation in gender.

Table 6.3: Income variation between male and female participants

Income Categories	*Male*	*Female*	*Df*	*X2*	*Sig.*
< Rs. 10,000	63	92			
Rs. 10,000-20,000	39	21	2	13.51	.01
>Rs. 20,000	28	17			
Total	130	130			

Note: Income categories = Monthly family income.

Results (Table 6.3) revealed that there was a significant ($\chi^2(2) = 13.51$, $p = .01$) variation of monthly family income between male and female participant. Higher number of male participants ($n = 28$) found with higher income (rupees 20,000 per month) in comparison to their female counterparts ($n = 17$). In order to understand that whether the income is affecting the attitude score of male and female participants and to rule out its impact as a confounding variable for the effect of gender and settlement on attitude towards substance abuse, Two Ways ANOVA was conducted (Tables 6.4 and 6.5).

Table 6.4 depicts that attitude scores of male participants and participants having family income above twenty thousand per month appeared high in comparison to other groups, at primary observation, on the basis of their mean and SD on attitude scores. For further analysis ANOVA was calculated. Before the calculation of ANOVA, data was checked for normality and homogeneity as there are unequal participants across the groups.

Levene's test [$F(5, 254) = .54, p > .05$] suggested the variance in attitude scores (error variance) is equal across the categories of monthly income

Table 6.4: Mean and standard deviation on attitude scale across the categories of monthly family income and gender

Income	*Gender*	*Mean*	*SD*
< Rs. 10,000	Male (n = 63)	71.92	12.54
	Female (n = 92)	67.29	12.47
	Total (n = 155)	69.17	12.67
Rs. 10,000-20,000	Male (n = 39)	69.54	13.94
	Female (n = 21)	69.38	10.51
	Total (n = 60)	69.48	12.75
>Rs. 20,000	Male (n = 28)	77.29	14.82
	Female (n = 17)	68.65	12.92
Total	Total (n = 45)	74.02	14.61
	Male (n = 130)	72.36	13.66
	Female (n = 130)	67.81	12.18
	Total (n = 260)	70.08	13.11

and genders. A test for normality of data distribution (Shapiro-Wilk) was also run to check whether the attitude scores of participants for substance were normally distributed. Results showed that attitude scores for all three categories of monthly family income i.e., below Rs. 10,000 W (155) = .98, p = .26, Rs. 10,000 to Rs. 20,000 W (60) = .98, p = .44 and above Rs. 20,000 W (45) = .95, p = .09 were normally distributed across the levels. Both test of normality and homogeneity of data allowed us to run ANOVA to see the effect of income on attitude score alone or/in relation to gender.

Table 6.5: Two ways ANOVA about the impact of monthly family income and gender on attitude towards substance use

Sources	*Sum of squares*	*Df*	*Mean Square*	*F*	*Sig.*
MFI	405.72	2	202.86	1.22	.29
Gender	926.21	1	926.21	5.58	.05
MFI* Gender	437.31	2	218.65	1.31	.26
Error (Within)	42129.92	254	165.86		
Total	1321650.00	260			

Note: MFI = Monthly family income.

Results in Table 6.5 revealed that there was no significant effect [F (2, 254) = 1.22, p > .05] of monthly family income on attitude score and there no significant interaction [F (2, 254) = 1.31, p > .05] between income and gender for the attitude. This result is suggesting that income is not a confounding variable for the effect of gender on attitude towards substance use.

In order to rule out the effect of monthly family income in combination with the settlements (rural and urban) further separate analysis (Table 6.6 and 6.7) was conducted.

Test of homogeneity and normality was carried for the data on attitude scale across the levels of gender and settlements. Levin's test [$F(5, 254) = 1.04$, $p = .39$] suggested that data on attitude scale is homogeneous

Table 6.6: Mean and standard deviation on attitude scale across the categories of monthly family income and settlements

Income	*Settlements*	*Mean*	*SD*
< Rs. 10,000	Urban (*n* = 54)	69.72	14.07
	Rural (*n* = 101)	68.88	11.91
	Total (*n* = 155)	69.17	12.67
Rs. 10,000-20,000	Urban (*n* = 36)	69.56	13.66
	Rural (*n* = 24)	69.38	11.55
	Total (*n* = 60)	69.48	12.75
>Rs. 20,000	Urban (*n* = 40)	74.50	15.31
	Rural (*n* = 05)	70.20	06.38
	Total (*n* = 45)	74.02	14.61
Total	Urban (*n* = 130)	71.15	14.42
	Rural (*n* = 130)	69.02	11.63
	Total (*n* = 260)	70.08	13.11

across the levels of monthly family income and settlements. Shapiro-Wilk $W(130) = .98, p = .15$ for urban and $W(130) = .99, p = .96$ for rural suggested that data on attitude scale is normally distributed within both type of settlements.

Table 6.7: Two ways ANOVA about the impact of monthly family income and settlements on attitude towards substance use

Sources	*Sum of squares*	*Df*	*Mean Square*	*F*	*Sig.*
MFI	148.01	2	74.05	.43	.65
Settlement	87.71	1	87.71	.51	.47
MFI*Settlement	58.82	2	29.41	.17	.84
Error (Within)	43612.72	254	171.70		
Total	1321650.00	260			

Results of ANOVA (Table 6.7) revealed that there is no significant impact of monthly family income [$F(2, 254) = .43, p > .05$], settlement [$F(1, 254) =$

$.51, p > .05$] and interaction between income and settlement [$F(2, 254) = .17$, $p > .05$] on attitude score of the participants. Hence, the data of participants (having varying monthly family income and two types of settlement i.e., rural and urban) on the attitude scale is not affected by either their family income or their residence locale. In other words these variables are not confounding the impact of gender and settlement on attitude towards substance abuse.

Table 6.8: Mean and standard deviation on attitude scale across the levels of gender and settlements

Gender	*Settlements*	*Mean*	*SD*
Male	Urban (*n* = 65)	74.17	15.73
	Rural (*n* = 65)	70.55	11.04
	Total (*n* = 130)	72.36	13.66
Female	Urban (*n* = 65)	68.12	12.37
	Rural (*n* = 65)	67.49	12.07
	Total (*n* = 1 30)	67.81	12.18
Total	Urban (*n* = 130)	71.15	14.42
	Rural (*n* = 130)	69.02	11.63
	Total (*n* = 260)	70.08	13.11

Results in Table 6.8 show the descriptive analysis of mean and SD across the levels of genders and settlements. In preliminary view of this descriptive data it seemed that settlements do not affect the attitude of the participants, whereas, male participants have obtained higher score on attitude scale than their counterparts showing that males possess higher positive attitude towards the substance abuse.

In order to check whether parametric statistics could be applied to analyze the impact of gender and settlements test for normality and homogeneity were run (Tables 6.9 and 6.10).

Table 6.9: Tests of normality for data on attitude scale across the levels of gender and settlements

Variables		*Shapiro-Wilk*		
		Statistic	*df*	*Sig.*
Gender	Male	.989	130	.428
	Female	.985	130	.182
Settlement	Urban	.985	130	.154
	Rural	.996	130	.964

Table 6.10: Test of homogeneity (Levin's test) for data on attitude scale across the levels of gender and settlements

F	*df1*	*df2*	*Sig.*
2.40	3	256	.06

The result outcomes in tables 6.9 and 7.10 represented that data on attitude scale is normally distributed and homogeneous across the levels of gender and settlement. These outcomes allowed the researchers to run ANOVA to see the impact of gender and settlement on attitude towards substance abuse.

Table 6.11: Two ways ANOVA showing the impact of gender and settlement on attitude towards substance use

Sources	*Sum of squares*	*Df*	*Mean Square*	*F*	*Sig.*
Gender	1347.93	1	1347.93	8.06	**.01**
Settlement	292.98	1	292.98	1.75	.18
Gender*Settlement	144.75	1	144.75	0.86	.35
Error (Within)	42782.46	256	167		
Total	1321650.00	260			

Results of ANOVA (Table 6.11) depicted that there is a significant impact of gender $[F(1, 256) = 8.06, p < .01]$ on attitude towards substance abuse. On other side, analysis revealed that there no significant impact of settlements $[F(1, 256) = 1.75, p > .05]$ and interaction between gender and settlement $[F(1, 256) = .86, p > .05]$ on attitude towards substance abuse. Post-Hoc t-test was run to further delineate which gender has significantly more positive attitude towards substance use.

Table 6.12: t-test showing the difference between mean scores of male and female on attitude scale

Gender	*Mean*	*SD*	*df*	*T*	*Sig.*
Male	72.36	13.66	258	2.83	.01
Female	67.81	12.81			

Results (Table 6.12) of t-test analysis showed that male participants ($M = 72$, $SD = 13.66$) had significantly higher $[t(258) - 2.83, p < 0.01]$ positive attitude towards substance abuse as compared to female participants ($M = 67.81$, $SD = 12.81$).

Discussion

Substance abuse/dependence has highly spread in different parts of India, especially in North-eastern states. North-eastern states including Mizoram are highest prevalent states in India for the use of opioids (opium, heroin and pharmaceutical opioids) and, sedatives and inhalants (Ambekar *et al.*, 2019). Substance abuse/dependence has many ill-effects on physical and mental health of the people. Injection drug use (IDU) contributes to great amount of global morbidity and mortality related to HIV/AIDS and other infections (Vlahov, Robertson, & Strathdee, 2010). Substance dependence also results in great amount of family burden. For example, interpersonal and social relationship, leisure time activities, and finance (Sharma, Sharma, Gupta, & Thapar, 2019). There are many research efforts to find out the different risk factors associated with the substance dependence. Researches came out with different internal (individual) and external (environmental) risk factors which are associated with the substance abuse. Comprehensive analysis by researchers emphasized that internal factors are relatively more responsible for the acts of substance abuse/dependence.

Taremian and associates (2018) found *attitude of individuals towards substance abuse was one of the key factors in determining their likelihood of substance abuse*. Attitudes are integral part of one's whole personality constitution. Although, it comprises of cognitive, affective and behavioural aspects, it is more visible in behavioural outcomes of individual towards specific and particular entities. These are persistent tendency prerequisites of feeling and acting towards any person, situation or things. Since they are persistent tendencies, they are resultants of various factors that surround an individual and interfere.

This study was intended to explore the attitude towards substance use (alcohol and drugs) and determinants of this attitude in the adolescents living in Aizawl District of Mizoram. Gender and residential locale were demographic determinants which were studied in the current research for their impact on attitude towards substance dependence.

It was found in the current research that about fifty per cent of adolescents had high favourable and around twenty-five per cent of adolescents had favourable attitude towards the use of substance. Only minor portion, i.e., around twenty-five per cent of adolescents had low favourable attitude towards substance dependence. It is quite alarming for the adolescents having such a favourable attitude, which is one of the key risk factor to develop the substance dependence.

In correspondence to another objective of the current study we could not see a significant impact of neither settlements nor combined impact of gender and settlement on attitude towards substance abuse. Though, we found a significant impact of gender on the attitude towards substance dependence, which further delineated that male participants were having sufficiently higher positive attitude towards substance dependence as compared to their counterparts. The findings of current research put forth that there is an attitudinal proximity towards substance use in male adolescents residing in rural and urban locales, which indicates that adolescents, especially male individuals are more prone to development of substance dependence in both the residential locale.

It is quite alarming for the adolescents in North-eastern states, here, particularly Aizawl District of Mizoram that they have positive attitude towards the consumption of substances and resultant is seen in national study by Ambekar *et al.* (2019) which illustrated that the prevalence of adolescent substance dependence individuals is quite high in this part of country. In order to control such a state of substance dependence in this part of country, we need to adopt all sorts of preventive strategies. Boogar, Tabatabaee and Tosi (2014) not only found in their study among youths that they have positive attitude towards the substance use but also attempted to find out the psychological and demographic factors predicting this positive attitude. They found that male gender, low socio-economic status, low agreeableness, decreased conscientiousness, higher neuroticism, diminished openness had major and significant role behind predicting the positive attitude towards the substance abuse among the college going youths. They suggested that these factors can be tailored into the rehabilitation and prevention programmes of substance abuse among the youth.

Ambekar *et al.* (2019) further enlisted certain advice to control the spread of substance abuse/dependence and to prevent its prevalence:

- Protecting the youth of nation is of paramount importance.
- Evidence for effectiveness of awareness programmes, which is a predominant prevention strategy, is very weak.
- Prevention programmes must address the risk and protective factors aimed at not just preventing substance use but ensuring that youth grow and stay healthy into their adulthood.

Preventive Approaches

Preventive approach is one of major approaches to control the occurrence of any condition. In context of present research positive attitude towards substance abuse should be the target and proper steps are required to be taken. CMSH (2003) has mentioned about four major prevention strategies:

1. School and public education campaigns to enhance knowledge about substances and present a negative view about their impact.
2. Skill training to enhance positive social coping, with a major emphasis on resisting peer pressure.
3. Multifaceted school programmes.
4. Multifaceted community programmes.

They have further described the skill training programmes that should include the following components:

a) Wide range of personal and social skills designed to enhance general competence and curtail interest in substance use.
b) Pursue the implementation in ways that ensure skills are learned.
c) And provide subsequent "booster inoculation."

Gray and Squeglia (2018) said that prevention of substance use in adolescent is a multimodal approach in which the focal points is reducing the risk factor and enhancing and/or reinforcing the protective or positive factors in the adolescents taking substance. As cited in Gray and Squeglia (2018) Allen *et al.* (2016) explained most of the programmes for prevention of substance abuse are implemented and evaluated in school, family, and community settings. They also found that are potential evidence for parenting focused programmes. Other authors as per in Gray & Squeglia (2018) advocates school based teacher-led (Lize *et al.*, 2017) and peer-led prevention programmes (MacArthur *et al.*, 2017).

From the finding of our current study it is intended that attitude among the adolescent (who are abusing or not) should be the target of the all above programmes applied. It important in the sense that internal factors are more important and external factors in the continuation of substance abuse. Although, attitude is a developmental factors in which different external factors play significant role.

Individual Focused Management

Above discussed preventive approach is for group conditions. However, when individual has already developed either positive attitude towards substance dependence or has developed substance dependence conditions, individualized tailored treatment approaches should be opted. Lesh, Benda, Gutierrez, & Walter (1997) described four stages to management of people suffering from addiction of drugs and/alcohol. The following are the four stages:

1. Detoxification, in which generally basic emphasis of clinician remain in handling withdrawal symptoms (primarily somatic in nature) and prepare the patient for preventing from taking drug. The duration for this programme mentioned as 5 days.
2. The second stage of this programme is basically focused on enhancing the level of self-confidence and self-esteem in the patient. Here clinician tries to enhance the motivation, to know or explore the areas of conflict and main emphasis remains on enhancing the existing coping skills. This stage of management runs around 10 days.
3. The third stage of the programme is an active phase in which clinician at first decide the goals of the management and different suitable psychotherapeutic strategies as per the goals, which he arrives at from second stage of programme. He also now focus on the nature of social support the patient receive and decide if any intervention required. This programme also runs around 10 days.
4. The fourth stage of is a long term outpatient programme. The main focus of this stage is relapse prevention. Clinician tries to find out and control different biological reasons of craving through pharmacotherapy. In addition various psycho-social factors responsible for craving and relapse are sought out and dealt with specific psychotherapy methods. This programmes is long term one, which goes around 1 year or longer.

Motivational Enhancement Therapy (MET)

Motivational enhancement therapy is one of the major choices of therapy for dealing with people with substance dependence conditions. The MET approach begins with the assumption that the responsibility and capability for change lie within the client. The therapist's task is to create a set of conditions that will enhance the client's own motivation for and commitment to change. Rather than relying upon therapy sessions as the primary locus of change, the therapist seeks to mobilize the client's inner resources, as well as those inherent in the client's natural helping relationships. MET seeks to support intrinsic motivation for change, which will lead the client to initiate, persist in, and comply with behaviour change efforts. Miller, Zweben, DiClemente, & Rychtarik (1995) have described five basic motivational principles underlying such an approach:

1. Express Empathy
2. Develop Discrepancy
3. Avoid Argumentation
4. Roll with Resistance
5. Support Self-efficacy.

Implication

The current study found that favourable attitude of adolescent, especially in males, put forth targets to modification in terms of attitudinal change. Adolescents in Mizo schools, community in addition to screening them, should be identified whether they are involving in such activities. Jiloha (2009) proposed signs through which people in family, community, school can identify through certain changes in their behaviours and appearance that may signal potential substance abuse. These behaviours can be extreme or lasting for more than few days and help early detection of problem that may help in further screening and assessment by professional.

- Sudden change in behaviour or personality without another known cause.
- Loss of interest in earlier hobbies, sports or other activities.
- Sudden decline in performance or attendance in school or work.
- Changes in friends and reluctance to talk about new friends.
- Deterioration in personal care in relation to earlier patterns.
- Difficulty in paying attention and forgetfulness.
- Increased secretiveness, heightened sensitivity to inquiry.

National Institute on Drug Abuse (2009) has proposed comprehensive drug/alcohol abuse or dependence programmes as shown in Fig.

Conclusion

The current study demonstrated that high percentage of adolescents in North-eastern states, here, particularly Aizawl District of Mizoram have found with positive attitude towards substance and male adolescents were found to have significantly higher positive attitude towards substance dependence. Residential locations did not influence the attitude towards

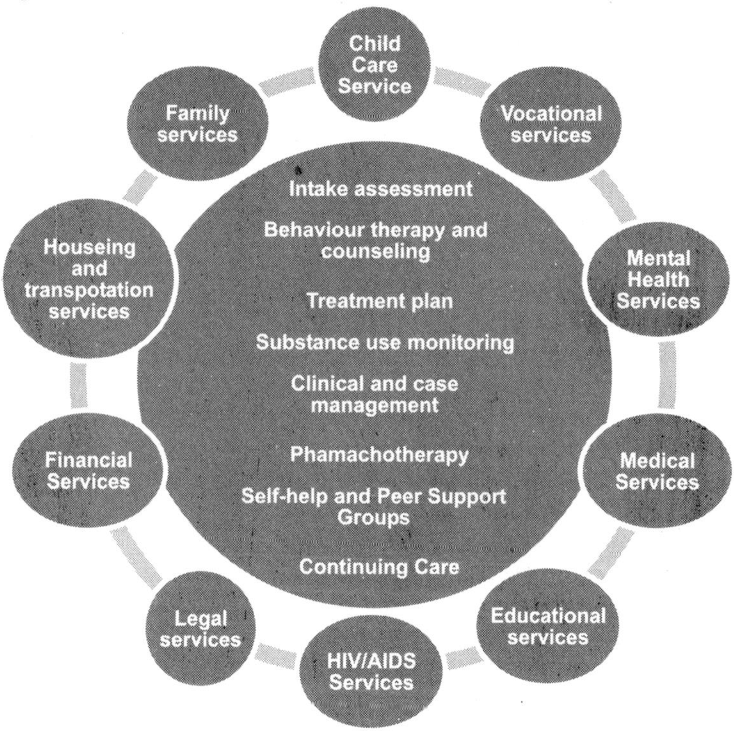

Source: Adapted from National Institute on Drug Abuse (2009).

drug abuse/dependence. The measures described in this chapter can be helpful in identifying, screening, rehabilitating and preventing such debilitating conditions.

References

Allen, M.L., Garcia-Huidobro, D., Porta, C., Curran, D., Patel, R., Miller, J., and

Borowsky, I. (2016). "Effective parenting interventions to reduce youth substance use: A systematic review". *Paediatrics*, 138(2) doi: 10.1542/peds.2015-4425.

Ambekar, A., Agrawal, A., Rao, R., Mishra, A.K., Khandelwal, S.K., Chadda, R.K. (2019). *"Magnitude of Substance Use in India"*. New Delhi: Ministry of Social Justice and Empowerment, Government of India.

American Psychiatric Association (2000). *Diagnostic and Statistical Manual of Mental Disorders* 4th Ed. Text Revision (DSM-IV-TR). Washington DC: American Psychiatric Association.

American Psychiatric Association (2013). *Diagnostic and Statistical Manual of Mental Disorders,* Fifth Edition. Arlington, VA, USA: American Psychiatric Association.

Boogar, I.R., Tabatabaee, M.S., and Tosi, J. (2014). "Attitude to Substance Abuse: Do Personality and Socio-demographic Factors Matter?" *International Journal of High Risk Behaviours and Addiction, 3*, 3, 1-12.

Centre for Mental Health in Schools (CMHS) at UCLA (2003). *Resource aid packet on Substance Abuse.* Los Angeles, CA: UCLA.

Chandran, U.K. (1998). "Attitudinal development." *Indian Journal of Training and Development, 28,* 1, 15-25.

Gray, K.M., and Squeglia, L.M. (2018). "Research Review: What have We Learned About Adolescent Substance Abuse?" *Journal of Child Psychology and Psychiatry, 59*(6), 618-627.

Hawkins, J.D., Catalano, R.F., and Miller, J.Y. (1992). "Risk and protective factors for alcohol and other drug problems in adolescence and early adulthood: Implication for substance abuse prevention", *Psychological Bulletin, 112,* 64-105.

Hohman, Z.P., Càrno, D.W., Siegel, J.T., and Alvaro, E.M. (2015). "Attitude Ambivalence, Friend Norms, and Adolescent Drug Use", *Prevention Science, 15*(1), 65-74. Retrieved from doi: 10.1007/s11123-013-0368-8.

Jiloha, R.C. (2009). "Social and cultural aspects of drug abuse in adolescents", *Delhi Psychiatry Journal,* 12, 2, 167-175.

Kastner, P. and Silbereisese, R.K. (1984). "Drogengebrauch Jugendlicher auaentwicklungs psychologischer Sicht." *BildunUnd Erziehung, 37,* 271-285.

Keane, R., Reaper-Reynolds, S., Williams, J., and Wolfe, E. (2005). *"Understanding Substances and Substance use—A Handbook for Teachers"*. Kildare, Ireland: South Western Area Health Board.

Lesch, O.M., Benda, N., Gutierrez, K., and Walter, H. (1997). "Craving in Alcohol Dependence: Pharmaceutical Intervention". In Judd, L.L., Saletu, B., and Filip, V. (Eds), *Basic and Clinical Science of Mental and Addictive Disorders* (pp. 136-147). Bangalore, India: Panther Publishers Private Limited.

Lize, S.E., Iachini, A.L., Tang, W., Tucker, J., Seay, K.D., Clone, S., DeHart, D., and Browne, T.A. (2017). "Meta-analysis of the effectiveness of interactive middle school cannabis prevention programmes", *Prevention Science, 18,* 50–60.

MacArthur, G.J., Harrison, S., Caldwell, D.M., Hickman, M., Campbell, R. (2016). "Peer-led interventions to prevent tobacco, alcohol and/or drug use among young people aged 11–21 years: A systematic review and meta-analysis", *Addiction, 111,* 391–407.

Miller, W.R., Zweben, A., Di Clemente, C.C. and Rychtarik, R.G. (1995). "Motivational Enhancement Therapy manual: A clinical research guide for therapists treating individuals with alcohol abuse and dependence (Vol. 2, Project MATCH Monograph Series)". Rockville, MD: National Institute of Alcohol.

Naeemi, N., Gheytarani, B. and Ghahari, S. (2016). "The Role of Early Maladaptive Schemas in Prediction of Dysfunctional Attitude toward Drug Abuse among Students of University", *International Journal of Medical Research and Health Sciences, 5,* 7, 571-575.

National Institute of Drug Abuse (1999). Sixth triennial report on Congress on drug use and drug and drug use research. Rockville, MD: National Institutes of Health.

National Institute on Drug Abuse (2009). *Principles of Drug Addiction Treatment: A Research-Based Guide*, 2nd Ed. NIH Publication: USA.

Oetting, E.R., and Beauvais, F. (1986b). "Peer cluster theory: Drugs and the adolescent", *Journal of Counselling and Development, 65,* 17-22.

Sharma, A., Sharma, A., Gupta, S., and Thapar, S. (2019). "Study of family burden in substance dependence: A tertiary care hospital-based study", *Indian Journal of Psychiatry, 61,* 131-138.

Taremian, F., Yaghubi, H., Pairvari, H., Hosseine, S.R., Zafar, M. and Moloodi, R. (2018). "Risk and protective factors of substance use among Iranian university students: A national study", *Substance Abuse Treatment, Prevention, and Policy, 13,* 46, 2-9.

Turk, J., Graham, P., and Verhulst, F.C. (2007). *Child and Adolescent Psychiatry: A Developmental Approach,* 4th Ed. Oxford University Press: New York, USA.

United Nations International Drug Control Programme (UNDCP) (2003). *Substance Use in Southern Africa: Knowledge, Attitudes, Practices and Opportunities for Intervention.* Switzerland: World Health Organization.

Vlahov, D., Robertson, A.M., and Strathdee, S.A. (2010). "Prevention of HIV Infection among Injection Drug Users in Resource-Limited Settings", *Clinical Infectious Diseases, 50,* 3, 114-121.

Vlahov, D., Robertson, A.M., and Strathdee, S.A. (2010). "Prevention of HIV Infection among Injection Drug Users in Resource-Limited Settings", *Clinical Infectious Diseases, 50,* 3, 114-121.

Vyey, M. (2010). "Steroids as pain relief adjuvants", *Canadian Family Physician, 56,* 12, 1295-129.

7

Teenagers, Adolescents and Children in Schools

Peer Group Pressure and Mental Health

Aradhana Shukla

It is a common and well accepted fact that man is a social animal that is why he always wants to be in touch with his supporting fellows who are near to him physically and mentally. This tendency is a basic instinct and always reflects in all across race, gender, SES or any other determinants. Children and adolescents are not exception of this fact and they also want to develop peer group and like to be with them. It is a truth that in the age of childhood and adolescence, people find them closer to their friends and class fellows sometime more than family members and sibling because they feel more safe, secure and confident under the underpinnings of their peers. Actually, this feeling of safety and security lies in the fact that the peers are non-judgmental and highly prone towards their friends. (Practice, 2015; Allen & Antonishak, 2008) Although parents are the biggest influence on children during the first few years of their life because young children do not get many opportunities to interact with the world outside their family (Maccoby, 2000). When the child grows older and starts school so many children of his age group meet him and their cognitive development starts with new framework and with united endeavour. Thus, the role of friends lays its' impact on the development of child. Actually, children want to behave like their similar aged peers because they have common interest, tasks and mental spectrum even they feel hatred and unsupportiveness to the parents and teachers who forbid them for school peers.

A peer can be any one of almost same age we look up to or someone with whom we should think and feel free. A peer can be a friend or a person (Hardcastle, 2002). While living in school peer group plays an important role and it directly influences the academic performance and academic success. A child or adolescent, surrounded by peers, acts many time as his peer group does and he cannot disregard the functioning and rules of the peers due to the insecurity or fear to be separated by them. This direct and indirect force that is produced by the peers and fore the child/adolescent to behave accordingly is termed as peer pressure. Children and adolescents in school see the negative role of peers. According to Kirk (2002), peers can lay their impact on friends school related performance but the extent is still a matter of debate.

Peer pressure, sometime provides a challenge or motivate the group. Not only it promotes deviant behaviour, but also it promotes academic performance and group related behaviour. It creates a good group dynamic and enhances the feeling of joint study or many good works that are useful for the society. One may slightly say that peer pressure is the emotional force. People of the same social group received through imposing of the group's norms of attitude or behaviour. But it is only one side of the coin, child selects the peers according to his own nature, demands and environmental circumstances.

In this way it is quite apparent that deviant and interrupting youth get more deviant when they openly interact with their more deviant peers (Thornberry & Krohn, 1997). So many skills of notoriousness and disruption appears in children when they meet and mix with their peers. Such plays of disruption show their outcome after some times when the child does not imagine to leave the group nor the habits (Dishion, McCord and Poulin, 1999; Smith, Dodge, Dision and McCord, 2005).

Theoretical Ground Work of Peer Influence

When we discuss about the pattern and impact of peer influence we simply remember and criticize the negative and socially rejected (disliked) values that are supposed to learned from their peers. We assume it although it is not printed or proved anywhere. In many homes where we can see very negative and unsupportive climate and distorted family network we blame on peer group for any indecency in behaviour. Studies on social behaviour have advocated the fact that deviant behaviour is concentrated in a specific group. If any member of the said group does any deviant behaviour others imitate it and the impact of peer behaviour can see through open eyes. There are many names of peer groups like, gang and cliques but their activities are more or less same (Cairns, Cairns, Neckerman Gest and Garietry, 1988; Dishion, Andrews and Crosby, 1995). Many longitudinal studies (Battin, Hill, Abbolt, Catalano and Howkins, 1998; Huizinga, 1995; Thornberry, 1998) have been made and it can be seen that gangs are found least in school or any settings. They are, although, least in numbers yet they are able to create highest level of disruption and neuscence. Also, they are found engaged in criminal behaviour. Moreover, affiliation in a gang is a sheer delinquent behaviour and seen in one of the most robust findings in the literature of juvenile delinquency (Thornberry & Krohn, 1997). Exposure to deviant peers is directly linked with a wide range of delinquent behaviour including drug use (Dishion & Medici Skagg, 2000; Thornberry & Krohn, 1997), violent behaviour (Elliot & Menard, 1996), overt antisocial behaviour (Keenan, Loeber, Zhang, Stouthamer, Loeber and Van Kamm, 1995), violent offenses (Elliot & Menaral, 1996) and early and high risk sexual behaviour (Dishion, 2000; Dishion, Andrew and Crosby, 1995). Deviant peer influence and their affiliation is a strong predictor than other variables like, family, school and community characteristics (Ellit & Menaid, 1996).

There is a disagreement between the advocates of peer group studies. One group of the psychologists think whether deviant peers make an increase in the delinquent behaviour (Burgess & Akers, 1996; Sutherland, 1936) or simply results in a common underlying factor i.e.; homophile among with a predisposition of crime behaviour (Glueck & Glnek, 1950; Hirashi, 1969). Before sometimes studies related to delinquent behaviour have permitted researcher to examine the temporal ordering of deviant peer involvement and delinquent behaviour more closely. It has been noted that such factors influence each other reciprocally during the course of delinquent career of the adolescent (Elliot, Huizinga and Ageton, 1985; Elliot and Menard, 1996; Thornberry, 1987).

The most important and apparent shortcoming of the researches have shared that most of the studies are based on single source of information (i.e. the self) to report about the peer's behaviour and the self-related behaviour (Gotlfredson & Hirschi, 1990; Kandel, 1996). However, the magnitude of the relation between deviant peer association and delinquent behaviour has been found to very across group and setting as affected by age of onset of delinquent behaviour (Cole & Miller-Johnson, 2001; Simons, Wu, Conger and Lorenz, 1994), The stage of criminal behaviour examined e.g. initiation, advice delinquency (Elliot & Menard, 1996), gender (Warr, 1996) and the nature of peer groups studies (gangs, informal peer groups, dyadic friends (Thornberry, 1998; Warr, 1996).

Origin of Peer Values: When we discuss about the origin of peer values we think the focal thought point or the place from where they emerged. In general we ask a question "from where do negative peer influences arise? Parents always blame the friends (of the child) responsible for the misconduct of their children (Davis & Kandel, 1996; Ide, Parkerson, Haertel and Walbog, 1981). The misconduct of their children means that negative values are the bane sources of the misbehaviour and are directly transmitted from the peers. It is neither logically sufficient nor particularly useful to state that adolescents as a group sometime behave badly because as a group they influence one another and force one another to be followed. It is true that peers transmit values to the others but it is not always true (Allen & Antoniskak, 2008). Classen and Brown (1985) have perceived students peer pressure and noted that peer pressure is multidimensional, differs in strength by domains, positive and negative both and not monolithic. So far as the management of the impact of peer groups is concerned, teacher and higher administrative authorities can make a watch over it (Cusick, 1973; Larkin, 1979). Johnson (1981) and Kaplon (1985) have stated that teachers and school administration, in case, make an eye over the activities and behaviour of school crowd, certainly control the students' indiscipline and unrest.

Johnson (1981) has stated that school environment can be more increased and become supportive with their positive and thoughtful approach. The student body is not a monolithic entity with a single system of values, attitudes and motivations" (Johnson, 1981). So many pressures are perceived by the adolescents between elementary and high school. It is a crucial time for development so, there is a need of peer group management and action can be rolled.

Adolescents' peer influence depends on the adolescents' culture and family background from where they have been brought up and it is merely based on the parental control. Sometimes parents think that all they are doing is good and anything which their children learn is the outcome of their external society. (Borzun, 2000; Bem, 1972; Dishionet *et al.,* 2001; Paulin *et al.,* 1999). Moreover, it is also seen that the parents impose unnecessary control on their children and implement unwanted restrictions. It also causes the attraction of children and adolescents towards peer groups. It has also been opined that nothing goes in vacuum but observing the development of adolescents social values in modern society, certainly pushes this thought to its' limit. To a remarkable extent, adolescents live in a vacuum vis-a-vis the norms of the larger adult world (Baumrind, 1988; Henggeler, 1991; Patterson *et al.,* 1989; Steinberg, 1987). Adults avoid adolescents, and adolescents in turn often reciprocate the same. We see many cases in which adolescents try to be more mature and feel free to take their own decision. Moffilt (1993) has noted that adolescents consider alcohol and drug use as minor forms of criminal behaviour.

Thus, we see two contrasts at one and these contrasts serve an important factors of adolescents' development (Allen & Philliber, 2001; Allen *et al,* 1997; Dishion and Mediciskaggs (2000), Dishion *et al.*, 1999, 2005). They are lack of access to adult values and their lack of access ability to adult like ways of engaging with the large society (Antonishaket *et al.,* 2006).

Keeping these views in consideration it is surely fair to say that there is very little direct intensive but friendly and extra-familial contact of adolescents with adults. Without proper interpersonal interaction we cannot expect normal adolescents and push them to absorb the values of larger society (Allen & Antonishak, 2008).

Determinants of Peer Pressure: Although peer group relation and pressure is determined by their personal attributes are circumstances yet, some may or determinants are as follows:

1. **Lack of time of parents to interact with their kids:** In this 21st century parents are so busy in work and earning. They do not have proper and quality time to devote for children this makes teenagers to get influenced more by peers and less by parents.
2. **Lack of guidance from teachers/parents:** Parents/teachers are not able to guide each and everything to teenagers. This may be because parents/teachers are unable to guide every phases of teenagers as they are forgotten their own problems of the time and unable to understand the problems of teenagers. So many a times teenagers feel that members of their peer groups are right persons to guide and support whenever there is any issue/ problems which leads to be more influenced by peers.
3. **Encourage bad behaviour and bad companies:** Parents unknowingly feel happy and proud when teenagers start friendship with many peers in a good sense but on contrary they forgot to check how many of the peers are on right track or wrong track such as smoking, drinking alcohol, gambling etc. Such kind of encouragement from parents may lead to influence by peers.
4. **Not listening what the teenagers want:** Many a times it is happened that parents/teachers do not listen or give proper attention to their child. This leads to feel a confidence in children/ teenagers that parents/teachers cannot understand their problems and it would be the wastage of time to them. This leads to feel more comfortable to share their feelings and views among their peer group and later on influence more by them.
5. **Age gap of parents and teenagers:** The experience which the

parents/teachers got and whatever they learnt in their early life are quite different to what the teenagers face. So, whatever the guidance provided by parents/teachers is not suitable for their children/teenagers and this leads to influence more by peer group.

6. **Unable to fulfill the demands of teenagers:** In the mainstream of simple middle class family parents are unable to afford the lavish lifestyle of the peers like costly smart phone bikes, dresses, eating lunch/dinner in big restaurants etc. Whenever teenagers experience some of their peers are having all those amenities which they like, that makes attractive and get influenced more by their peers as compared to the parents.
7. **Emotional insecurity:** Parents/teachers cannot be all the time with teenagers and also not possible to secure them when and where needed. So teenagers feel more secured towards their peers because peers can be all the time with them and support them.
8. **Negligence of teachers and parents**: Sometimes willingly or unwillingly it is happened that parents/teachers are unable to care and console teenagers. This leads to more influence by their peers as they require some support being a human being.
9. **Feeling that parents or teacher cannot understand their problems**: After prolonged negligence, continues avoidance and care teenagers start to feel that their problems are impossible to be understood by parents/teachers and possibly can be understood by their peers as they have the same traits and age group.
10. **Seeking to get liberty and free from all boundations:** Many teenagers are not happy with does and don't of their parents/teachers. They want to get some new experiences which is different than the routine activities in life. They want to get more liberty and to live freely likewise some of their peers do. So this gives more inclination towards peer influence than parents/teachers.
11. **Curious to know some new experience of life:** Teenagers feel very curious to know and want to experience to have hetero-sexual trend, go for dating, watching movie, smoking etc. If some of their friends share the experience of having heterosexual companionship and what had happened in dating such kind of information are very luring to teenagers and that makes to incline more towards the peer influence.
12. **Same age group and need of companionship:** It is the human nature and tendency that one cannot live alone. In order to feel

secure and get support they need someone who is/are in the same age and same traits. These factors makes the teenagers to get influence more by peer group, rather than parents and teachers.

13. **Believe and accept easily what peers told:** As the peers groups are in the same age, same education, and they have same problems etc., whatever the information provided by their peers whether it is right or wrong it does not matter, but the informations are more acceptable and believable in teenagers. This leads to influence and more towards peer.
14. **To pass time:** Teenagers as they grow up, they require someone to be with them and it is possible only with their peers. This makes influence by peers.
15. **Impress by their looks and style:** Teenagers prefer new looks, dressing style which looks something different from the old and traditional style. This may be in terms of hair cutting, dressing, ways of talking, working, eating etc. These kind of feelings and impressions are more towards the peers.

Although it is necessary and even after adverse, peers group impacts negatively many times. So it is the challenges of parents to watch the activities of their children. There are some warning signs of peer pressure which parents require to know. They are as follows:

- Low moods, tearfulness or feelings of hopelessness.
- Aggression or antisocial behaviour that not usual for the child.
- Sudden changes in behaviour, often for no obvious reason.
- Trouble falling asleep, staying asleep or waking early.
- Loss of appetite or over-eating.
- Reluctance to go to school.
- Withdrawal from activities the child used to like.

Positive Impact of Peer Group on the Development of Adolescents

Although peer group is blamed to spoil the nature and career of their team yet everything is not wrong. Adolescents can learn many good qualities and develop well accepted and socially desirable traits in them. They are as follows:

1. **Learning through imitation:** Children and adolescents get to learn by imitation each other whatever good or bad, they see

how to behave, how to talk, how to dress and work (Schunk, 1987). Even they learn the way to express their feeling, emotions and aggression. If they got good company, they learn many good things in their lives from their friends and lead to great achievement in academics, sports, extra-curricular activities which are very much required for a person in their survival. It is vice versa if they get bad companion and imitates bad behaviour and activities (Apesteguia, Huck, Oechssler, Weidenholzer and Weidenholzer, 2018).

2. **Sense of belongingness:** Many times adolescents feel comfort to share their experiences to their close friends who are of their age group or having certain similar traits like classmates, studying in same school, belong to the same place, being neighbours etc. Many times we do not deny the fact that children or adolescents not share everything to their parents or teachers as they do not feel a sense of comfort. There are many things in life which they feel comfort sharing their experience only to their peers and not to their parents and teachers. For instance, liking of some hetero-sexual friend, comments about a teachers, or making fun of someone, inappropriate jokes or pet jokes which they don't feel comfortable sharing with teachers and parents and even siblings and can only be shared with their peers and that develops a sense of belongingness (Newman, Lohmna and Newman, 2007).
3. **Become more assertive, try new activities:** Young adolescents develop more confidence and belief in themselves confining with their peers. If the group members encourage them for certain activities, for instance, academic homework, sports, seminars, topic discussion and feel support whenever got insecure from their peer groups and feel happy. At times when they are in distress and feel insulted they get emotional support from their peers and it becomes one of the coping mechanism in their life (Padma, 2014).
4. **Choosing the same clothes, hairstyle or jewellery as their friends:** Adolescents feel matured by wearing the same clothes, changing their hairstyle and wearing jewellery as their friends do. They feel a sense of updating themselves according to time and new generation. Wearing outdated clothes, traditional hairstyle, jewellery makes them feel a sense of old traditional people. They want to get change and do something different which was not the old tradition. By doing so they feel a sense of individuality and

identity and also want to show that they are different now and also can perform more better than the older generation. These kind of activities is encouraged and accepted by their peer group (Padma, 2014).

5. **Listening to the same music or watching the same TV shows as their friends:** Youngsters prefer to listen to the same music particularly western songs, pop, rock and roll, metallica and rap. By doing so they feel they are different and feel proud of themselves. They feel a sense of belongingness to each other and also indirectly convey the message to their parent and teachers that they are more stylish, fashionable and up to date with the current trends of society (Victoria, *et al.,* 2019).
6. **Changing the way they talk, or the words they use:** Youngsters are impressionable and copy language and style of talking which they hear in movies and role models in the form of movie stars. By doing so their command in language changes and improves. They have common role models like film stars, actors and actresses which are acceptable by their group. They are so much influenced by their role models that they copy and start speaking among themselves and derive a sense of pride (Victoria *et al.,* 2019).
7. **Working harder at school:** Peer influence are very necessary in the life of everyone. They imitate and learn among themselves. They also learn to contest in academics, sports, extra-curricular activities etc. By doing so they start competition and try to achieve more better than others do. This in turn improves their skills, knowledge, efficiency which are important in their future life (Victoria, *et al.*, 2019).

Negative Impact of Peer Pressure: Although the peers impact positively yet they lay their negative impact also. They are given below:

1. **Mobile addiction:** Young adolescents used to have mobile of their own as fashion Smart and android phones in particular is very impressive to them as it has multiple facilities, they keep on playing video games like PUBG, Blue Whale etc. which has the potential to pose risk in their life. Whenever they get free time they keep on watching movies, YouTube, adult pictures for hours on end. Binge watching is also a factor which leads to mobile addiction.

2. **Smoking cigarettes and drinking alcohol:** Youngsters in order to conform to group norms engage in health risk behaviour such as smoking and drinking. They feel proud, matured, independent and feel equal to adults.
3. **Bunking classes/truancy:** Bunking classes can be common amongst adolescents. They feel proud and happy as it accepted by their peer group. Usually they bunk classes which are not interesting to them and prefer to go to theatre for watching movies. Slowly and gradually, this kind of activity turns into a habit and dramatically harms their career and future progress in the domain of academics.
4. **Peer and romantic relationship:** Young adolescents learn of indulging in romantic relationship from their peers. They become so much curious of knowing what is romance and also feel happy of discussing about their opposite sex. They feel excited to share their experience in the group as this is the first experience of their life. They learn about how the opposite sex talk, dress and his/her socializing attributes etc. They also learn to maintain friendship with the opposite sex and learn about dating.
5. **Pornography and Sexual activities:** Young adolescents at this stage start watching pornographic films and videos and develop curiosity about sexual activity. Even some if one is not interested in pornography they start indulging in such activities due to peer pressure to oblige the group.
6. **Disobedience towards teacher and parents:** At this stage they learn to disobey parents and teachers and more accepting of what their peer group suggest and decide. They are highly influenced by the opinions of the peers and less influenced by their elders in the form of parents and teachers. They are of the opinion that their elders are only there to give advice and suggestion and not more.
7. **Bullying:** Bullying is a major concern amongst adolescent youth. They learn bullying behaviour from their peers to gain acceptance within their peer group. Their fear and apprehension of being isolated from their peer group compels them to indulge in bullying behaviour.
8. **Eve-teasing:** They learn how to pass negative comments towards the opposite sex (specially females) from their peers and derive pleasure from it. They indulge in hooting and pass derogatory comments in order to feel a sense of belongingness with their peer group.

9. **Delinquency:** Delinquent behaviour amongst adolescent youth is a growing concern which manifests in aberrant behaviour such as stealing, cheating and destruction of public property. Often behaviour is learned from peer group members who provide encouragement which in turn fuels a vicious cycle of destructive and socially unacceptable behaviour.
10. **Parent avoid the peer group at home:** Sometimes parents do not welcome the trends/peer of the child at home. It is job a parents to encourage the childs' friend to come at home so that they can get a chance to check on whether negative peer pressure and influence is an issue for him/her or not the child. Good communication and a positive relationship with child might also encourage the child to talk to parents if he/she is feeling negative influence from peers.
11. **Lack of assertiveness of the parents towards the child:** Parents should be assertive while communicating the child about the behaviour they do not like rather than criticizing others because it is possible to change their own child rather than changing others child but talking and communicating in such a way that teenagers should accept it instead of getting negativism or vice-versa must be followed by parents.

Techniques to Overcome Peer Pressure

Peers pressure is not so impossible that it cannot be solved. If people think and act confidently, it can be solved. There some techniques following which peer pressure can be overcome. They are given below:

1. **Build up self-esteem and confidence:** Children who have strong self-esteem are better at resisting negative peer pressure and influence. They should be encouraged and taught to say if they feel something unwanted that are going to happen. They should be encouraged to do something new. Parents and teachers are required to motivate teenagers to develop more confidence and self-esteem by which they can take their own decisions.
2. **Keep the lines of communication open:** Parents and teacher should not show teenagers as they are busy and do not have time to concern and discuss about their problems. Parents should show curiosity to know about them more, ask what is going on in school, friend, student etc. every day. Also, they have should

to them and be frank and open so that they can open up their feeling and start sharing to them.

3. **Give teenagers a way out:** Parents should always ready to give time to teenagers and try to solve their issues and problems they face. Once parents and teachers start helping and trying to show some way out then definitely.teenagers will build confidence and will start sharing their problems whenever they are under trap. They will start believing that their parents or teacher will solve their problems and start believing them as a good friend on the earth.
4. **Encourage a wide social network**: If the teenagers are confining only in one group then the scope of changing and thinking broadly will be limited and the support will also be limited but if teenagers have the chance to develop friendship from many sources, like from gym, club, sports, family friends then they will get lots of support from many sources in case of deviation.
5. **Peer Pressure and peer influence:** Whenever it is thought that teenagers friendship is more and over then what is required? We should devote more time to the family, spend time with our kids ask what are the negative pressure from friends or anything unwanted asked by friends etc. It will definitely help to resolve and guide them in right direction.
6. **Positive relationship:** Parents should maintain good relationship with teenagers and also stop criticizing them all the time. If parents criticize them teenagers will not open up their feelings and will scare to share to parents. If parents maintain positive relationship then teenagers will share their peer pressure freely and openly so as to seek help from parents.
7. **Judgment:** If the parents are judgmental then teenagers will not share their problems of peer pressure or may be more influenced by peers. Parents should always keep the opinion broad and non-judgmental and suggest the reality and need of time. Also, the parents should tell them clearly what is right and what is wrong and what is desirable and undesirable. It is their moral duty to make them realize and give an opportunity to choose of their own.
8. **Talk to students:** Teachers should talk to students just like a friend, should show them they are capable enough to resolve any issue. They should ask to open up whatever peer pressure is there and assure that confidentiality will be maintained.

9. **Make a plan:** It is the responsibility of parents and teachers to help the teenagers to get rid of peer pressure and teach, them the ways to out with little consequences. Parents or teacher should guide them to contact them whenever they are in problem. It will help them to get out of peer pressure without facing much problems.
10. **Applying own positive pressure**: Teenagers basically get pleased from parents or teacher through little affection or care. Therefore, parents and teachers should remember that if they keep on pleasing them then they will not progress much in life.
11. **Provide information they need:** Parents and teachers should not expect that teenagers know everything, they need to know many things in life. It is the duty of parents and teachers that they should teach moral of life to them. Also, they should provide knowledge about drugs, alcohol and heterosexual relationship and its deleterious effect on future. Although, the adolescents may not like such conversation but still parents or teacher need inform so as to get knowledge and able to take their own decision.
12. **Making boundaries:** Parents and teachers require to make certain limitations for teenagers like when they go out from home, bully the youngers and drop the class. Teenagers should be taught when to come back home and follow the rules of home and school.
13. **Confidence on the teenagers:** It is important for parents and/ or teacher to show confidence towards teenagers. They should let the teenagers to play their own path. Parents and teachers encourage, believe them and motivate them that they can do the most difficult task.
14. **Ask for help if necessary:** Teenagers should be asked to seek help if someone bullying them. They should simply wait to go away the situation because it may worsen later. They should reach out to parents, teacher or counselor for help.
15. **To make a watch on the trends:** Parents and/or teachers should encourage teenagers to choose friends carefully as teenagers are inclined more towards bad companies than good but dry companies. At this stage they are impressed towards new learning and test like smoking, drinking alcohol etc. They should be taught all these habits are bad and not good for health and better to leave those friends who have the habits of smoking and substance use.

16. **It is okay to be alone:** It is the human nature that a person can not stay alone without friend but if the friends are pressurizing to smoke or drink or to do some untoward activities then it is okay to be alone instead of making friends and spoiling the career and health. It is also the duty of parents and teachers to make a watch on them and observe their activities.
17. **Walking Away:** From the circumstance parents and teachers should teach teenagers to say "No". Even though it is very hard to do so but it can be done once. It will promote inner strength and confidence which will enable the teenagers to enhance the capabilities and restrict to avoid unwanted activities. Inner strength and confidence will make you firm in your belief and your capabilities. These will help them to resist from doing unwanted activities.

Future Recommendations

There are so many investigations on peer group behaviour and they reveal the fact that for which type of peer intervention is needed? In order to answer the query three types of researches are required.

1. **Studying and reporting the benefits and side effects:** It is true that there are many intervention strategies that can be used but they may have their positive and negative impact (Kelly, 1987). In this direction McCord's endeavour is worth to be mentioned (McCord, 1992). Before intervention we should keep the cognitive efficiency, situational demands, intensity of peer group relation and level of pressure in our mind which will facilitate the intervention (Pittman, 2019; Boyd-Bale *et al.*, 2014; Leshargie *et al.*, 2019).
2. **Measuring and analyzing multiple levels of intervention strategies:** In order to give proper intervention in adequate setting proper testing tools and kits are required. There is a need to record the data and observe the facial expression of the child/ adolescent. One measure having broad and dealing with multiple situations can be used and with due course of time the measure must be updated to incorporate required changing contexts and values of society (Muthen & Muthen, 2001; Raudenbush & Bruk, 2001).
3. **Studying the family environment and family pressure:** In many

studies it was found that peer pressure and family environment certainly plays a very important role in determining the inclination, initiation and practices towards alcohol consumption parents toward future of children, parental satisfaction with academic performance, approval of career choice by father, use of any other substance by a family member, working status of the mother, bullying at school, peer pressure, use of internet, duration of internet use, use of social sites and involvement in sexual activity to be risk factors for depression among adolescents (Singh, Gupta & Grover, 2017; Kaur *et. al*, 2015) in Bishwalata & Raleng (2014). There is a need to rethink over them.

4. **Studying existing programmes, institutions and various intervention practices:** It is very glittering to provide interventions to the needy population but deep knowledge and before-practices is always required. Therefore, study the post-intervention strategies, institutional practices and existing programme is warranted to avoid side-effect of intervention. A general sets of principles and exercises can be developed that may apply to an emerging theory of intervention that is grounded in both developmental theory and accumulative experience of efforts to change the behaviour of children and adolescents.

References

Allen, J.P., Philliber, S., Herrling, S. and Kuperminc, G.P. (1997). "Preventing teen pregnancy and academic failure: Experimental evaluation of a developmentally based approach", *Child Development, 68*, 729-742.

Allen, J.P. and Philliber, S.P. (2001). "Who benefits most from a broadly targeted prevention programme? Differential efficacy across populations in the Tee Outreach Programme", *Journal of Community Psychology, 29*, 637-655.

Allen, J.P. and Antonishek. J. (2008). "Adolescent Peer influences: Beyond the dark side" In: M.J. Primtein and K.A. Dodge (Eds.) *Understanding Peer influences in Children and Adolescents*, New York. Gilford.

Antonishak, J.; Allen, J.P. and McFarland, F.C. (2006). "Social Competencies and Peer Relationships: Longitudinal Associations with Peer Group and Adolescent Aggression", Paper presented at the Biennial Meetings of the Society for Research on Adolescence, San Francisco, California.

Apesteguia, J., Huck, S., Oechssler, J., Weidenholzer, E. and Weidenholzer, S. (2018). "Limitation of peers in children and adolescents", *Games*, 9, 1, 11.

Barzun, J. (2000). *From Dawn to Decadence: 500 Years of Western Cultural Life 1500 to the Present*, London: Harper Collins.

Baumrind, D. (1988). "Effective parenting during the adolescent transition", In *Advances in Family Research*, Vol. 2, Hillsdale, NJ: Lawrence Erlbaum Associates.

Battin, S.R., Hill, K.G., Abbott, R.D., Catalano, R.F. and Hawkins, J.D. (1998). "The contribution of gang membership to delinquency beyond delinquent friends", *Criminology*, *36*, 93–112.

Bem, D.J. (1972). "Self-perception theory", *Advances in Experimental Social Psychology*, *6*, 1–62.

Bishwalata, R., and Raleng, I. (2014). "Inhalant substance abuse among adolescents in Manipur, India: An upcoming issue", *International Journal of Medicine and Public Health* 4 (3), 237-242.

Boyd-Ball, A.J., Veronneau, M.H., Disgion, T.J. and Kavanagh, K. (2014). "Monitoring and peer influences as predictors of increases in alcohol use among American Indian youth", *Preventive Science*, 15, 4, 526-535.

Burgess, R.L. and Akers, R.L. (1966). "A differential association—reinforcement theory of criminal behaviour", *Social Problems*, *14*, 128–147.

Cairns, R.B., Cairns, B.D., Neckerman, H.J., Gest, S.D. and Gariépy, J.L. (1988). "Social networks and aggressive behaviour: Peer support or peer rejection", *Developmental Psychology*, *24*, 815–823.

Coie, J. and Miller-Johnson, S. (2001). "Peer factors and interventions", In R. Loeber and D.P. Farrington (Eds.), *Child Delinquents: Development, intervention, and service needs*, (pp. 191–210). Thousand Oaks, CA: Sage.

Clasen, D.R. and Brown, B.B. (1985). "The multidimensionality of peer pressure in adolescence", *Journal of Youth and Adolescence*, H. 451-468.

Cusick, P. (1973). *Inside High School*, New York: Holt, Rinehart and Winston.

Davies, M. and Kandel, D. (1981). "Parental and peer influences on adolescents' educational plans: Some further evidence", *American Journal of Sociology*, li, 87, 363-387.

Dishion, T.J., McCord, J. and Poulin, F. (1999). "When interventions harm: Peer groups and problem behaviour", *American Psychologist*, *54*, 755-764.

Dishion, T.J. and Burraston, B. and Poulin, F. (2001). "Peer group dynamics associated with iatrogenic effects in group interventions with high-risk young adolescents", In: D.W. Nangle and C.A. Erdley (Eds.), *The Role of Friendship in Psychological Adjustment. New Directions for Child and Adolescent Development*, *No. 91*. (pp. 79-92). San Francisco, CA: Jossey-Bass Inc.

Dishion, T.J. (2000). "Cross-setting consistency in early adolescent psychopathology: Deviant friendships and problem behaviour sequelae", *Journal of Personality*, *68*, 1109–1126.

Dishion, T.J., Andrews, D.W. and Crosby, L. (1995). "Antisocial boys and their friends in early adolescence: Relationship characteristics, quality and interactional process", *Child Development*, *66*, 139–151.

Dishion, T.J., McCord, J. and Poulin, F. (1999). "When interventions harm: Peer groups and problem behaviour", *American Psychologist*, *54*, 755–764.

Dishion, T.J. and Medici Skaggs, N. (2000). "An ecological analysis of monthly "bursts" in early adolescent substance use", *Applied Developmental Science*, *4*, 89–97.

Dishion, T.J. (2000). "Cross-setting consistency in early adolescent psychopathology: Deviant friendships and problem behaviour sequelae", *Journal of Personality*, *68*, 1109–1126.

Dishion, T.J., Andrews, D.W. and Crosby, L. (1995). "Antisocial boys and their friends in early adolescence: Relationship characteristics, quality and interactional process", *Child Development*, *66*, 139–151.

Dishion, T.J., McCord, J. and Poulin, F. (1999). "When interventions harm: Peer groups and problem behaviour", *American Psychologist*, *54*, 755–764

Dishion, T.J. and Dodge, K.R. (2005). "Peer contagion in interventions for children and adolescents: Moving towards and understanding of the ecology and dynamics of change", *Journal of Abnormal and Child Psychology*, 33,3, 395-400

Dishion, T.J. and Medici Skaggs, N. (2000). "An ecological analysis of monthly "bursts" in early adolescent substance use", *Applied Developmental Science*, *4*, 89–97.

Elliott, D.S., Huizinga, D. and Ageton, S.S. (1985). *Explaining Delinquency and Drug Use*, Beverley Hills, CA: Sage.

Elliott, D.S. and Menard, S. (1996). "Delinquent friends and delinquent behaviour: Temporal and developmental patterns", In Hawkins, J. David (Ed.), *Delinquency and Crime: Current Theories. Cambridge Criminology Series*. New York: Cambridge University Press.

Gottfredson, M.R. and Hirschi, T. (1990). *A General Theory of Crime*, Stanford, CA: Stanford University Press.

Glueck, S. and Glueck, E.T. (1950). *Unraveling Juvenile Delinquency*, New York: Commonwealth Fund.

Hardcastle, M. (2002). *Beating. Peer Group: Your Guide on Teen Advice*, California: Advice Books.

Henggeler, S.W. (1991). *Multidimensional Causal Models of Delinquent Behaviour and Their Implications for Treatment*, Hillsdale, NJ: Erlbaum.

Hirschi, T. (1969). *Causes of Delinquency*, Berkeley: University of California Press.

Huizinga, D. (1995). "Developmental sequences in delinquency: Dynamic typologies", In: L.J. Crockett and A.C. Crouter (Eds.), *Pathways through adolescence: Individual development in relation to social contexts. The Penn State series on child and adolescent development*, Mahwah, NJ: Erlbaum.

Ide, J., Parkerson, J., Haertel, G. and Walberg, H. (1981). "Peer group influences on educational outcomes: A quantitative synthesis", *Journal of Educational Psychology*, 73, 472-484.

Johnson, C. (1981). "Subcultures in the high schools", *The Education Digest*, 47(2), 60-62.

Kandel, D.B. (1996). "The parental and peer contexts of adolescent deviance: An algebra of interpersonal influences", *Journal of Drug Issues*, *26*, 289–315.

Kaplan, L.S. (1985). *Coping with Peer Pressure*, New York: Rosen.

Kammen, W.B. (1995). "The influence of deviant peers on the development of boys' disruptive and delinquent behaviour: A Temporal Analysis", *Development and Psychopathology*, *7*, 715–726.

Kaur, N., Chaudhary, R.K., Gupta, P., Devgun, P. and Khurana, B.S. (2015). "Alcohol in Teenagers of Amritsar District: A KAP Study", *Journal of Indian Academy of Forensic Medicine*, 33 (2), 152-154.

Kelly, J.G. (1987). "An ecological paradigm: Deferring mental health consultation as a preventive service", In: J.G. Kelly and R.E. Hess (eds.). *The Ecology of Prevention: Illustrating Mental Health Consultation*, New York, Haworth.

Keenan, K., Loeber, R., Zhang, Q., Stouthamer-Loeber, M., and Van Rammen, W.B. (1995). "The influence of deviant peers on the development of boys' disruptive and delinquent behaviour: A temporal analysis", *Development and Psychology*, 7,715-726.

Kirk, A.J. (2002). "The peer effect on academic achievement among public elementary school students was hengton: Centre for Data Analysis Report.

Larkin, R.W. (1979). "Suburban youth in cultural crisis", New York: Oxford University Press.

Leshargie, C.T., Alebel, A., Kibret, G.D., *et al.* (2019). "The impact of peer pressure on cigarette smoking among high school and university students in Ethiopia: A systemic review and meta-analysis", Plos one. Retrieved from https://journals.plos.org/plosone/article?id =.10.1371/journal.pone.0222572on 20/10/2019

Maccoby, E.E. (2000). "Parenting and its effects on children: on reading and misreading behaviour genetics", *Annual Review of Psychology*, 51: 1-27.

McCord, J. (1992). "The Cambridge-Somerville Study: A Pioneering Longitudinal-Experimental Study of Delinquency Prevention", In: J. McCord, J. and R.E. Tremblay (eds). *Preventing Antisocial Behaviour: Interventions from Birth Through Adolescence*, New York: Guilford.

Muthén, L.K. and Muthén, B.O. (2001). *Mplus Statistical Analysis with Latent Variables*, Los Angeles: Muthén & Muthén1.

Moffitt, T.E. (1993). "Adolescence-limited and life-course-persistent antisocial behaviour: A developmental taxonomy", *Psychological Review*, *100*, 674-701.

Newman, B.M., Lohman, B.J. and Newman, P.R. (2007). "Peer group membership and a sense of belonging: Their relationship to adolescents behaviour problems", *Adolescence*, 42.166

Padma (2014). "The teacher digest", Retrieved from http://theteachersdigest.com/6-ways-in-which-children-are-negatively-affected-by-peer-pressure/ on 12/10/2019

Patterson, G.R., DeBaryshe, B.D. and Ramsey, E. (1989). "A developmental perspective on antisocial behaviour", *American Psychologist*, *44*, 329-335.

Pittman, A.F. (2019). "Implications of peer pressure for Adolescent Nursing Research: A concept Analysis Approach", *Journal of Comprehensive Child and Adolescent Nursing*. 42(1). Retrieved from http://www.tandfonline.com/doi/abs/10.1080/24694193.2017.1387829 on 10/10/2019

Poulin, F., Dishion, T.J. and Haas, E. (1999). "The peer influence paradox:

Friendship quality and deviancy training within male adolescent friendships", *Merrill-Palmer Quarterly*, 45, 42-61.

Practice, I. (2015). IELTS Essay: Friends have a greater influence than parents on young people", Retrieved from https://www.ielts-practice.org/ielts-essay-friends-have-a-greater-influence-than-parents-on-young-people/on 18/10/2019

Raudenbush, S.W. and Bryk, A.S. (2002). *Hierarchical Linear Models: Applications and Data Analysis Methods*. Thousand Oaks: Sage.

Schunk, D.H. (1987). "Peer models and children's behavioural change", *Review of Educational Research*. 57(2). 149-174

Simons, R.L., Wu, C., Conger, R.D. and Lorenz, F.O. (1994). "Two routes to delinquency: Differences between early and late starters in the impact of parenting and deviant peers", *Criminology*, *32*, 247–275.

Singh, M.M., Gupta, M., and Grover, S. (2017). "Prevalence and Factors associated with depression among school going adolescents in Chandigarh", North India *J Med Res* Retrieved from http://www.Indiaecvironmentportal.org.in//files/file/depression%20 adolescents%20Chandigarh.pdf on 23/10/2019

Singh, M.M., Gupta, M. and Grover, S. (2017). "Prevalence and factors associated with depression among school going adolescents in Chandigarh, North India", *Indian J Med Res*. Retrieved from http://www.indiaenvironmentportal.org.in/file/depression%20adolescents%20chandigarh.pdf on 23/10/2019

Smith, M.G., Dodge, K.A., Dishion, T.J. and McCord Soan. (2005). "Peer influence in children and adolescents: Crossing the bridge from developmental to intervention Science", *Journal of Abnormal and Child Psychology*, 33.3.255-265

Sutherland, E.H. (1936). *Principles of Criminology* (3rd ed.). Philadelphia: Lippincott.

Steinberg, L. (1987). "Familial factors in delinquency: A developmental perspective", *Journal of Adolescent Research*, *2*, 255-226.

Thornberry, T.P. (1987). "Toward an interactional theory of delinquency", *Criminology*, *25*, 863–891.

Thornberry, T.P. and Krohn, M.D. (1997). "Peers drugs use and delinquency", In: D.M. Shiff, J. Breiling and J.D. Maser (eds). *Handbook of Antisocial Behaviour*, John Wiley & Sons, USA.

Thornberry, T.P. (1998). "Membership in youth gangs and involvement in serious and violent offending", In: R. Loeber and D.P. Farrington (Eds.), *Serious and Violent Juvenile Offenders: Risk Factors and Successful Interventions*, Thousand Oaks, CA: Sage.

Vitoria, P., Pereira, S.E., Muinos, G., Vries, H., Lima, M.L. (2019). "Parents modelling". Peer influence and peer selection impact on adolescents smoking behaviour: A longitudinal study in two age cohorts. Addict Behave, Retrieved from http://www.nebi.nlm.nih.gov/pubmed/31614308on 20/10/2019

Warr, M. (1996). "Organization and instigation in delinquent groups. *Criminology*, *34*, 11–37.

8

Conjunction of Spirituality, Mental Health and Happiness in Adolescents with Special Reference to PERMA Model

Shivangi Pandey and *Anubhuti Dubey*

Introduction

Studies indicate that spiritual people are happier and mentally healthy than those who don't believe in a supreme power. There are substantial evidences that religion and spirituality are strongly associated with mental health and psychological wellbeing (e.g., Chamberlain & Zika, 1992; Hill & Pargament, 2003). Spirituality provides meaning, coherence, and purpose to life. Religion and spirituality have been shown to be efficient in confront with impairment, ill-health, and unfavourable life circumstances. It has also been found that spiritual engagement provides both meaning to death and optimism at the end of life cycle (Glick, Weiss and Parkes, 1974; Pruiser, 1986). Social support from people in the spiritual community plays a strong role in positive coping and socializing. Spiritual commitment is negative predictor of drug habit and addiction (Gorsuch, 1995). According to Poloma and Pendleton (1989), "Prayer can be an effective coping mechanism."

Spirituality is helpful in positive development of youth. It has been found as a protector for adolescents in opposing to dangerous attitudes such as anxiety, suicidal tendency, substance abuse, delinquency and sexual promiscuity. Researchers have also delineated that spirituality is undoubtedly correlated with indicators of subjective prosperity, positive emotions, personal welfare and more life satisfaction in adolescents. Researchers have advocated that spirituality may be developmental assets for young people (Crawford, Wright & Masten, 2006). Moreover, spirituality promotes greater mental health, more positive family relationships and academic success. Adolescence is a precise period to the development of spirituality. So, it is essential for researchers to understand how spiritual thoughts develop in adolescents and which techniques are helpful in increment of spirituality among adolescents.

This paper reveals that how spiritual engagement is beneficial for mental health and happiness in adolescents by the reflection of literature.

Conceptualization of Spirituality

The interpretation of spirituality has grown and extended with time, and numerous definitions can be found. Spirituality has two basic characteristics; first, spirituality is a faith in a greatest power, that guide the whole world and nature; Second, spirituality is an eagerness to attain the intention in one's life in order to live an efficient life. Spirituality is associated with personal experience of transcendent. It is described as an inner personal knowledge that makes an individual able in understanding the significance of events in life (Ellens, 2008, p. 1). Tart (1975) delineates spirituality as an extensive dimension of human ability that includes divinity, affection, devotion, respect for everyone, and tenderness.

Tanyi (2002, p. 506) described that spirituality is a subjective investigation for the sense and significance of life. This significance of life motivates individuals to accomplish their best existence. This situation increases belief, hope, harmony, unity, and empowerment. Spirituality is also a connection between a people and supreme power. This connection brings joy, compassion for oneself and others, consciousness and acceptance for difficulties of life, and the competence to transcend beyond the infirmities of existence.

On the basis of above description it is clear that spirituality is a complex phenomenon, multidimensional in nature, and any single definition is likely to reflect a limited viewpoint and perspective.

Spilka (1993) contends that spirituality can be categorised into three sections: 1) God-oriented spirituality, where understanding and practice are predicted in religious theory; 2) world-oriented spirituality, which deals the strong connection between humanity and nature; 3) humanistic spirituality stresses on human achievement or potential.

Piedmont (1999) attempted to measure spirituality on the substructure of three dimensions: (1) prayer fulfilment, where prayer provide inner happiness and mental peace that results from personal confrontation with God; (2) universality, a belief that there is a supreme power that binds all people; (3) connectedness, faith that one is component of larger humanity. Many researchers (e.g. Beck, 1986; Elkins, Hedstrom, Hughes, Leaf,

& Sunders, 1988; Lopierre, 1994; Helminik, 1986) have also proposed multidimensional framework of spirituality. For example, Lapierre noted that spirituality includes six components—(1) an exploration for purpose of life; (2) an encounter with transcendence; (3) a sense of community; (4) an exploration for extreme reality; (5) a dignity and honour for the creation; and 6) a personal transformation.

Hill *et al.* (2000) contend that central to the involvement of both religion and spirituality is 'a search for sacred', 'sacred' being defined as ultimate truth. Hill and his colleagues also refer to the term 'search' which includes the endeavour to identify what is sacred, to articulate, to maintain the sacred within the individual's religious or spiritual experience, and finally to modify the sacred through search process. Oldnall (1996) states that the association between self, others, and God is pivot of spirituality. Hay (1989) clearly states that spiritual wellbeing is the improvement of one's inner resources. Hay (1989) further says that spirituality occur with the connection of others. Sodestrom and Martinson (1987) said that a natural link with others is a main feature of spirituality. The third element of spirituality is 'God'. Stoll (1979 p. 1574) says that whatever a person takes to be highest value in life can be regarded as his 'God'. These three main components of spirituality provide a force which activates individual towards his/her goal. Therefore, self, others, and God and the strong relationship between these elements are a central point to spirituality. So, it is necessary to study each component separately and all components collectively within a multidimensional framework for better understanding of spirituality (Spilka & McIntosh, 1996).

In Indian culture spirituality means expression of potential divinity within people by duty (*karma yoga*) or prayer (*bhakti yoga*) or philosophy (*gyana yoga*) or physical control (*raja yoga*). Through this expression people can control their internal and external character and they can achieve entire liberation. The *Vedas* convey spiritual predisposition to the Indians providing them the essentials of spiritual and honourable life. So, the *Vedic Rishis* acclaimed as the earliest master of the spirituality on earth. In India, spirituality is also defined as a science of soul or *adhyatmavidya*, the great understanding which helps people to lift high from worldly suffering. The Indians prefer spiritual pursuits to other pursuits of human life—*artha* and *kama*— which are much subordinate to it, as the same leads them to attain *moksha,* a state of existence of a *jeevana mukti* or liberated soul. Hence, spiritualism in India is absolute philosophy of life, the accurate manner of thinking and appropriate way of living. A spiritual person is one who is isolated from the duel effect of *karma* (victory or defeat); sees God every all around; keeps himself in stable communication of God. Therefore, according to Indian tradition spiritual people are the ambassador of God and the protector of mankind.

The above description reveals that spirituality is very significant portion of human life. Spirituality creates some questions about life and identity. In other words, spiritual thought forces a person to find precise answer of some questions about life and identity, such as: who am I and what is the meaning of my life; how can I live my life in the finest way; What is my relation to the world around me; what are the specific reasons behind events; how can I monitor my life circumstances and adjust with them. The exact answer of these questions promotes emotional wellbeing, mental health, and happiness.

Conceptualization of Mental Health

Mental health is apart from absence of mental disorders. Concept of the mental health encompasses subjective wellbeing, perceived self-efficacy, competence, and the ability to become aware of one's intellectual and inner capacity. According to Keyes (2003), mental health has two aspects—positive and negative. Its positive aspect includes emotional wellbeing (e.g. positive affect), psychological wellbeing (e.g., self-regard, consideration, good relation with others), and social wellbeing (e.g., positive attitude towards others). Its negative aspect includes depression, anxiety, anger, substance abuse etc. Mentally healthy people can recognize their abilities and they can manage with the normal pressure of life. Mentally healthy people are also helpful for their communities. Such people are also able to attain their life goals.

The WHO (World Health Organization) defined mental health as state of wellbeing in which the individual realizes his or her own abilities, can cope with normal stresses of life, can work productively and fruitfully, and is able to make a contribution to his or her own community. The WHO stresses that mental health "is not just the absence of mental disorder."

The Mental Health Foundation (2001) focuses some attributes of children's mental health (e.g. self-esteem; physical, emotional, social, and spiritual growth; resilience; the capability to develop better personal relationships; understanding that what is right and what is wrong in the world; the inspiration to fight with setbacks and learn from them; a sense of belonging; and a repertoire of problem-solving approaches). The Mental Health Association describes ten attributes of mentally healthy people: they have positive feelings for themselves; they do not become overwhelmed by emotions such as fear, anger, love, jealousy, guilt or anxiety; they have satisfying personal relationships; they feel comfortable with other people; they can laugh at themselves and with others; they can adjust easily with other people; they always keep in mind their prestige and give respect to others; they can accept their failure and can improve their practice for success; they are able to make their own resolutions.

Mental Health Issues

Mental health problems influence society as a whole, not only those, who suffer from a mental disorder. So, we should think about the solution of this problem because it is a major challenge for global development. No person and society are immune to mental disorder, but risk is higher among the poor, sick, homeless, the unemployed, victims of violence, migrants, children and adolescents, abused women, and neglected elderly. It is not possible to reliably tell whether someone has mental problem, however if certain signs (e.g. abnormal sleeping and eating; consistently low energy; using drugs or alcohol more than normal; unable to complete quality work; hearing voices; harming one's self or others) appear in a person, it may be beginning of mental problem.

Maintenance of Mental Health

Mental health is a condition in which individual is less likely to succumb with illness and adversity and more likely to recover rapidly and successfully. External support and practice are very helpful to maintain one's mental health. Environmental factors also influence mental health. To sustain mental health people should protect themselves from emotional abuse and trauma. It is necessary for a person to maintain their sense of being in control. Spiritual qualities and attributes are also necessary to increase mental health, because these qualities and attributes decrease the effect of bad genetic and environmental factors. Mental health undermines by the sense of loneliness and helplessness. Therefore, social affiliation and gaining help from others are also crucial for mental health. It helps people to overcome with adversity.

Some manners for maintenance of positive mental health are—staying positive, connecting with others, helping others, getting physically active, developing coping skills, getting help from others etc. Mental health can affect ordinary life, relationship with others, and even physical fitness. Mental health also includes a person's ability to gain equilibrium between life tasks, and efforts to attain psychological resilience. Positive mental health encourages people to cope with stresses of life and work successfully, realize their potentials, and make a significant contribution to their family and community.

Conceptualization of Happiness

In the present time individuals, institutions, decision-makers and strategist are focusing much more on the concept of happiness and wellbeing. Evidence indicates that happiness, subjective wellbeing, optimism, and mental health are associated with many advantageous results including successful marriage life, educational and occupational success, good social relationships, and physical health (e.g. Diener & Chan, 2011; Huppert, 2009; Lubomirsky, King, & Diener, 2005). Lyubomirsky *et al.* (2005) define happy person as someone who experiences always positive emotions such as happiness, pleasure, and contentment and rarely negative emotions such as fear, depression, and anger. It means that nobody is immune to life stressors, but the question is whether they see these stressors as moments of opposition or moments of opportunity.

Happiness emerges within people. They cannot get it from external world. Veenhoven (2006) makes a difference between common happiness and what are the major components of happiness. Common happiness is an extent to which people estimate the quality of life as delightful condition. Components of happiness include a well-balanced attitude to one's life and its related sensation and faith. Haller and Hadler (2006) delineate five ways to characterize happiness: happiness as a permanent character of a person, happiness as an outcome of objective life event, happiness as a valuable function, and happiness as a result of comparison with other groups of individuals, happiness as a continuing cultural trait.

Ancient Indian sacred writings, such as: *Vedas, Upanishads, Bhagavad Gita* have analyzed the nature of happiness, and the insights gained from these writings are still relevant to Indian people, influencing their conceptions of happiness and guiding them on how to lead a happy life (e.g. Bhawuk, 2011). *Bhagavad Gita* verse (5.21) indicates that "He, who is unattached to the external world and its objects and is attached to the inner-self, will attain supreme happiness which is everlasting." In *Bhagwad Gita* the notion of the *nishkama karma* (activity without wish of its fruits) and *sthitaprajna* (reliable wisdom and balanced mind) delineated as the central point to happiness. Giving up the fruits of one's efforts (*nishkama karma, or karma yoga*), is recommended by *Gita* as intervention to avoid unhappiness resulting from the pursuit of desire (e.g., verse 12.12) and leads to peace of mind and *sthitaprajna* (Bhawuk, 2011). *Sthitaprajna*—a situation of total equilibrium and harmony happens when a person gives up all the wishes of his *manas* and remains satisfied within himself (verse 2.55). According to Bhawuk, 2011 "Spirituality is a situation of equanimity in which a person goes beyond cognition, emotion and behaviour even beyond happiness—to bliss."

In Indian texts, it is also described that people should search the inner source of happiness called *satchitananda*—*sat* means 'being truthful', *chit* means 'being aware', and *ananda* means 'bliss' (Srivastava & Misra, 2011). Salve (2010) states that living in present is an essential key for happiness and stress-free life. Further Salve says that if a person eliminates all preconceptions, creeds and assumptions, lives in present moment, and gives credit for result to supreme power, he can definitely experience bliss—a state that is beyond happiness. Therefore, happiness is the considerable and prevalent theme in India. It is a meaningful psychological experience in Indian tradition.

Many scholars have regarded happiness as something whose value is supreme. Happiness is the most dominant predictor of success in various domains of life. There are some questions that are strongly related with happiness, such as: what makes people happy; what are the causes of individual differences in happiness level; what these differences are able to predict regarding success in various life domains, for example—social relationships and connections, achievement in life, gaining the purpose of life, success in profession, and better health. There are some theories of happiness that try to find precise answer of these questions.

In the sustainable happiness model, Lyubomirsky *et al.* (2005) suggested that three types of variables may influence happiness. These are: happiness relevant life circumstances (marriage and employment status); a genetically determined set point for positive mood/happiness; the extent to which people engage in happiness increasing strategies, such as: physical exercise, making positive relationship with others, involving in spiritual activities (Lyubomirsky, 2007). This model is similar to Seligman's happiness prescription. Seligman described that permanent happiness is the sum of one's set range for happiness; life circumstances; factors under one's spontaneous control (Seligman, 2002). These three sources of happiness provide a precise and reliable schema to understand happiness.

Some scholars used the term wellbeing and flourishing for happiness. Keyes (2002) suggested that flourishing requires "symptoms of high emotional, psychological and social wellbeing". Rusk and Waters (2015) experimentally obtained a five-domain model of happiness (knowledge and confront, consideration and consciousness, objective and practices, goodness and positive emotion, affiliation). Ryan and Deci (2001) characterize wellbeing as hedonic and eudemonic domains. The hedonic domain focuses on emotion, whereas eudemonic domain emphasizes the good life, with a focus on meaning and related wellbeing constructs.

The above described theories reveal that happiness is not only the presence of some positive emotions and absence of some negative emotions, but rather is something more. Real happiness emerges within individuals when they adopt these components in practice. While distinct theories describe separate dimensions, theorists have recognized that multifaceted models needed to appropriately understand the optimal psychological happiness (e.g. Forgeard *et al.,* 2011; Friedman & Kern, 2014; Huppert & So, 2013; Ryff & Keyes, 1995). In this way happiness is an active ideal condition of psychological functioning that comes to light from working well in different psychosocial domains. There is no single best model of happiness, but various approaches can be advantageous for providing concrete elements of happiness that can be realized, measured and developed. The present paper focuses here on the five domains of happiness defined by Seligman's (2011) PERMA theory: positive emotion (P), engagement (E), relationships (R), meaning (M), and accomplishments (A). Martin Seligman (2011) declares that these five elements can helpful for people to attain a life of fulfilment and happiness:

P	Positive Emotion
E	Engagement
R	Relationships
M	Meaning
A	Accomplishments

Fig. 8.1: The PERMA Model: Wellbeing Theory by Martin Seligman

The five elements of Seligman's theory are as follows:

Positive Emotion: Positive emotions are more than just smiling. It is the ability to be optimistic and view the past, present and future with a positive perspective. Frederickson (2001) said that positive emotions produce flourishing and worth cultivating. According to 'Broaden and Build' model of positive emotions, positive emotion can be broad on individuals thought—action repertoire, which will in turn build enduring personal resources for the individual (Frederickson, 1998). Positive emotion helps people in relationships and works and motivates them to take more chances and to be creative. There are advantages and disadvantages in everyone life, focusing on disadvantages increase the chances of developing depression and anxiety. Therefore, people should focus on the positive aspects of life to sustain positive emotion.

Engagement: It is essential in life to do some activities that require full engagement. Engagement in the activities is important for people to learn, grow, and nurture personal happiness. Engagement is a psychological connection (e.g. being compelled and absorbed) to a specific activity. Complete levels of engagement have been defined as a state of flow. Csikszentmihalye (1990, 1997) defines the flow state as a single-minded immersion, an excellent condition of attention in intrinsically motivated tasks. This type of 'flow' of engagement is crucial to extend person's intelligence, skills, and capabilities.

Research on engagement has taken place across several relatively disparate domains. Student engagement comprises educational, intellectual, and developmental domain (Appleton & Furlong, 2008). Positive psychology has been focused maximum on cognitive and emotional domain that involves severe concentration (Csikszentmihalyi, 1990). Departmental domain focused on vigour devotion and concentration for work (Schaufeli, Bakker, & Salanova, 2006). In this way engagement motivates a person to carrying out his activities with passion and commitment. It brings a prominent output in the end.

Relationships: Relationships and social connections are very important aspects of human life. Berscheid and Reis (1998) say that social relationships are crucial to life. Social support directly link with less depression, less anxiety, less frustration, good physical health, and other positive result (Tay *et al.*, 2012; Taylor, 2011). Taga (2006) describes sub-domains of relationship. These sub-domains are—social networks, quality of those networks, gaining support from others, giving support to others, satisfaction with support. Social relationships provide techniques for chronic illness self-management and decrease the suicidal tendencies (Tay, Diener, and Gonzalez, 2013). Some researchers expose that pain centres of brain become activate when person is at risk of being isolated. Building positive relationships with parents, siblings, and peers are important to spread friendship, affection, and enjoyment. Strong relationships provide support when a person is in difficult situation.

Meaning: Steger (2012) states that a sense of meaning has been defined in terms of having direction in life, connecting to something larger than oneself, feeling that one's life is valuable and worthwhile, and that there is a purpose to what one does. Life of meaning increases physical health, reduces mortality risk, provide higher achievement and gratification in life (Ryff, Singer, and Love, 2004; Steger, 2012).

Frankl's Logotheory delineates that how a purposeful life is necessary to live a happy life and long life. During the World War II, Frankl found that, in spite of some physical deprivation, the prisoners, who were able to find the meaning of events happening to them, were able to stay alive. But Prisoners, who were not able to find the meaning of events, experienced damage of physical strength, vigour, and stamina (Frankl, 1962). Frankl said that a life meaning motivates people to analyze and search for a purpose of the events in which they participate. Thus, having a purpose and meaning of life is crucial for living a life of happiness and fulfilment. Such meaning provides to people a reason for their life and that there is a great purpose in life.

Accomplishments: Making progress towards one's goals and gaining higher level results can lead to a personal sense of accomplishment. Accomplishment is about a sense of performance and success, about challenging oneself, and the opportunity to strengthen one's skill. Although accomplishment can be defined in objective terms, it is also subject of personal ambition and drive. Conditions and opportunities influence objective success. Subjective accomplishment is gaining one's own goal and attaining competence and potency to complete responsibility. "Self-Determination Theory" presents that competence is essential human need (Ryan & Deci, 2000). Accomplishment is often pursued for its own sake. For example, research shows that expert bridge players are driven to play to the best of their ability; even if they lose, they feel a sense of accomplishment in the knowledge that they played well (Seligman, 2011).

Seligman's (2011) PERMA model can help in improvement of people consciousness. When people focus on these constructs, (positive emotion, engagement, relationship, meaning, and accomplishment), they experience more happiness and wellbeing than people who have not managed all these PERMA constructs. Seligman (2011) states that these five constructs can be defined and measured as separately but correlated constructs.

Outcomes of Happiness

Diener and Oishi (2006) conducted a study and found that respondents rated the importance of happiness 8.03 on a 9-point scale, higher than the importance of any of the other 11 attributes involved in the survey, such as success, intelligence, or material wealth. Happiness scholars found that it plays an innovative role in bringing individually and socially beneficial outcomes. Evidences reveal that subjective wellbeing and happiness affect physical health and longevity. This idea supports the biblical notion that "a merry heart does good like a medicine" (Cohen and Pressman, 2005). It is also well-known fact that high level of negative emotions (e.g., stress, anxiety, anger, depression) are associated with lower immune system functioning and coronary heart disease.

People with positive mood have been observed to judge persons in more positive light, to become more interested in social interaction, and more prone to self-disclosure (Berry & Hansen, 1996; Mayer, Mamberg & Volanth, 1988). According to Brehm and Rahn (1997), the people who reported higher life satisfaction, exhibited more trust in others. Inglehart and Klingemann (2000) said that general wellbeing is a harbinger of democratic government. Tov and Diener (2008) found in their study that on a national level, happier countries were higher in generalized faith, volunteerism, and democratic attitudes. These findings reveal that happiness is not a self-indulgent hedonism. There is a strong connection between happy life and pro-social behaviour.

Happiness has been linked with superior acquirement in professional life. In previous researches it has been found that happier individuals are able to get academic success, better job, and favourable evaluation from their directors. (e.g. Borman, Penner, & Allen, 2001; Diener, Nickerson, Lucas, & Sandvic, 2002; Roberts, Caspi, & Moffitt, 2003). Positive emotions allow individuals to make strong their intellectual, psychological, and social resources. They use these resources for themselves and for others. Therefore, the above description makes it clear that happiness leads people to better use of all kind of skills.

Review of literature reveals that happiness is excessively crucial in life. Happiness functions as a resource that increases health, kindness, compassion, and other positive attributes. Therefore, happiness is beneficial not only for people, but also for societies. Oishi, Diener, and Lucas (2007) found in their study that people, who experienced the highest levels of happiness to be more successful in the domain of close relationships and volunteering. People who reported slightly lower levels of happiness, on the other hand, were more successful in the terms of income, education, and political participation.

Lyubomirsky (2007) delineated the techniques that have been experimentally examined to be adequate in growing happiness. These strategies are—expressing obligation, nurturing good social relationships, practicing spirituality, taking care of others and own-self, doing act of compassion, commitment for ambitions, developing new manners for coping. If people follow these strategies in their life, they find themselves happy.

Review of Empirical Evidence Regarding Spirituality and Mental Health in Adolescents

Spiritual issues are clearly important to adolescents. Spirituality is usually delineated as a protective factor for adolescents against negative health outcomes. In general, adolescents, who are highly spiritual, get success than their less spiritual peers. They have lower rate of unhealthy behaviour and fewer mental health problems because they use spiritual coping to handle their physical and mental problems. Several studies suggest that spirituality has been confidently related with positive behaviours, attitudes, and outcomes and negatively related with risky health behaviours among adolescents.

A review research paper on spirituality and mental health introduced by *Canadian Journal of Psychiatry* (2008) concluded that spiritual involvement is related with happiness, better coping with stress, and less depression. Pearce *et al.* (2003) conducted a cross-sectional survey on adolescents to examine the relationship between depressive symptoms and religiousness and to examine the moderating influences of gender and ethnicity upon this relationship. They found that being spiritual/ religious and having had positive interpersonal religious experiences were associated with lower levels of depressive symptoms, whereas having had negative experiences were associated with greater levels of depressive symptoms. Davis *et al.* (2003) found in their study that spiritual wellbeing decreased the possibility of anxiety among adolescents. Frydenberg *et al.* (2003) conducted a cross-sectional survey to determine how adolescents cope with concerns. They measured seeking spiritual support as a coping mechanism and found that Colombian and Palestinian adolescents were most likely to seek spiritual support to cope with concerns. Smith and Faris (2002) found that spiritual involvement provides positive life attitudes, satisfaction, and hope for future. According to National Centre on Addiction and Substance Abuse at Columbia University (2001), spirituality has been negatively related with alcohol and drug use. Hodge *et al.* (2001) conducted a study to explore the relationship between spirituality, religious participation, and substance use among adolescents, aged 12-17 years. In this study they measured the tentative interconnection with God and found that spiritual involvement was related negatively with using marijuana and hard drugs. Furrow, King, and Wagener said that spirituality improves internal and external developmental resources that contribute to risk reduction, wellbeing, and thriving. Johnson, Jan, Larson, and Li (2001) concluded that spirituality reduces the probability of crime-violence and delinquency among adolescents.

Holder *et al.* (2000) conducted a cross-sectional study on adolescents to determine the association between certain dimensions of spirituality and voluntary sexual activity. They found that higher levels of spirituality were associated with a lower possibility of engaging in voluntary sexual activity. Regnerus (2000) found that religious and spiritual involvement improves school success. Religious involvement is also helpful in positive identity formation in adolescents (Donelson, 1999; Youniss *et al.,* 1999). Benson, Larson, and Masters (1997) revealed that spirituality improves resiliency and coping behaviour among adolescents. Spirituality reduces the possibility of depression (Wright, Frost, & Wisecarver, 1993).

Balk (1991) conducted a study on adolescents, aged 14-19 years. He measured religious coping and found that religion provided a source of coping with death. Elifson and Hadaway (1983) examined association between delinquency and religiosity in a random sample of 360 white adolescents. They found that multiple indicators of adolescent religiosity, such as religious salience, belief that God answers, and prayers were negatively associated with delinquency measures.

Indian researchers also found evidence that spirituality is helpful in reducing various mental illness because spiritual framework improve hope and individuals are able to locate meaning within their sufferings. Spiritual and religious organizations provide social support to adolescents, which protect them from social isolation and provide them a sense of attachment and self-esteem. In Indian studies, it has also been found that Meditation focusing on a mantra (word with spiritual significance) is effective in reducing the symptoms of anxiety, anger, stress, depression and in improving spiritual wellbeing and quality of life. Studies also indicate that spiritual reliance and tradition improve aspiration and relaxation in schizophrenic patients. Indian researchers found in their study that pranic healing meditation activity reduced the behaviour problems including aggression, nail-biting, bullying, absenteeism from school, and enhanced the scholastic performance in adolescents.

The above findings certify that the scholars found positive relationships between spirituality and mental health and inverse association between mental health risk behaviours (e.g., drug and alcohol use, depression, anxiety, suicide attempts, and voluntary sexual activity) among adolescents.

Theoretical accounts are also suggesting that spirituality is a preceding factor for mental health. Frankl proposed the theory of logo therapy. This theory asserted that when there is existential vacuum (loss of meaning in life), mental problem emerge to fill this vacuum. The spirituality provides personal meaning and purpose of life. Thus, there is no possibility of existential frustration and mental health problems in a spiritual person.

The review of literature suggests that spiritual people realizes greater life meaning and greater wellbeing and feels less psychopathology. Emmons also contended that religion and spirituality provide life meaning and significance, which shapes various facets of a person's life. Ryff and Singer revealed that the purpose of life and self understanding are two main components of positive mental health where purpose of life provides crucial intellectual capability for optimal functioning. Therefore, it is crucial to enhance personal meaning through spirituality that promotes mental health and psychological wellbeing.

Review of Empirical Evidence regarding Spirituality and Happiness among Adolescents

Spirituality is helpful for enhancement of happiness also among adolescents. Studies of spirituality have been reported positive correlations between spirituality and subjective wellbeing including happiness (Argyle, 2001; Francis *et al.* 2000, 2003a; French and Joseph, 1999) and life-satisfaction (Kelley & Miller, 2007; Zulling *et al.*, 2006). Holder (2014) conducted a study on 320 children, aged between 8-12 years. He measured the correlation between spirituality and happiness through wellbeing questionnaire and found that more spiritual children were happier. Pearce *et al.*, found that middle school students who evaluated themselves as being spiritual and attended church regularly expressed less depressive symptoms than students who did not evaluate themselves as being spiritual or did not attend church regularly. The researchers have also suggested that spirituality provides high self-evaluation (Steger & Frazier, 2005), hope (Wnuk, 2010), optimism (Park, 2007; Wnuk *et al.*, 2009, Steger & Frazier, 2005) subjective sense of health (Zulling *et al.*, 2006) which in result, lead to an improved happiness and wellbeing. Furthermore, spiritual belief enhances healthy lifestyle among children, adolescents, adult, and elderly.

According to Argyle (2001), a meta-analysis of 56 studies indicated that overall spirituality, religiousness, and happiness are positively but weakly correlated (r = .16). MacIntosh, Poulin, Silver, and Holman focused their attention on efficacious component of subjective wellbeing in connection with religiosity and spirituality, in which religiosity and spirituality permanently anticipated higher positive effect. Several people prefer material goods for pleasure, happiness, and life satisfaction although it is known that the deeper layers of happiness is fewer affected by external conditions and more influenced by internal feeling of spirituality. Modern consumer society is causing anxiety and frustration in people because there is lack of morality and proper value system. Moreover, internalization of deviant behaviour is resulting in crime from the intention of gaining material benefit. The above description suggests that material goals do not provide long lasting happiness, but spiritual involvement enables a person to gain actual pleasure through a deep meaning of life.

In India, since ancient times it is believed that spiritual engagement takes a person towards happiness, mental health, ideal life and a sense of well-being. Contemporary Indian psychologist found similar result in their researches. They have been found in their study that people who have had spiritual experiences report immense positive feelings as compared to others. It is also found that spiritual engagement may help people to deal better with negative life events and stress. Adolescents with spiritual engagement reported higher levels of satisfaction, greater personal happiness and less negative effect and contentment with the meaning and purpose they find in their lives.

Theories have also suggested that spirituality promote happiness with some ways (Ellison, 1991). One of the major functions of spirituality is that it provides the sense and meaning to life. This meaning is helpful in handling with life stressors. The bad impact of a stressful situation can be confined by finding the meaning of events and with faith that no destructive situation can occur without God permission. Spiritual people try to evaluate the stressful situation through consent, spiritual reattribution, acceptance, and positive reinterpretation of events (Park, 2005). Therefore, meaning of life is a significant variable that mediate between spirituality and happiness and increase the quality of life among adolescents. So, happiness is the consequence of efficacious discovery of meaning in various situations of life.

Conclusion

The real intention of this review paper was to explore the correlation of spirituality on mental health and happiness among adolescents.

The theoretical reviews presented above delineate average to strong relationship between spirituality and different components of purposeful and meaningful life, mental health, and happiness. It has been observed in the studies that adolescents, who were more spiritual, perceived themselves connected with higher power, with other people, and with natural environment. They tried to find peace and harmony in their life through spiritual involvement. They also experienced contentment with life. All eminent philosophical scholars found in their study that people who were connected with transcendent beyond the realms of physical world and believed in higher power, realized themselves happy and solved their mental conflicts easily.

The present paper provides evidence that five elements of Seligman's (2011) PERMA model contribute to sustain and improve happiness. Subsequently, PERMA provide a key-element for spending a better life. Furthermore, the present paper reveals the importance of meaning of life to enhance mental health and happiness among adolescents. Researchers have recognized several techniques in which spirituality may promote subjective wellbeing (Worthigton *et al.*, 1996). These techniques include expressing kindness for others, obtaining approval and acceptance from others, acts of altruism, and volunteering. These techniques enhance personal meaning through spirituality and this personal meaning promote mental health and happiness. The idea that personal meaning promotes wellbeing is consistent with the finding that the meaning of life was related with lower levels of anxiety, frustration, and risk-taking behaviours in adolescents, who reported highly spiritual (Cotton *et al.*, 2005).

This brief review of extant research linking spirituality, mental health, and happiness shows positive connections. It is also essential for the researchers to search appropriate answer of some questions: such as, what are the forms of the spirituality that emerge in adolescence? How spiritual developments contribute to achievement of life meaning among adolescents? How social environment shapes spiritual development in adolescents? How adolescents can improve their mental health and happiness through spiritual involvement? A large number of viewpoints and approaches are necessary to find accurate answer for these questions.

The wideness of the contribution in the field of the spirituality reflects the broad interest that is produced by the notion that spirituality increases happiness and mental health. The modern materialistic and money-oriented society creates mental health risk behaviours (anxiety, depression, restlessness, nervousness, and impatience) and reduces happiness and quality of life. The modern society is also ragged by cultural and racial hostility. In this situation, spiritual involvement assists to find connectedness with self and with everything that is other than self. It promotes mental health and happiness in adolescents. Therefore, it is necessary to encourage further attention, research and study in the field of spirituality.

References

Babincak, P. and Parkansha, A. (2016). "Religiosity and spirituality as predictors of subjectively perceived happiness in university student in Slovakia", *IAFOR Journal of Psychology and Behavioural Sciences, 2*(1), 33-43.

Balk, D.E. (1991). "Sibling death, adolescent bereavement, and religion", *Death Studies, 15*(1), 1-20.

Cotton, S., Zebracki, K., Rosenthal, S.L., Tsevat, J., and Drotar, D. (2006). "Religion/Spirituality and adolescent outcomes: A review", *Journal of Adolescent Health*, 38, 472-480.

Csutora, M. and Zsoka, A. (2012, September). Relation of spirituality to happiness, life satisfaction, and sustainable life style", In *Annals of International Conference on Spirituality and Sustainability: A New Path for Entrepreneurship,* pp. 1-33.

Dyson, J., Cobb, M., and Forman, D., (1997). "The meaning of spirituality: A literature review", *Journal of Advanced Nursing*, 26, 1183-1188.

Eaude, T. (2009). "Happiness, emotional wellbeing and mental health—what has children's spirituality to offer", *International Journal of Children's Spirituality*, 14:3, 185-196.

Frydenberg, E., Lewis, R., Kennedy, G., Ardila, R., Frindte, W., and Hannoun, R. (2003). "Coping with concerns: An exploratory comparison of Australian, Colombian, German, and Palestinian adolescents", *Journal of Youth and Adolescence, 32*(1), 59-66.

Goswami, S. (2014). "Spiritual dimensions of Indian culture", *Journal of Sociology and Social Work, 2*(1), 241-256.

Hill, P.C., Pargament, K.I., Hoad, R.W., Mccullough, M.E., Swyers, J.P., Larson, D.B., and Zinnbauer, B.J. (2000). "Conceptualizing religion and spirituality: Points of commonality, points of departure", *Journal for Theory of Social Behaviour*, 30, 1, 0021.8308.

Hodge, D.R., Cardenas, P., and Montoya, H. (2001). "Substance use: Spirituality and religious participation as protective factors among rural youths", *Social Work Research, 25*(3), 153-161.

Holder, M.D., Coleman, B., and Wallace, J.M. (2010). "Spirituality, religiousness and happiness in children aged (8-12) years", *Journal of Happiness Studies, 11*(2), 131-150.

Holder, D.W., Durant, R.H., Harris, T.L., Daniel, J.H., Obeidallah, D., and

Goodman, E. (2000). "The association between adolescent spirituality and voluntary sexual activity", *Journal of Adolescent Health, 26*(4), 295-302.

Ivtzan, I., Chan, C.P. L., Gardner, H.E. and Prashar, K. (2013). "Linking religion and spirituality with psychological wellbeing: Examining self-actualization, meaning in life, and personal growth initiative", *Journal of Religion and Health, 51*(3), 915-929.

Kern, M.L., Butler, J. (2016). "The PERMA profiler: A brief multidimensional measure of flourishing", *International Journal of Wellbeing, 6* (3), 1-48.

Khaw, D. and Kern, M. (2014). "A cross-cultural comparison of the PERMA model of well-being", *Undergraduate Journal of Psychology at Berkeley, University of California, 8*(1), 10-23.

Khoddam, R. (2015). "What's your definition of happiness? *Psychology Today.*

Miller, M., Devis, M., and Greenwald, S. (2000). "Religiosity and substance use and abuse among adolescents in the National Comorbidity Survey", *Journal of the American Academy of Child and Adolescent Psychiatry, 39*(9), 1190-1197.

Prajapati, S.N. (2018). "The concept of happiness in India", *International Journal of Research and Analytical Reviews, 5*(4), 395-396.

Pearce, M.J., little, T.D. and Perez, J.E. (2003). "Religious and depressive symptoms among adolescents", *Journal of Clinical Child and Adolescent Psychology, 32*(2), 267-276.

Sauza, M.D. (2009). "Spirituality and wellbeing", *International Journal of Children's Spirituality,* 14.3, 181-184.

Shah, H., Romani, M., Gopal, A., and Mukhopadhyay, S. (2017). "Spirituality and happiness among youth: A correlative study", *International Journal of Technical Research and Applications*, *5*(3), 43-46

Sharma, P., Charak, R., and Sharma, V. (2009). "Contemporary perspective on spirituality and mental health", *Indian Journal of Psychological Medicine, 31* (1), 16.

Sharma, S.K. and Sharma, O.P. (2016). "Spirituality leads to happiness: a correlative study", *International Journal of Indian Psychology*, *3*(2), 50-54.

Shekh, D.T. L. *et al.* (2012). "Spirituality as a positive youth development construct: A conceptual review", *The Scientific World Journal,* Article Id 458953.

Warner, R.M. and Vroman, K.G. (2011). "Happiness including behaviours in everyday life: An empirical assessment of "The how of happiness". *Journal Happiness Study*, 12, 1063-1082.

Wnuk, M. and Marcinkows, J.T. (2012). "Do existential variable mediate between religious-spiritual facets of functionality and psychological wellbeing?, *Journal of Religion and Health,* 53, 56-67.

9

Genetic Predispositions for Stress, and Depression in Adolescents

Madhumita Roy, Shobhna Joshi, and *Madhu G. Tapadia*

Introduction

The adolescent group is characterized by physical transition marked by growth spurts, hormonal changes and the onset of puberty (sexual maturation) which include changes in sex organs, height, weight, and muscle mass, as well as major changes in brain structure, organization and termination of physical growth which is a result of simultaneous release of growth hormone, thyroid hormone and androgen during this period. The characteristic positive features of adolescents are reasoning, self-determination, positivity, capability of exercising self-control and confidence in sexual behaviours. Combination of heredity, childhood experiences and adolescent's experiences determines the course of their development and thus, adolescence is a combination of biological, cognitive and socio-emotional processes which are intricately interwoven. Adolescents undergo a quest for independence, conflict with parents and a desire to spend more time with peers, increased sexual maturation that produces greater interest in romantic relationships, aggression towards peers, assertiveness, and enjoyment of social events.

If we see human brain development then we find that it is critically influenced by various factors at four stages: First, prenatal by mother's thyroxin; second, post-natal by thyroxin supplements in food that helps in proper growth of brain as the brain attains almost its full size by 2 years of age (Howdeshell, 2002); the third, childhood stage where, brain development is dependent on growth hormones and the fourth, when a person attains puberty (early to middle adolescent stage), where the remaining part of brain development occurs under the influence of sex hormones (Raisman & Field, 1973) when it undergoes substantial anatomical changes (changes in folds especially in cortex region) that have important implications on behaviour (Casey *et al.,* 2008). During adolescence, synaptic pruning and myelination in the pre-frontal cortex increases, improving the efficiency of information processing and neural connections between the pre-frontal cortex and other regions of the brain are strengthened, which leads to better evaluation of risks and rewards, as well as improved control over impulses (Giedd *et al.,* 1999).

Along with brain, the body also develops in many steps called as stages of life, viz., infancy (till 1 year), childhood (up to 10 years, from toddler to primary school going stage), pre-adolescence (10 to 12 years), adolescence (early adolescence from 13 to 15 years when the changes in the body starts, middle adolescence from 16 to 18 years of age when there is quest for identity formation, independent thinking, late adolescence or early adulthood from 19 to 21 years of age when the thinking becomes mature), adulthood (early from 22 till 30 years, mid from 31 till 45 years and late from 46 till 60 years of age) and at last the old age (beyond 60 till death) (Santrock, 2007).

All organisms reciprocate to changing environment. This reciprocation over-ruling the resistance to change causes stress (Selye, 1936), giving rise to two variants, eustress and distress (Le Fevre *et al.,* 2003). Eustress is associated with the kind of stress that gives an impetus to perform better, but continuous stress may result in distress. Still, when the cause of stress is reversed, the person can return back to normal life. Thus, stress is considered as a reversible process. But, continuous stress leads to complications and ultimately results in sadness. Sadness is a normal reaction to life's struggles, setbacks and disappointments but if this makes semi-permanent changes in routine life, then it is considered as depression (Horowitz and Wakefield, 2007).

The Depression is a feeling of sinking down from where there is no come back. In biological terms, it is a mood disorder featuring gloomy mood, sadness, loss of interest in daily activities and with sometimes thoughts of suicide. A report from WHO has revealed that approximately 322 million people in the world irrespective of age are depressed and nearly half of them are from south-east Asia and west pacific region (WHO report, 2017). Also depression has become the third leading global disease and may become the leading cause of disease burden by 2030 (Pattanayak & Sagar, 2014). India is an amalgamation of vast diversity in geographical, religion, linguistic, cultural and with approximately 1.37 billion people, the prevalence of depression reaches a maximum of 39.6 per cent (WHO report, 2017).

Potential Causes for Stress and Depression

Some of the potential sources of stress are—environmental (economic, political, technological); organisational (role conflicts, interpersonal relationships, peer pressure, organisation's life stages); individual factors (family problems, economic problems) and personality (perception, experiences of oneself, social support, belief in locus of control, self-efficacy, hostile behaviour). Few of the examples of environmental stress specifically for adolescents are—changes in living area (city/state/country) due to parental occupation transfer; change from one school to another resulting in change of friends; failure of performing well with new technologies introduction which may lead to frustration later; Other factors (organizational) such as limited time for performance, work load, studying conditions at school or home, behaviour of classmate, peer pressure, behaviour of teacher (leader), excessive rules and being deficient in participation in decision-making and finally, the individual make up, where the genetic factor plays an important role, that is difference from individual to individual, in experiences, perception of things, their own nature, efficiency of performing, individual behaviour, and persons' belief in his own self (Santrock, 2007). These all affect the body by affecting the hypothalmo-pituitary-adrenocortical axis (HPA). Also there are hormonal, sometimes physical and emotional changes which adversely affect the health. For example, during high stress, cortisol is majorly produced by adrenal glands to combat the situation. So salivary cortisol was thought to be a reliable test for measuring severity of depression (Mannie *et al.* 2007) but negative results have also been obtained by few groups of researchers. Mannie *et al.,* also observed that those adolescents (16-20 years) who have increased level of cortisol in saliva in morning generally have a risk of depression (Mannie *et al.* 2007).

Depression has a close association with stress and is affected by environmental as well as genetic factors, and these factors are inter-linked with each other. Environmental factors include condition at home, condition in school or work place, diet being taken, hormonal conditions, etc. It has been observed that, the hypothalamo-pituitary axis (HPA) regulates hormone levels through certain gene function which in turn affects environmental conditions in the body affecting mood, and may cause depression. The environment provides the raw materials for the biochemical synthetic processes controlled by genes. It is known that genes comprises dominant element which determines the fate of an organism but the environment determines the actual course of development. There is a difference in individuals in environment it encounters but complexity arises with the sequence in which environment interactions are encountered by an individual. Therefore, genes playing role in an individual is called the genotype and environment interaction with genes determine the phenotype.

Also stress and depression are expressed differently in different ages of life in a person's lifetime. In childhood these feelings are expressed in the form of decreased appetite, changes in eating habits, headaches, stomach pain with other physical illness, sleep disturbances, new fears, stubborn or aggressive behaviour, recurrent bedwetting, crying, not participating in school activities. In adolescents the expressions are: feelings of tension, frustration, sadness and withdrawal, worry, poor self-worth, blaming, feeling ugly and humiliated. Lack of communication with parents aggravates the problem in adolescents. Adult stress is a continuation of teenage stress. Handling pressure in adult lives depends greatly on what kind of personalities an individual has formed. Much of the adult stress results from rigid self-image. Dealing with adult stress by conscious decision-making is helpful for reducing everyday stress. In elderly people it is expressed as insomnia, loss of appetite, palpitation, frequent urination, fear, frustration, restlessness, forgetfulness, which all can lead to other health problems. Therefore, an early intervention of stress and/or depression can prevent the damaging consequences especially during adolescents as they are in a transition period from childhood to adult and the most vulnerable group for stress and depression.

Depression is considered one among the 10 most threatening diseases with India being the major victim. As stated above the situation is also alarming with 70 per cent suicide cases out of the world's total suicide happens in India and usually within the highest literacy rates. Hence understanding the cause at the root level is need of the hour. The studies available on stress and depression, especially on the genetic predisposition are by and large from the subjects of other countries which may not affect the same way in Indian context. Also India being a vast country with varied environment, the studies on stress and depression are needed to be undertaken from different parts of the country.

Molecular Pathways in Stress and Depression

Brain is the most sophisticated and precious organ of our nervous system co-ordinating the entire behavioural spectrum. Brain is made up of neurons that are involved in sensory and motor activities and the glial cells for nourishment of the neurons. The sensory and the motor activities occur as neuron relays a signal from one neuron to other through release of neurotransmitter. Neurotransmission is the process by which the signalling molecules/neurotransmitters are released in the synaptic cleft from the presynaptic neuron and are absorbed by the receptors therefore activating them on the post-synaptic neuron (Graybiel, 1990). The excess neurotransmitter is later taken back in the pre-synaptic neuron by the transporters. There are three basic pathways of neurotransmission, viz., Glutamate, Dopamine and Serotonin pathways. These pathways are operational in the nervous system and all of them affect the behavioural spectrum of an individual. All the neurotransmitters are produced in the brain and none are imported from outside because of presence of Blood-Brain-Barrier (BBB). Only amino acids are absorbed from the blood by active transport, Glutamate is formed from amino acid glutamine, dopamine form tyrosine, and serotonin from tryptophan.

A cartoon depicting different regions of brain is presented below. This will serve as a reference when the different molecular pathways associated with brain are being described.

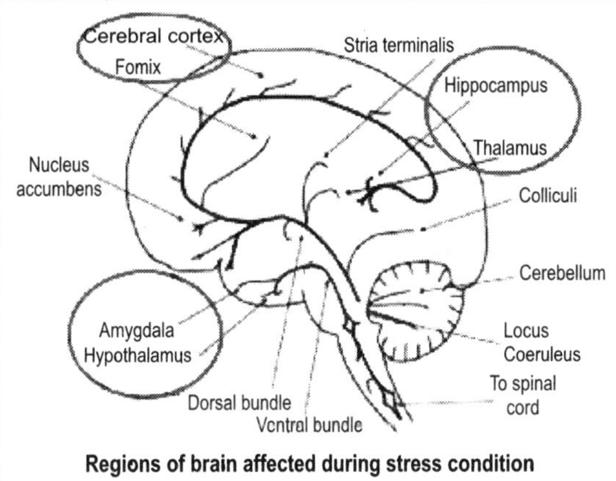

Regions of brain affected during stress condition

Fig.: Regions of brain: Affected regions during stress/depression are encircled

Glutamate Pathway

Glutamate is the major excitatory neurotransmitter, acting on three key cell compartments, i.e., pre-synaptic, post-synaptic and glial cells; so called tripartite glutamatergic synapse, in the nervous system and forming a complex mesh work with other pathways (Rothman *et al.,* 2003). Its receptors are found throughout the brain and spinal cord, controlling many physiological functions. More than 20 glutamate receptors have been identified in mammals and these are of two types—ionotropic (voltage sensitive; fast acting) and metabotropic (ligand sensitive; slow acting). Ionotropic receptors are namely *N*-methyl-D-aspartate (NMDA), α-amino-3-hydroxyl-5-methyl-4-isoxazole-propionate (AMPA), and kainic acid (KA). Activation of ionotropic receptors causes depolarisation of neural membrane by inward flow of sodium which in turn frees Mg^{++} from receptor therefore allowing influx of calcium. It is found that NMDA antagonist have antidepressant like effects. On the other hand, metabotropic receptors exert their effect through G-protein activation, which in turn triggers a second messenger system and through a series of activation causes specific gene expression. Metabotropic glutamate receptors are also of 3 types: Group I, expressed on the postsynaptic membrane, associated with learning and memory as well as motor regulation (Niswender & Conn, 2010). Group II, expressed on pre as well as post-synaptic neurons and whose dysfunction have been shown to cause anxiety and schizophrenia (Lesage & Steckler, 2010). Group III are expressed on pre-synaptic neurons within the hippocampus and hypothalamus and inhibit neurotransmitter release. Their dysfunction may cause Parkinson's disease and anxiety disorders (Swanson *et al.,* 2005).

Glutamate transporters, called as excitatory amino acid transporters (EAATs) are located at a near vicinity on pre-synaptic and post-synaptic neurons and also on astrocytes. Astrocytes are a type of glial cell for regulation of glutamate concentrations to prevent excitotoxicity (Kanai *et al.,* 1994). Five excitatory amino acid transporters (EAATs) are known, in which EAAT-2 mainly expressed on cells in brain regions rich in glutamate (Eulenburg & Gomeza, 2010).

Under normal conditions, glutamate is continuously recycled between neurons and glia through glutamate-glutamine cycle. Excess of glutamate present in the synapse is taken up by glial cells, where it get converted to glutamine. Glutamine is then transported back into neurons, where again it is reconverted to glutamate (Rothman *et al.,* 2003).

GABAnergic Pathway

GABA is synthesized from glutamate by the enzyme L-glutamic acid decarboxylase and this is the main inhibitory neurotransmitter in the brain. When GABA is released in near vicinity, it does not allow any other neurotransmitter to act. It acts by blocking the activity of other neurotransmitters and itself binds to receptor, therefore inhibiting any other neurotransmitter to act at that time point. Similar to glutamate receptors

(GluRs), GABA receptors are ionotropic (GABA-A) or metabotropic (GABA-B). GABA-A receptors mediate the majority of fast synaptic inhibition. Metabotropic GABA-B receptors are G protein-coupled heterodimers of GABA-B1 and GABA-B2 and expressed on both the presynaptic and postsynaptic terminals where they inhibit neurotransmitter release and induce cell membrane hyperpolarization. GABA is produced more in the brain by yoga, exercises, etc. and is inhibited by coffee or caffeine like substances keeping the brain over-stimulated.

Dopaminergic Pathway

Dopamine (3-hydroxytyramine; DA) is a catecholamine neurotransmitter that is synthesized from tyrosine in a two step process by rate limiting tyrosine hydroxylase. In 1958, Carlsson showed for the first time dopamine has signaling properties. In that study catecholamines were depleted by reserpine, and then added DOPA (3,4-dihydroxyphenylalanine) and it was found that: (i) reserpine effects were reversed, (ii) Dopamine concentration increased (Carlsson *et al.,* 1958). Later work pointed to enrichments of DA in certain brain regions, e.g., basal ganglia (Bertler & Rosengren, 1959). Dopamine neurons are mainly situated in mid-brain and get sub-divided according to location, projection and behaviour. There are four main types of dopaminergic pathway (Fuxe, 1965; Ungerstedt, 1971): (i) the tuberoinfundibular pathway—a group of dopamine neurons in the arcuate nucleus of the hypothalamus that project to the median eminence, controls prolactin secretion from the anterior pituitary gland (Weiner & Ganong, 1978), (ii) the nigrostriatal pathway—consists of neurons whose cell bodies originate in the substantianigra and terminate in the dorsal striatum and is responsible in movement and feeding behaviour (Volkow *et al.,* 2002; Sotak *et al.,* 2005; Robinson *et al.,* 2007); degeneration of these projections has been shown to cause Parkinson's Disease (Barbeau, 1962), (iii) the mesocortical pathway-neurons project from the ventral tegmental area (VTA) to the frontal lobes of the cerebrum, particularly the prefrontal cortex, and are involved in cognition and emotion, and iv) the mesolimbic pathway originate in the ventral tegmental area (VTA) innervate the ventral striatum and is involved in reward and pleasure. It is unique among the modulatory system because it has discrete projections to specific brain regions involved in motor, cognition and emotion therefore, abnormalities leads to several neuropsychiatric diseases, as Parkinson's disease, attention-deficit hyperactivity disorder (ADHD), schizophrenia, bipolar disorder, eating disorder and addictions (Wise, 1998; Horschitz *et al.,* 2005; Kienast & Heinz, 2006; Volkow *et al.,* 2007; Davis *et al.,* 2008; Koob & Le Meal, 2008). So nigrostriatal system is thought to give us the motivation for basic needs, e.g., food, while the mesolimbic pathway enables us to feel pleasure from them (Palmiter, 2007). Therefore, dysfunction in DA signaling has been linked to eating disorders and obesity (Wang *et al.,* 2001; Shinohara *et al.,* 2004; Chen *et al.,* 2008).

Nor-epinephrine Pathway

Nor-epinephrine (NE) is formed from dopamine (3-hydroxytyramine; DA) and transfers messages in the sympathetic nervous system, as part of the autonomic nervous system's fight-or-flight response. Secondly, norepinephrine prepares the brain to encounter and respond to stimuli. So in both roles, norepinephrine mediates arousal (Torres *et al.,* 2003; Moret & Briley, 2011).

Neurons in the *loci coerulei*, a pair of structures located within the pons of the brain stem synthesize norepinephrine (Moret and Briley, 2011). These are blue coloured due to melanin. A single neuron in the locus coeruleus can innervate tissue in wide-ranging areas involved in emotion regulation. The branching axons of norepinephrine innervate the frontal cortex, brain stem, spinal cord, and cerebellum, as well as the limbic system (implicated in emotion and cognition) includes—hypothalami, hippocampus, thalamic relay nuclei, amygdalae, and neocortex (Moret and Briley, 2011). Reduced nor-epinephrine is associated with decreased alertness, low energy, problems of attention, concentration problems and cognitive ability (Marin & Menza, 2005).

Serotonin Pathway

Serotoninor 5-hydroxytryptamine (*HT*) is a monoamine neurotransmitter produced in the raphe nuclei of brain stem region, and is known as a contributor to feelings of well-being and happiness. This brain region regulates behaviour, cognition and mood. Serotonin does not directly excite other neurons but instead modulates the responses of neurons to other neurotransmitters. There are approximately one lakh serotonergic neurons in the human brain and fourteen types of serotonin receptors have been discovered so far in the brains of mammals. Serotonin in the human body is found in two places: (i) enterochromaffin cells in the gastrointestinal tract, (ii) neurons of the *raphe nuclei.* Serotonin is made from the amino acid tryptophan which is obtained by the digestion of proteins in the gut and is transported in the blood plasma to the brain, where it is converted to serotonin. Axons of neurons in the lower raphe nuclei terminate in the spinal cord and also in the cerebellum's deep nuclei and cortex, while axons of neurons in the higher raphe nuclei terminate in: (1) subcortical nuclei including the centrally located thalami; the surrounding corpus striata including the nucleus accumbens; the hypothalamus, hippocampus, and amygdala, (2) the cingulate cortex, including the cingulum, a tract of association fibers connecting the corpus callosum with the hippocampus, and (3) the neocortex. The 5HT released by the serotonergic neurons into the synaptic cleft, is removed by 5-hydroxytryptamine transporter (5HTT) of the pre-synaptic neuron. A serotonin deficiency is related to anxiety, obsessions and compulsion and fatigue.

Summarising all the pathways it appears that not only one system but pathophysiology is related to disruption within the systems. In schizophrenia there is deficit in hippocampus and prefrontal cortex, whereas in depression deficit arises in medial frontal cortical region and amygdala. Interneurons are last component to be incorporated in developing brain, and they migrate to final positions to stabilize excitatory networks. Interneurons are also critical for generation of rhythmic activity within brain circuits. Therefore in pathological condition they can get disrupted. Interneurons are highly susceptible to oxidative stress or glutamatergic drive especially early in postnatal development before the protective perineuronal nets are formed.

Genetic Predisposition

Copy number variation (CNV) in a given gene or more genes is a factor which causes variability in the genome (Redon *et al.*, 2006). A study in 2010 by Saus *et al.*, found approximately 14 genes with CNVs which had a correlation with psychiatric disorder. Largest study of CNV in depression was done recently by Kendall *et al.*, in 2019 on UK biobank data, and found neuro-developmental CNVs association with depression especially 1q21.1 duplication (duplication of G-band 2, sub band 1, sub-sub band 1 on chromosome 1), PWS duplication, 16p13.11 deletion and 16p11.2 duplication. Another approach is by performing linkage analysis study. Linkage analysis studies carried out in earlier years have identified several loci to be associated with depression, however, in 2011 through a genome wide study by Breen *et al.* found that 3p25-26 was a significant locus for severe recurrent depression. This was the first report of depression association on linkage analysis. Then later in 2012 a study conducted by

Wong *et al.* in Mexican-American patients with Major depressive disorder (MDD) identified significant association with multiple MDD genotype clusters. Another study in 2016 by Knowles and their group on Mexican American individuals identified a single genome wide Quantitative trait loci (QTL) on 10q26.13. Several genome wide association studies conducted after 2012 identified different genetic loci (Ripke *et al.*, 2013), for instance tSNARE1 (proteins which mediates docking of synaptic vesicle with the pre-synaptic membrane) (Sleiman, 2013); MAD1L1 (a component of mitotic spindle assembly checkpoint that ensures proper alignment of chromosome at metaphase and does not allow next phase to occur without proper alignment) (Su *et al.*, 2016); and few of the molecular pathways involved in membrane scaffolding and neuronal cell adhesion (O'Dushlaine *et al.*, 2011). Hyde and their group identified 15 genetic loci associated with depression in European subjects (Hyde *et al.* 2016). Recently, Howard and their group identified 17 independent loci association with depression in a genome wide association study which are expected to contain approximately 78 genes in 3,22,580 UK biobank participants (Howard *et al.*, 2018). Role of micro RNAs in gene regulation has provided a new insight in the understanding of the complexities of gene function. Micro RNA-132 has shown consistent evidence as biomarker for depression in few studies (Yu *et al.,* 2018).

Gene Polymorphisms and its Association with Stress and Depression

Of the entire behavioural spectrum, genetic studies are mainly concentrated with major depressive disorders, schizophrenia and suicidal cases mainly on genes for neurotrophic factors, brain signalling molecules, their receptors and transporters were. Very few studies are available with stress. Among those genes which were associated with depression, we are considering only two of them viz., Brain derived neurotropic factor (BDNF) and a gene of solute carrier (SLC) transporter protein family, SLC1A3, as we worked on these in our laboratory and the finding will be described in the following section.

BDNF

BDNF translation and folding into pro-BDNF (a precursor protein) takes place in the endoplasmic reticulum and ultimately get packed in secretary vesicles (Lu, 2003). A replacement of valine amino acid with methionine at 66th amino acid position located in the pro-domain affects BDNF sorting and secretion (Martinowich and Lu, 2007). Such replacement occurs due to mutation, called as single nucleotide polymorphism (SNP). This polymorphism was shown to be associated with deficits in short-term episodic memory and neuropsychiatric disorders (Guerini *et al.*, 2009; Pivac *et al.*, 2011) and affects synaptic plasticity of NMDA and GABArgic neurons (Egan *et al.*, 2003; Chen *et al.*, 2005, 2006; Neves-Pereira. *et al.*, 2002; Sklar *et al.*, 2002; Schumacher *et al.* 2005; Strauss *et al.* 2005; Okada *et al.*, 2006; Patwell *et al.*, 2012). In normal condition BDNF binds to Trk-B (Nakagawara *et al.*, 1994), however, the polymorphism alters BDNF binding and in turn activates a set of signalling cascade (Huang and Reichardt, 2001; Gentry *et al.*, 2004; Teng *et al.*, 2005) leading to cell cycle arrest, activation of apoptotic pathway and also initiation of N-methyl-D-aspartic acid (NMDA) receptor dependent synaptic depression (Ibanez, 2002; Lu & Je, 2003; Barker, 2004; Lu *et al.*, 2005).

A valine amino acid at 66th position in the BDNF protein has been generalized with extraversion while a methionine at this position (Met66Met) (mutated allele) in homozygous condition or Val66Met (heterozygous) were shown to be associated with introversion (Terracciano *et al.*, 2010). Experiments on animal models indicated BDNF to be a modulator of brain reward system. Absence of BDNF or its ectopic presence causes depression and cognitive dysfunctions and memory deficit (Nestler & Carlezon, 2006; Monteggia *et al.*, 2007; Pattwell *et al.*, 2012).

Solute Carrier (SLC) Family

There are approximately 350 transporters organised into 55 families of SLC series, namely SLC1, SLC2, etc. (Hediger *et al.*, 2004; for overview see Fredriksson *et al.*, 2008; He *et al.*, 2009). SLC1 family consists of high affinity glutamate and neutral amino acid transporters, namely, SLC1A1, SLC1A2, etc., that mediate the cellular uptake of glutamate coupled co-transportation of Na^+, H^+ and antiport of K^+. On the other hand, SLC6 family is among the largest consisting of 20 genes encoding proteins, namely SLC6A1, SLC6A2, etc., that perform transport of amino acid into the cells along with the transport of Na ions. SLC6 transporters have again been classified into 4 subclasses based on four types of substrate specificity (monoamines, amino acids, GABA and orphan amino acids) and sequence similarity (Bröer, 2006).

Solute Carrier Family 1 Member 3 (SLC1A3)

SLC1A3 is a member of a family of high-affinity sodium-dependent glutamate transporter (Gegelashvili & Schousboe, 1997). SLC1A3 protein regulates excitatory glutamate neurotransmitter at synapse and transports it back to presynaptic neuron and glial cells (Kirschner *et al.*, 1994; Winter *et al.*, 2012) as accumulation of extracellular excitatory glutamateis cytotoxic. Thegene is located on 5th chromosome at one-three G-band position. Shashidharan *et al.* (1994) first time found this transporter mainly in substantianigra, red nucleus, and hippocampus, and in cerebral cortical layers. Stoffel *et al.* (1996) referred to it as GLAST1 and found to consist of 542 amino acids. Matsugami found that mice lacking Glast died on 17 to 18th embryonic day and exhibited cortical, hippocampal, and olfactory bulb disorganization leading to several essential aspects of neuronal development impairment as stem cell proliferation, radial migration, neuronal differentiation, and survival of subplate neurons (Matsugami *et al.*, 2006; Turic *et al.*, 2005).

Only two polymorphisms, G replaced by C in 869 nucleotide position (G869C) and C replaced by T at 3590 nucleotide position (C3590T) in the *SLC1A3* gene are known for this gene and they have not been related to stress or depression. C/T has been related with suicidal behaviour where T allele has been found as protective allele (Murphy *et al.,* 2011).

A Study Conducted by Us on Adolescents Evaluating the Known Polymorphisms in BDNF and SLC1A3

All the studies conducted in the last decade on the association of polymorphisms mentioned above in BDNF and SLC1A3 were on participants from countries other than India. Hence an endeavour was made by us to evaluate whether the polymorphism G196A on *BDNF* and C3590T on SLC1A3 are associated with stress and depression among school going adolescents in the population from Varanasi and adjoining areas (eastern Uttar Pradesh of India).

The Methodologies followed in Our Studies

Evaluation of the Status of Stress and Depression

Adolescent participants aged 16 and 19 years were recruited for the study. More than 300 samples, nearly 100 were cases having variable degrees of stress and depression and nearly 200 were controls having no stress and depression were chosen for this study after taking their written consent and with approval from Ethical Committee. All participants were clinically examined by a psychiatrist and were asked to fill a questionnaire developed for this purpose (Cohen *et al.,* 1983; Radloff, 1977) according to *DSM-5* guidelines towards assessing the level of stress and depression.

Isolation of DNA from Cells Present in Saliva and Evaluation of Polymorphisms in the Chosen Genes

Saliva samples collected from the participating adolescents in phosphate buffered saline, cells were pelleted down by centrifuging at 4°C, lysed by SDS (a detergent) and proteinase K treatment at 65°C. By this treatment the membranes are disrupted and all components of the cell are released in the buffer solution. They were then extracted with phenol-chloroform extraction method to remove proteins, and finally DNA was precipitated using ethanol. The precipitated DNA was air dried at 37°C, dissolved in Tris-EDTA (pH = 8.0) buffer or in distilled water and stored at 10°C. The quality and quantity of DNA was verified by using a spectrophotometer.

Further, genotyping is a method to locate the differences in the genetic makeup of individuals by analysing individual's DNA sequence and comparing it to a reference sequence. For this specific region of the DNA was amplified by Polymerase Chain Reaction (PCR) and subjected to endonuclease digestion to evaluate the presence of changed base. In this technique a few hundred basepair (bp) region is selected for which primers (approximately 15 to 20 bp short DNA sequences) were designed to amplify a selected region of DNA. In the present study Primer 3 (v.0.4.0) and Primer-BLAST tools were used to design region specific primers. These primers get annealed at given temperatures. PCR is carried out in three steps—denaturation was done at 95°C, primer annealing at specific temperature (lower than denaturation temperature), and final elongation at 72°C. Denaturation is a step to separate the double stranded DNA helix into single stranded, after which short sequences of DNA (called primers) are allowed to bind to the DNA, and finally the short strands were extended to form the double helix, in the elongation step. These three steps were repeated for 35 cycles to increase the amount of DNA under observation. Final extension is carried out for a longer time, i.e., 3 to 5 min. at 72°C to ensure complete DNA strand synthesis. A control sample is chosen without DNA along with the samples as negative template to ensure no contamination.

The PCR products were finally checked on 2 per cent agarose gel by electrophoresis, a method used for separation of macromolecules on the basis of size. Agarose is obtained from a sea algae, which on dissolution in hot water forms a gel having intermolecular spaces which allows small molecules to pass.

The PCR products were subjected to restriction endonuclease digestion, a process of cutting DNA molecule using molecular scissors and the sizes of fragments obtained were evaluated after electrophoresis. The pattern of bands obtained indicates the base present at the polymorphic site.

Statistical Analysis

Hardy-Weinberg equilibrium is a statistical equation to check whether the genetic variation is constant from one generation to another in a population in absence of disturbing factors. Hardy-Weinberg equilibrium was checked for both the polymorphisms, *BDNF* G196A and *SLC1A3* C3590T, in cases and controls (p value > 0.05).

The Results obtained in Indian Context

BDNF G196A

In normal population a guanosine (G) base is found at nucleotide position 196 in *BDNF* gene (the counting is done from the transcription initiation site). Since humans are diploids so it has two copies of *BDNF* gene is present in an individual. Therefore, individuals having G at 196 position in both copies of *BDNF* constitute GG genotype. An individual having G in one copy of *BDNF* and adenine (A) in another copy, then the individual is GA (heterozygous). While, individuals having A in both copies, have a genotype AA. As the frequency of A is low and the frequency of individuals having both copies AA is further lower, therefore A is considered as minor allclc.

BDNF G196A polymorphism has been known to reduce the expression of the gene and has been shown to be associated with depression cases in the population from other countries (Jiang *et al.,* 2005; Chen *et al.* 2006; Hwang *et al.* 2006), Also several psychiatric disorders have been shown to be associated with this polymorphism, such as anxiety, obsessive compulsive disorder, schizophrenia, psychosis, eating disorder, etc. (Hong *et al.,* 2011; Notaras*et al.*, 2015). The minor allele A carrying individuals have shown to have reduced activity dependent secretion of

BDNF and because of this reason this allele has been considered as the risk factor. But few studies have reported association of G allele (major allele) with increased BDNF activity (Tsai, 2007; 2018), substance use (Cheng *et al.,* 2005; Simet *et al.,* 2010) and also with bipolar disorder (Neves-Pereira *et al.,* 2002; Sklar *et al.,* 2002). In contrast to the previous work in Mexican-American population GG genotype (Valhomozygote) has shown association with increased chance of depression (Ribeiroet *et al.,* 2007). Moreover, a significant association of G allele was shown with bipolar in Europeans in a meta-analysis on different ethnic groups (Li *et al.,* 2016). On the other hand, allele A carriers were found to show an increased disposition towards Parkinson's disease in only Europeans but not in Asians.

In contrast to these observations, the present study on an Indian population did not find association of G196A with stress and depression. Strikingly in the controls the minor allele frequencies (AA) of *BDNF* G196A was more than in cases. A relevant report that the frequency of allele A 0 per cent in Africa and almost upto72 per cent in Asia is also available (Petryshen *et al.,* 2010). Such observations of allelic frequency distribution may have some role to play in specific populations and needs a wider study.

SLC1A3 C3590T

In normal population a cytosine base is found at position 3590 in *SLC1A3* gene. Since humans are diploids so it has two copies of *SLC1A3* gene, so individuals having C at 3590 position in both copies of *SLC1A3* constitute CC genotype. An individual having C in one copy of *SLC1A3* and T in another copy, then the individual is said to be heterozygous, and their genotype is CT. Individuals having T in both copies, have a genotype TT. As the frequency of T is low and both copies having T is further lower, therefore T is considered as minor allele.

In the present study, T allele of *SLC1A3* C3590T polymorphism was found to be associated with stress and depression in the population from Varanasi (an eastern region of Uttar Pradesh). The study suggests a contribution of the minor allele (T) in *SLC1A3* C3590T as a risk factor of stress and depression both individually as well as when they are together. In contrast to this, a significant association of *BDNF* G196A was not found in cases with reference to controls when calculated for stress or depression.

As it is already known that SLC1A3 is a glial high-affinity transporter molecule which regulates glutamate concentration after synaptic transmission. Therefore, its abnormal expression may show impairment in synapses and reuptake of glutamate, leading to prolonged activation of synapses; neuronal and glial cell death due to cytotoxicity (Choudary *et al.,* 2005). Also it was shown in a study by Bechtholt-Gompf (2010) on rats that prolonged activation of glutamate, due to disruption of glutamate uptake, shows depressive symptoms as reduced sensitivity to reward.

MDD (Major depressive disorder) patients have been shown to have downregulated SLC1A3, also suicide victims have shown reduced expression of *SLC1A3* gene (Coyle & Schwarcz, 2000; Kim *et al.,* 2007). In the present study it was found that 3'UTR polymorphism *SLC1A3* (C3590T) is associated with stress as well as depression.

A family based study done in 2005 on Caucasian samples supports our observation as they had found significant association of the same polymorphism, i.e., T allele of *SLC1A3* (C3590T) with attention deficit hyperactivity disorder (ADHD) (Turicet *et al.,* 2005). The association of this polymorphism was later shown by Murphy *et al.* (2011) in suicidal victims where they had also shown highly reduced SLC1A3 expression (Murphy *et al.,* 2011; Medina *et al.,* 2013).

Hence, from the present study C allele or the major allele could be said to act as a protective allele whereas the T allele acts as a risk factor and was associated with stress and depression. Therefore, from the present observation it could be hypothesised that presence of T allele, may have a role in the expression of the gene and predisposing the individuals to stress and/or depression.

We consider these findings significant in Indian context which opens an avenue to explore this aspect further in different populations in India. A consensus on the allelic predisposition not only in the genes discussed above but with all other genes associated with stress and depression will greatly help in modulating the cases and in preventing the occurrence of this disorder in future.

References

Barbeau, A. (1962). "The pathogenesis of Parkinson's disease: A new hypothesis", *Canadian Medical Association Journal*, 87, 802-807.

Barker, D.J. P. (2004). "The developmental origins of adult disease", *Journal of American College of Nutrition*, 23, 588S-595S.

Bechtholt-Gompf, A.J., Walther, H.V., Adams, M.A., Carlezon Jr., W.A., Ongur, D. and Cohen, B.M. (2010). "Blockade of astrocytic glutamate uptake in rats induces signs of anhedonia and impaired spatial memory",

Neuropsychopharmacology, 35, 2049.

Bertler, Å. and Rosengren, E. (1959). "Occurrence and distribution of dopamine in brain and other tissues", *Experientia*, 15, 10-11.

Breen, G., Webb, B.T., Butler, A.W., van den Oord, E.J., Tozzi, F., Craddock, N. and Mors, O. (2011). "A genome-wide significant linkage for severe depression on chromosome 3: The depression network study", *American Journal of Psychiatry*, 168, 840-847.

Bröer, S. (2006). "The SLC6 orphans are forming a family of amino acid transporters", *Neurochemistry International*, 48, 559–567.

Carlsson, G. (1958). *Social Mobility and Class Structure* 1, London C.W. K. Gleerup.

Casey, B.J., Jones, R.M. and Hare, T.A. (2008). "The adolescent brain", *Annals of the New York Academy of Sciences*, 1124, 111-126.

Chen, Z.Y., Ieraci, A., Teng, H., Dall, H., Meng, C.X., Herrera, D.G. and Lee, F.S. (2005). "Sortilin controls intracellular sorting of brain-derived neurotrophic factor to the regulated secretory pathway", *Journal of Neuroscience*, 25, 6156-6166.

Chen, Z.Y., Jing, D., Bath, K.G., Ieraci, A., Khan, T., Siao, C.J. and Hempstead, B. (2006). "Genetic variant BDNF (Val66Met) polymorphism alters anxiety-related behaviour", *Science*, 314, 140-143.

Chen, P.S., Yang, Y.K., Yeh, T.L., Lee, I.H., Yao, W.J., Chiu, N.T. and Lu, R.B. (2008). "Correlation between body mass index and striatal dopamine transporter availability in healthy volunteers: A SPECT study", *Neuroimage*, 40, 275-279.

Cheng, C.Y., Hong, C.J., Yu, Y.W., Chen, T.J., Wu, H.C. and Tsai, S.J. (2005). "Brain-derived neurotrophic factor (Val66Met) genetic polymorphism is associated with substance abuse in males", *Molecular Brain Research*, 140, 86–90.

Choudary, P.V., Molnar, M., Evans, S.J., Tomita, H., Li, J.Z., Vawter, M.P., Myers, R.M., Bunney, W.E. Jr, Akil, H., Watson, S.J. and Jones, E.G. (2005). "Altered cortical glutamatergic and GABAergic signal transmission with glial involvement in depression", *Proceedings of National Academy of Sciences USA*, 102, 15653–15658.

Cohen, S., Kamarck, T. and Mermelstein, R. (1983). "A global measure of perceived stress", *Journal of Health and Social Behaviour*, 24, 386-396.

Coyle, J.T. and Schwarcz, R. (2000). "Mind glue: implications of glial cell biology for psychiatry", *Archives of General Psychiatry* 57, 90–93.

Davis, C., Levitan, R.D., Kaplan, A.S., Carter, J., Reid, C., Curtis, C., Patte, K., Hwang, R. and Kennedy, J.L. (2008). "Reward sensitivity and the D2 dopamine receptor gene: A case-control study of binge eating disorder", *Progress in Neuro-Psychopharmacology and Biological Psychiatry* 32, 620-628.

Egan, M.F., Kojima, M., Callicott, J.H., Goldberg, T.E., Kolachana, B.S., Bertolino, A. and Lu, B. (2003). "The BDNF val66met polymorphism affects activity-dependent secretion of BDNF and human memory and hippocampal function", *Cell*, 112, 257-269.

Eulenburg, V. and Gomeza, J. (2010). "Neurotransmitter transporters expressed in glial cells as regulators of synapse function", *Brain Research Reviews* 63, 103-112.

Fredriksson, R., Nordström, K.J., Stephansson, O., Hägglund, M.G. and Schiöth, H.B. (2008). "The solute carrier (SLC) complement of the human genome: Phylogenetic classification reveals four major families", *FEBS Letter*, 582, 3811–3816.

Fuxe, K. (1965). "Evidence for the existence of monoamine neurons in the central nervous system. IV The distribution of monoamine terminals in the central nervous system", *Acta Physiologuca Scandinavica* 247, 39-85.

Gegelashvili, G. and Schousboe, A. (1997). "High affinity glutamate transporters: Regulation of expression and activity", *Molecular Pharmacology*, 52, 6-15.

Gentry, J.J., Barker, P.A. and Carter, B.D. (2004). "The p. 75 neurotrophin receptor: Multiple interactors and numerous functions", *Progress in Brain Research*, 146, 25-39.

Giedd, J.N., Blumenthal, J., Jeffries, N.O., Castellanos, F.X., Liu, H., Zijdenbos, A. and Rapoport, J.L. (1999). "Brain development during childhood and adolescence: A longitudinal MRI study", *Nature Neuroscience*, 2, 861.

Graybiel, A.M. (1990). "Neurotransmitters and neuromodulators in the basal ganglia", *Trends in Neuroscience*, 13, 244-254.

Guerini, F.R., Beghi, E., Riboldazzi, G., Zangaglia, R., Pianezzola, C., Bono, G. and Clerici, M. (2009). "BDNF Val66Met polymorphism is associated with cognitive impairment in Italian patients with Parkinson's disease", *European Journal of Neurology*, 16, 1240-1245.

He, L., Vasiliou, K. and Nebert, D.W. (2009). "Analysis and update of the human solute carrier (SLC) gene superfamily", *Human Genomics*, 3, 195–206.

Hediger, M.A., Romero, M.F., Peng, J.B., Rolfs, A., Takanaga, H. and Bruford, E.A. (2004). "The ABCs of solute carriers: Physiological, pathological, and therapeutic implications of human membrane transport proteins", *Pflugers Archives*, 447, 465–468.

Hong, C.J., Liou, Y.J. and Tsai, S.J. (2011). "Effects of BDNF polymorphisms on brain function and behaviour in health and disease", *Brain Research Bulletin*, 86, 287–297.

Horowitz, A.V. and Wakefield, J.C. (2007). "The loss of sadness: How psychiatry transformed normal sorrow in to depressive disorder", p. 312, Oxford University Press.

Horschitz, S., Hummerich, R., Lau, T., Rietschel, M. and Schloss, P. (2005). "A dopamine transporter mutation associated with bipolar affective disorder causes inhibition of transporter cell surface expression", *Molecular Psychiatry*, 10, 1104.

Howard, D.M., Adams, M.J., Shirali, M., Clarke, T., Davies, G., Coleman, J.R. I., ZAlloza, C., Shen, X., Barbu., M.C., Wigmore, E.M., Gibson, J., Hagenaars, S.P., Lewis, C.M., Ward, J., Smith, D.J., Sullivan, P.F., Haley, C.S., Breen, G., Deary, I.J. and McIntosh, A.M. (2018). "Genome-wide association study of depression phenotypes in UK biobank identifies variants in excitatory synaptic pathways", *Nature Communications*, 9, 1-10.

Howdeshell, K.L. (2002). "A model of the development of the brain as a construct of the thyroid system", *Environmental Health Perspectives*, 110, 337.

Huang, E.J. and Reichardt, L.F. (2001). "Neurotrophins: Roles in neuronal development and function", *Annual Review of Neurosciences*, 24, 677-736.

Hwang, J.P., Tsai, S.J., Hong, C.J., Yang, C.H., Lirng, J.F. and Yang, Y.M. (2006). "The Val66Met polymorphism of the brain-derived neurotrophic-factor gene is associated with geriatric depression", *Neurobiology of Ageing*, 27, 1834-1837.

Hyde, C.L., Nagle, M.W., Tian, C., Chen, X., Paciga, S.A., Wendland, J.R. and Winslow, A.R. (2016). "Identification of 15 genetic loci associated with risk of major depression in individuals of European descent", *Nature Genetics*, 48, 1031.

Ibáñez, C.F. (2002). "Jekyll–Hyde neurotrophins: The story of proNGF", *Trends in Neurosciences*, 25, 284-286.

Jiang, X., Xu, K., Hobabman, J., Tian, F., Marko, A.J., Waheed, J.F. and Lipsky, R.H. (2005). "BDNF variation and mood disorders: A novel functional promoter polymorphism and Val66Met are associated with anxiety but have opposing effects", *Neuropsychopharmacology*, 30, 1353.

Kannai, Y., Stelzner, M., Nussberger, S., Khawaja, S., Hebert, S.C., Smith, C.P. and Hediger, M.A. (1994). "The neuronal and epithelial human high affinity glutamate transporter. Insights into structure and mechanism of transport", *Journal of Biological Chemistry*, 269, 20599-20606.

Kendall, K.M., Rees, E., Bracher-Smith, M., Legge, S., Riglin, L., Zammit, S., O'Donovan, M.C., Owen, M.J., Jones, I., Kirov, G. and Walters, J.T. R. (2019). *JAMA Psychiatry*, 76, 818-825.

Kienast, T. and Heinz, A. (2006). "Dopamine and the diseased brain", *CNS and Neurological Disorders-Drug Targets*, 5, 109-131.

Kim, S., Choi, K.H., Baykiz, A.F. and Gershenfeld, H.K. (2007). "Suicide candidate genes associated with bipolar disorder and schizophrenia: An exploratory gene expression profiling analysis of post-mortem prefrontal cortex", *BMC Genomics*, 8, 413.

Kirschner, M.A., Copeland, N.G., Gilbert, D.J., Jenkins, N.A. and Amara, S.G. (1994). "Mouse excitatory amino acid transporter EAAT2: isolation, characterization, and proximity to neuroexcitability loci on mouse chromosome 2", *Genomics*, 24, 218-224.

Knowles, E.E., Kent Jr., J.W., McKay, D.R., Sprooten, E., Mathias, S.R., Curran, J.E., Carless, M.A., de Almeida, M.A., Harald, H.H., Dyer, T.D., Olvera, R.L., Fox, P.T., Duggirala, R., Almasy, L., Blangero, J. and Glahn, D.C. (2016). "Genome-wide linkage on chromosome 10q26 for a dimensional scale of major depression", *Journal of Affective Disorders*, 191, 123-131.

Koob, G.F. and Le Meal, M. (2008). "Addiction and the brain anti-reward system", *Annual Review of Psychology*, 59, 29-53.

Le Fevre, M., Matheny, J. and Kolt, G.S. (2003). "Eustress, distress and interpretation in occupational stress", *Journal of Managerial Psychology*, 18, 726-744.

Lesage, A. and Steckler, T. (2010). "Metabotropic glutamate mGlu1 receptor stimulation and blockade: Therapeutic opportunities in psychiatric illness", *European Journal of Pharmacology*, 639, 2-16.

Li, M., Chang, H. and Xiao, X. (2016). "BDNF Val66Met polymorphism and bipolar disorder in European populations: A risk association in case-control, family ased and GWAS studies", *Neuroscience and Biobehavioural Reviews*, 68, 218–233.

Lu, B. (2003). "Pro-region of neurotrophins: role in synaptic modulation", *Neuron*, 39, 735-738.

Lu, B. and Je, H.S. (2003). "Neurotrophic regulation of the development and function of the neuromuscular synapses", *Journal of Neurocytology*, 32, 931-941.

Mannie, Z.N., Harmer, C.J. and Cowen, P.J. (2007). "Increased waking salivary cortisol levels in young people at familial risk of depression", *American Journal of Psychiatry*, 164, 617-621.

Marin, H. and Menza, M.A. (2005). "The management of fatigue in depressed patients", *Essential Psychopharmacology*, 6, 185-192.

Martinowich, K., Manji, H. and Lu, B. (2007). "New insights into BDNF function in depression and anxiety", *Nature Neurosciences*, 10, 1089.

Matsugami, T.R., Tanemura, K., Mieda, M., Nakatomi, R., Yamada, K., Kondo, T. and Tanaka, K. (2006). "Indispensability of the glutamate transporters GLAST and GLT1 to brain development", *Proceedings of National Academy of Sciences USA*, 103, 12161-12166.

Medina, A., Burke, S., Thompson, R.C., Bunney Jr, W., Myers, R. M., Schatzberg, A., Akil, H. and Watson, S. J. (2013). "Glutamate transporters: a key piece in the glutamate puzzle of major depressive disorder", *Journal of Psychiatric Research*, 47, 1150-1156.

Monteggia, L.M., Luikart, B., Barrot, M., Theobold, D., Malkovska, I., Nef, S., Parada, L.F. and Nestler, E.J. (2007). "Brain-derived neurotrophic factor conditional knockouts show gender differences in depression related behaviours", *Biological Psychiatry*, 61, 187-197.

Moret, C. and Briley, M. (2011). "The importance of norepinephrine in depression", *Neuropsychiatric Disease and Treatment*, 7, 9.

Murphy, T.M., Ryan, M., Foster, T., Kelly, C., McClelland, R., O'Grady, J. and Brown, K. (2011). "Risk and protective genetic variants in suicidal behaviour: Association with SLC1A2, SLC1A3, 5-HTR1B and NTRK2 polymorphism", *Behavioural and Brain Functions*, 7, 22.

Nakagawara, A., Azar, C.G., Scavarda, N.J. and Brodeur, G.M. (1994). "Expression and function of TRK-B and BDNF in human neuroblastomas", *Molecular and Cellular Biology*, 14, 759-767.

Nestler, E.J. and Carlezon Jr, W.A. (2006). "The mesolimbic dopamine reward circuit depression", *Biological Psychiatry*, 59, 1151-1159.

Neves-Pereira, M., Mundo, E., Muglia, P., King, N., Macciardi, F. and Kennedy, J.L. (2002). "The brain-derived neurotrophic factor gene confers susceptibility to bipolar disorder: Evidence from a family-based association study", *American Journal of Human Genetics*, 71, 651–655.

Niswender, C.M. and Conn, P.J. (2010). "Metabotropic glutamate receptors: Physiology, pharmacology, and disease", *Annual Review of Pharmacology and Toxicology*, 50, 295-322.

Notaras, M., Hill, R. and Van Den, B.M. (2015). "The BDNF gene Val66Met polymorphism as a modifier of psychiatric disorder susceptibility: Progress and controversy", *Molecular Psychiatry*, 20, 916–930.

O'Dushlaine, C., Kenny, E., Heron, E., Donohoe, G., Gill, M., Morris, D. and Corvin, A. (2011). "Molecular pathways involved in neuronal cell adhesion and membrane scaffolding contribute to schizophrenia and bipolar disorder susceptibility", *Molecular Psychiatry*, 16, 286.

Okada, T., Hashimoto, R., Numakawa, T., Iijima, Y., Kosuga, A., Tatsumi, M. and Kunugi, H. (2006). "A complex polymorphic region in the brain-derived neurotrophic factor (BDNF) gene confers susceptibility to bipolar disorder and affects transcriptional activity", *Molecular Psychiatry*, 11, 695.

Palmiter, R.D. (2007). "Is dopamine a physiologically relevant mediator of feeding behaviour?", *Trends in Neurosciences*, 30, 375-381.

Pattanayak, R.D. and Sagar, R. (2014). "Depressive disorders in Indian context: A review and clinical update for physicians", *Journal of Association of Physicians of India*, 62, 827-832.

Pattwell, S.S., Bath, K.G., Perez-Castro, R., Lee, F.S., Chao, M.V. and Ninan, I. (2012). "The BDNF Val66Met polymorphism impairs synaptic transmission and plasticity in the infralimbic medial prefrontal cortex", *Journal of Neurosciences*, 32, 2410-2421.

Petryshen, T.L., Sabeti, P.C., Aldinger, K.A., Fry, B., Fan, J.B. and Schaffner, S.F. (2010). "Population genetic study of the brain-derived neurotrophic factor (BDNF) gene", *Molecular Psychiatry*, 15, 810–815.

Pivac, N., Nikolac, M., Nedic, G., Mustapic, M., Borovecki, F., Hajnsek, S. and Seler, D.M. (2011). "Brain derived neurotrophic factor Val66Met polymorphism and psychotic symptoms in Alzheimer's disease", *Progress in Neuro-psychopharmacology and Biological Psychiatry*, 35, 356-362.

Radloff, L.S. (1977). "The CES-D Scale: A Self-Report Depression Scale for Research in the General Population", *Applied Psychological Measurement*, 1, 385-401.

Raisman, G. and Field, P.M. (1973). "Sexual dimorphism in the neurophil of the preoptic area of the rat and its dependence on neonatal androgen", *Brain Research*, 54, 1-29.

Redon, R., Ishikawa, S., Fitch, K.R., Feuk, L., Perry, G.H., Andrews, T.D., Fiegler, H., Shapero, M.H., Carson, A.R., Chen, W. and Cho, E.K. (2006). "Global variation in copy number in the human genome", *Nature*, 444, 444.

Ribeiro, L., Busnello, J.V., Cantor, R.M., Whelan, F., Whittaker, P. and Deloukas, P. (2007). "The brain-derived neurotrophic factor rs6265 (Val66Met) polymorphism and depression in Mexican-Americans", *Neuro Report*, 18, 1291–1293.

Ripke, S., Wray, N.R., Lewis, C.M., Hamilton, S.P., Weissman, M.M., Breen, G. and Heath, A.C. (2013). "A mega-analysis of genome-wide association studies for major depressive disorder", *Molecular Psychiatry*, 18, 497.

Robinson, S., Rainwater, A.J., Hnasko, T.S. and Palmiter, R.D. (2007). "Viral restoration of dopamine signaling to the dorsal striatum restores instrumental conditioning to dopamine-deficient mice", *Psychopharmacology*, 191, 567-578.

Rothman, D.L., Behar, K.L., Hyder, F. and Shulman, R.G. (2003). "In vivo NMR studies of the glutamate neurotransmitter flux and neuroenergetics: Implications for brain function", *Annual Review of Physiology*, 65, 401-427.

Santrock, J.W. (2007). *Adolescence*", McGraw Hill, 11th Edition, India.

Saus, E., Brunet, A., Armengol, L., Alonso, P., Crespo, J.M., Fernandez-Aranda, F., Guitart, M., Martin-Santos, R., Menchon, J.M., Navines, R., Soria, V., Torrens, M., Urretavizcaya, M., Valles, V., Gratacos, M. and Estivill, X. (2010). "Comprehensive copy number variant (CNV) analysis of neuronal pathways genes in psychiatric disorders identifies rare variants within patients", *Journal of Psychiatric Research*, 44, 971-978.

Schumacher, J., Jamra, R.A., Becker, T., Ohlraun, S., Klopp, N., Binder, E.B. and Zobel, A. (2005). "Evidence for a relationship between genetic variants at the brain-derived neurotrophic factor (BDNF) locus and major depression", *Biological Psychiatry*, 58, 307-314.

Selye, H. (1936). "A syndrome produced by diverse nocuous agents", *Nature* 138, 32.

Shinohara, M., Mizushima, H., Hirano, M., Shioe, K., Nakazawa, M., Hiejima, Y. and Kanba, S. (2004). "Eating disorders with binge-eating behaviour are associated with the s allele of the 3'-UTR VNTR polymorphism of the dopamine transporter gene", *Journal Psychiatry and Neuroscience*, 29, 134.

Sim, M.S., Mohamed, Z., Hatim, A., Rajagopal, V.L. and Habil, M.H. (2010). "Association of brain-derived neurotrophic factor (Val66Met) genetic polymorphism with methamphetamine dependence in a Malaysian population", *Brain Research*, 1357, 91–96.

Sklar, P., Gabriel, S.B., Mcinnis, M.G., Bennett, P., Lim, Y. and Tsan, G. (2002). "Family-based association study of 76 candidate genes in bipolar disorder: BDNF is a potential risk locus", *Molecular Psychiatry*, 7, 579–593.

Sleiman, P., Wang, D., Glessner, J., Hadley, D., Gur, R.E., Cohen, N. and Kim, C. (2013). "GWAS meta analysis identifies TSNARE1 as a novel Schizophrenia Bipolar susceptibility locus", *Scientific Reports*, 3, 3075.

Sotak, B.N., Hnasko, T.S., Robinson, S., Kremer, E.J. and Palmiter, R.D. (2005). "Dysregulation of dopamine signaling in the dorsal striatum inhibits feeding", *Brain Research*, 1061, 88-96.

Stoffel, W., Sasse, J., Düker, M., Müller, R., Hofmann, K., Fink, T. and Lichter, P. (1996). "Human high affinity, Na+-dependent L-glutamate/L-aspartate transporter GLAST-1 (EAAT-1): gene structure and localization to chromosome 5p11-p12. *FEBS*", *Letters*, 386, 189-193.

Strauss, K.M., Martins, L.M., Plun-Favreau, H., Marx, F.P., Kautzmann, S., Berg, D. and Wolburg, H. (2005). "Loss of function mutations in the gene encoding Omi/HtrA2 in Parkinson's disease", *Human Molecular Genetics*, 14, 2099-2111.

Su, P.H., Gasic, M., Mrksic, N., Rojas-Barahona, L., Ultes, S., Vandyke, D. and Young, S. (2016). "Continuously learning neural dialogue management", *arXiv:1606.02689.*

Swanson, C.J., Bures, M., Johnson, M.P., Linden, A.M., Monn, J.A. and Schoepp, D.D. (2005). "Metabotropic glutamate receptors as novel targets for anxiety and stress disorders", *Nature Reviews Drug Discovery*, 4, 131.

Teng, H.K., Teng, K.K., Lee, R., Wright, S., Tevar, S., Almeida, R.D. and Kraemer, R.T. (2005). "Pro-BDNF induces neuronal apoptosis via activation of a receptor complex of p75NTR and sortilin", *Journal of Neurosciences*, 25, 5455-5463.

Terracciano, A., Sanna, S., Uda, M., Deiana, B., Usala, G., Busonero, F. and Distel, M.A. (2010). "Genome-wide association scan for five major dimensions of personality", *Molecular Psychiatry*, 15, 647.

Tsai, S.J. (2007). "TrkB partial agonists: Potential treatment strategy for major depression", *Medical Hypotheses*, 68, 674–676.

Tsai, S.J. (2018). "Critical Issues in BDNF Val66Met Genetic Studies of Neuropsychiatric Disorders", *Frontier in Molecular Neuroscience*, 11, 156.

Torres, G.E., Gainetdinov, R.R. and Caron, M.G. (2003). "Plasma membrane monoamine transporters: Structure, regulation and function", *Nature Reviews Neuroscience*, 4, 13.

Turic, D., Langley, K., Williams, H., Norton, N., Williams, N.M., Moskvina, V., van den Bree, M.B., Owen, M.J., Thapar, A. and O'Donovan, M.C. (2005). "A family based study implicates solute carrier family 1-member 3 (SLC1A3) gene in attention-deficit/hyperactivity disorder", *Biological Psychiatry*, 57, 1461-1466.

Ungerstedt, U. (1971). "Postsynaptic supersensitivity after 6 hydroxy-dopamine induced degeneration of the nigrostriatal dopamine system", *Acta Physiologica Scandinavica*, 82, 69-93.

Volkow, N.D., Wang, G.J., Fowler, J.S., Logan, J., Franceschi, D., Maynard, L. and Swanson, J.M. (2002). "Relationship between blockade of dopamine transporters by oral methylphenidate and the increases in extracellular dopamine: therapeutic implications", *Synapse*, 43, 181-187.

Volkow, N.D., Wang, G.J., Newcorn, J., Telang, F., Solanto, M.V., Fowler, J.S. and Wong, C. (2007). "Depressed dopamine activity in caudate and preliminary evidence of limbic involvement in adults with attention-deficit/hyperactivity disorder", *Archives of General Psychiatry*, 64, 932-940.

Wang, G.J., Volkow, N.D., Logan, J., Pappas, N.R., Wong, C.T., Zhu, W. and Fowler, J.S. (2001). "Brain dopamine and obesity", *The Lancet*, 357, 354-357.

Weiner, R.I. and Ganong, W.F. (1978). "Role of brain monoamines and histamine in regulation of anterior pituitary secretion", *Physiological Reviews*, 58, 905-976.

Winter, N., Kovermann, P. and Fahlke, C. (2012). "A point mutation associated with episodic ataxia 6 increases glutamate transporter anion currents", *Brain*, 135, 3416-3425.

Wise, R.A. (1998). "Drug activation of brain reward pathways", *Drug and Alcohol Dependence* 51, 13-22.

Wong, M.L., Dong, C., Andreev, V., Arcos-Burgos, M. and Licinio, J. (2012). "Prediction of susceptibility to major depression by a model of interactions of multiple functional genetic variants and environmental factors", *Molecular Psychiatry*, 17, 624.

World Health Organization. *Depression in India Let's talk.* Copyright 2017

Yu, H. and Chen, Z.Y. (2011). "The role of BDNF in depression on the basis of its location in the neural circuitry", *Acta Pharmacologica Sinica*, 32, 3.

10

Adolescent Mental Health

Cognitive Styles and Academic Achievement

Madhurima Mukherjee and *Purnima Awasthi*

Introduction

In the present competitive world, quality education is one of the key determinants of success. A major interest of parents, teachers and societal agencies lies in determining the factors that influence the success of education to guide the children towards a desirable future. One of the performance measures of any educational system is the student's academic achievement. Academic achievement refers to the ability of an individual to reach the academic milestones within the stipulated period. It reflects the brilliance in curricula such as mathematics, language and science as well as extracurricular activities such as sports, art, and communication skills. Although it is a self-evaluated measure of one's objective success, societal norms regard high academic achievement to be one of the major parameters of a successful life. Therefore, academic achievement holds an important place in the life of the learner and is influenced by the efficiency of the teachers, pedagogy, and the students' individual characteristics.

On one hand, education nurtures the innate abilities of children to lead them towards a brighter future. On the other hand, it is a potential source of stress and poor mental health among students although the stress is not due to education itself but due to the improper management of academics. A number of researches have identified academics to be a continuous source of both chronic and sporadic stress for adolescents in both Western and Asian counties and it is significantly associated with mental health problems such as anxiety, depression, substance abuse, and suicidal ideation (Fawzy, 2017; Latiff *et al.*, 2016). These findings highlight the need for further research to study the interplay between the predictors of academic achievement and their impact on adolescent's mental health and wellbeing.

Mental health is a major determinant of one's overall health, and it influences how one handles stress, relates to others and makes choices. It is, therefore, an important indicator of human functioning. It is important at every stage of life, with adolescence being a crucial period of study. Adolescence is a critical period in human life that marks the transition from childhood to adulthood. It marks the period between 10-19 years of age, with girls generally achieving puberty before boys.

A number of developmental milestones are achieved during adolescence. It is a period of physical, emotional, psychological and personality change, which can lead to emotional and behavioural problems in the individual. This period is not limited to bodily changes but it reflects in social and institutional changes as well, making the adolescents more vulnerable to stress. For instance, shifting to high school and even the beginning of college requires a lot of change and adjustment. The demanding nature of the academic field today is compromising the mental health of more and more adolescents. Academic stress refers to the conflicts, frustration and anxiety experienced by students with respect to their academics. It takes away normalcy from the life of adolescents.

Academic Stress and Mental Health

The concept of stress has existed in psychological literature since 1950s. It is still an important area of research because it is no longer related to health psychology but has found its implications in physiological psychology, organizational psychology, educational psychology and the like. The present conception of stress sees it as a "lifestyle crisis" (Masih and Gulrez, 2006) and affects anyone and everyone irrespective of the stage of life they are in (Banerjee & Chatterjee, 2016). Overcoming stress primarily depends on individual's coping resources as well as individual's characteristics.

Poor mental health is both a cause and effect of low academic achievement. High performance expectations, work overload, poor performance, lack of interest in a subject, inadequate resources, and low support from teachers or parents are potential sources of stress (Chiang, 1995). Studies have reported few other sources of academic stress such as the vastness of syllabus (Agrawal & Chahar, 2007), long hours and expectations of rote-learning (Deb *et al.*, 2015), difficulty balancing personal and academic life, and hindrances in social interaction due to fear of failure (Chernomas & Shapiro, 2013).

In the recent years, academic learning has emerged as the most important source of stress among young students worldwide and more specifically in Eastern countries. Academic achievement was consistently found to be significantly correlated with depression and self-expectations. In adolescents, parent and teachers' expectations were the main source of stress with girls facing more stress than boys (Jayanthi, Thirunavukarasu, & Rajkumar, 2015). Depression was found to be linked to inability to concentrate, fear of failure and a negative evaluation of the future (Busari, 2012). Suicide, which is a major cause of adolescent deaths, is often preceded by unrevealed depression.

Kadapatti and Vijayalaxmi (2012) have reported academic stress as a "career stopper" as students with high levels of stress exhibited signs of depression, anxiety, phobia, school refusals, irritability, poor concentration, and reduced interest in academics. The incidence of stress is not stream-specific. It is reported across all streams of education. Medical and engineering students reported highest levels of stress (Behere, Yadav & Behere, 2011). Moreover, a number of adolescents spend their crucial academic years in hostels to prepare for future exams. Some studies have identified staying away from home and adapting to a new environment a major source of stress (Hall *et al.,* 2006). A related source of anxiety in adolescents is the uncertainty about securing a good rank in competitive examinations. Eastern students were found to have more academic burden, high performance expectations, and lower satisfaction with performance. As a result, they suffer from more stress than their Western counterparts. A probable cause of this finding lies in the socialization process of children from the East as well as the collectivistic culture. Since childhood, high performance expectations are set in accordance with societal expectations. Societal expectations and conditioning with respect to parameters of achievement imposed upon them from an early age puts the mental health and future of adolescents in jeopardy.

Mental health has a significantly positive relationship with scholastic achievement. Tomar *et al.* (2014) studied stress and coping strategies among private and government high school children in Karnataka. Results revealed that 3 per cent student in private schools and 2 per cent in government schools were likely to suffer from severe mental disorders. They outlined the cause to be academic burden and relationship with parents and peers. Anxiety was also found to be negatively correlated with academic achievement. Safree, Yasin and Dzulkifli (2011) investigated the differences in mental health problems between low and high achieving students. The results reported significant differences in the levels of depression, anxiety and stress. Low achieving students or students who failed reported high levels of psychological problems. Further, there were gender differences in perception of anxiety with females reporting more anxiety than males in similar situations.

Adolescents constitute 23 per cent of Indian population (India, UNDAF Report, 2013-2017). The atmosphere of rat race poses a significant threat to the wellbeing of the society. Academic stress causes distress not only to the student but also to their parents and the institution. In light of this, it becomes important to identify the factors that influence one's academic achievement. Additionally, research on academic achievement is important due to its direct policy interventions for education.

There are a number of constructs contributing to academic achievement such as the student's background, interests, habits, personality, cognitive abilities, cognitive style, and the like. In the present chapter, we discuss the cognitive domain related to the acquisition of knowledge, concept formation and applications of ideas and skills. Learning of this type has great emphasis in the classroom where information processing plays a major part.

While learning, students gather information, process and organize them in the memory, remember, recall and utilize them in problem-solving and decision-making. Even though the basic psychological processes may be the same universally, each individual has a unique style that guides overall psychological processes and behaviour. Organization of information in memory, speed and accuracy of decision-making, the choice of problem-solving strategies, are some of the instances where individuals demonstrate their distinctiveness in processing information.

This preferred mode to behave in a distinct manner characteristic to the individual has been termed 'style'. These individual differences in information processing approach while dealing with a single task is often not due to differences in intelligence or abilities but rather individual preferences for reaction to environmental stimuli (Noroozi, 2003). For instance, some people have quick reactions in most circumstances, while others are reflective and react slowly; some students write answers in complete accordance with the textbook, while others write their own understanding of the topic.

This suggests that much of an individual's cognitive activity is guided by cognitive styles. Cognitive styles are a subset of the broad construct of 'style'. Although cognitive style is distinct from cognitive ability, it has been associated with performance in different cognitive domains where performance matters, such as creativity, problem-solving and intelligence as well as academic achievement, choice of educational and work fields, leadership and the like.

Cognitive Style

The construct of cognitive style refers to the ways one processes information, the strategies used to organize and handle the information, one's typical way of thinking and one's tendency to behave in a certain manner. For years, psychologists, as well as educationists, have been interested in this construct. Cognitive styles are observed when different individuals with similar cognitive competence react differently to the same cognitive problem (Dasen & Mishra, 2010). The choice of a specific cognitive style is not a voluntary, conscious choice, but rather unconscious like values and beliefs, and it is greatly influenced by age, gender, previous experiences, socialization, ecology, and cultural factors. Different areas of psychological activities such as attention, memory, problem-solving, and creativity as well as values, beliefs, and general perception towards life are often guided by cognitive styles.

Kumar (2011) defined cognitive style as a holistic process beginning with perception, mediated by information processing, and resulting in retrieval. It varies from person to person and is affected by various personality factors. Cognitive styles develop slowly and there is a general development from field-dependence to field-independence with increasing age. They do not seem to be easily modifiable through specific training. They remain stable across different spheres of behaviour and they are interlinked with one's temperament, affect, personality, and motivation.

Despite its controversial usage along with the terms thinking style and learning style, cognitive style remains a key concept in the field of education and psychology.

The research on field-dependence-independence as a stylistic construct began in 1954 with the work of Witkin and his associates. Field-dependence-independence was conceptualized as a bipolar construct representing the degree of autonomous functioning in assimilating information from the self and the field. The primary difference between FI and FD individuals lies in their cognitive restructuring abilities. Cognitive restructuring is the ability to break up the organized field into its elements to give an alternate organization or to give a structure to an ambiguous stimulus (Riding & Cheema, 1991). Field dependence or independence is derived on the basis of the ability of an individual to draw upon internal referents in cognitive restructuring. FI individuals are better at cognitive restructuring, that is, they are more able to see objects or details as discrete from their background. In the presence of unclear, ambiguous situations, FI individuals impose structure on field and analyze the information following a hypothesis-testing approach (Witkin & Goodenough, 1981). They are better able than FD individuals to focus their attention on task-relevant information and ignore distractions and better cognitive restructuring.

However, when it comes to social skills, FI individuals are more demanding, inconsiderate, manipulative, cold and maintain more personal distance in communication. They are less sensitive to social cues and thus, there exists an inverse relationship between cognitive differentiation and social skills (Witkin & Goodenough, 1981). FD individuals, on the other hand, are more socially efficient as they draw cues from their external referents. FI individuals rely on their bodily cues and are generally less oriented towards social engagement with others. FD individuals are better in interpersonal competency but poorer in cognitive restructuring. On the other hand, FI people are likely to have poorer interpersonal skills but much greater cognitive restructuring ability. In short, FIs are more skilled in tasks of cognitive restructuring while FDs are more skilled in interpersonal competencies (Bertini, Pizzamiglio & Wapner, 1986). Thus, it is difficult as well as incorrect to conclude which cognitive style may be more preferred or advantageous. However, as for any psychological dimension, only a few individuals fall at the extreme ends, most fall in the middle range of these dimensions.

One's cognitive style may be measured either on visual or verbal domain. Most studies on cognitive styles have used Group Embedded Figures Test (GEFT) where the task was to locate a previously seen simple figure within a more complex design. Few other measures are available such as the Portable Rod and Frame Test (where the task is to ignore a visual or postural context to locate a true vertical), Hidden Words Task, and Story Pictorial Embedded Figures Test (SPEFT). SPEFT was developed by Sinha (1988) to assess field-dependence-independence in Indian context. Although field-dependence-independence was initially proposed as a perceptual experience, gradually the study of its impact was broadened to include other cognitive and social behaviours.

Due to the importance of academic achievement in contemporary life and the contribution of cognitive styles to it, we review the literature on the association between cognitive style and academic achievement in students. There has been a lack of consensus regarding the influence of cognitive styles on academic achievement. While some studies found the two constructs to be related, others found no significant relationship between the two (Yeatts & Strag *et al.*, 1971; Zhang, 1982). One possible reason for this disagreement is that the samples for each of these studies ranged greatly from preschoolers to university students, which also included studies specifically on gifted children, students of a specific grade or studying a specific subject such as mathematics or language. A comprehensive study of literature also reveals that most researchers have studied the vastly critiqued but still most common dimension of cognitive style that is field-dependence-independence. In general, it has been demonstrated that field-dependence-independence is positively related to academic achievement and field-independent (FI) students are better achievers than field-dependent (FD) students.

In one of the initial studies on these constructs, Swanson (1980) examined the relationship between birth order, intelligence, academic achievement and cognitive styles on a sample of eighth-grade science students. Field-dependence-independence was measured using Group Embedded Figures Test (Witkin, Oltman, Raskin & Karp, 1971) and academic achievement was assessed by achievement in science. They obtained a significant low positive correlation between field-dependence-independence and achievement after controlling the influence of intelligence and family size. Helen, Walt, and Clifford (1987) investigated the relationship between cognitive style and achievement in mathematics. GEFT was administered on 44 students to categorize them into Field Dependence-Independence groups. They found that low achievers were more frequently grouped as FD. They concluded a significant positive relationship between cognitive style and academic achievement (Helen, Walt & Clifford, 1987; Martinettie & Raymond, 1995). Bal (1988) studied the relationship between cognitive styles and achievement with a sample of 150 female students from various colleges of Delhi. Field-dependence-independence was measured using the Embedded Figures Test and field-independence was found to be significantly related to academic achievement. Significant associations also existed between achievement levels and cognitive style. Adeyemi (1992), Kiranmayi et al. (1996), Kirk (2000), Muhammad (2001), Verma (2001), Malathi and Malini (2006), and Kenth (2009) reported similar findings.

Kumar (2006) studied the differences between tribal and non-tribal children with respect to their cognitive styles. On comparing 12th-grade students, it was found that non-tribal students were more FI than tribal students. In general, FI students can separate the elements from a general pattern and analyze it from their own perspective. They apply this style to studies as well, where they take out concepts from the text and understand it from their own perspective. Contrarily, FD students are unable to separate the elements. They perceive the pattern from a holistic view which they apply to studies as well. To understand a concept, they understand it as a whole and not by breaking it into details. A significant relationship was also found between cognitive style and career-choice of students (Frank, 1986; Onyekuru, 2015), which is consistent with the field-dependence-independence theory. FD students are strong in interpersonal skills needed for excellence in behavioural sciences and education.

In a study where the performance of FI and FD students were compared according to their field of study, it was found that FI students had higher achievement in Science while FD students performed better in Arts (Onyekuru, 2015). FI students are significantly better at problem-solving which is crucial in studying mathematics and science. On the other hand, Ndudi and Mkpa (2003) who found FD to have greater achievement scores than FI individuals in Social Studies supported the better performance of FD students in arts. This finding can be explained by the fact that FD students possess better social and interpersonal skills and prefer situations requiring direct communication with others.

In a cross-cultural investigation of field-dependence-independence, Utley (1983) found gender differences in cognitive styles. Male students were more FI than female students because cultural stereotypes lead to males being more independent than females in everyday life. While examined the role of gender in cognitive styles, the results showed that women are more likely to be FD and men are more likely to be FI. Further, FI females were more achievement oriented than FD females. Females in most societies hold an inferior position and their actions are more strictly guided by social norms. Therefore, they draw their motivation from their environment and society's judgment of them, making them more FD than males. Panda (1991) studied the influence of age and gender on cognitive styles of preschool children and its relationship with achievement striving. There were no significant gender differences, but with increase in age, there was an increase in field-independence. This finding was explained that at such early developmental stages, sex roles are not clearly and strongly fixed. They are in the process of development and therefore, slight methodological variations will not highlight these differences.

Jantan (2014) examined the relationship between cognitive styles and mathematics achievement among 150 six-year-old students selected from primary schools in Malaysia. GEFT was used to identify the cognitive stylea dnit was found that 112 students were of FD cognitive style. There was a low positive correlation between cognitive styles and mathematics achievement and there were significant gender differences in the results. It was suggested by the researcher that mathematics teachers should consider cognitive styles of students while preparing their lesson plans, teaching aids and examination questions.

In another study, the effect of cognitive styles and achievement motivation on academic achievement was studied (Sharma & Pooja, 2018). 64 students from 9th grade were selected from Sonepat, India and their cognitive style was assessed using GEFT. Achievement Motivation Scale by Deo and Mohan (2011) was used and academic achievement was measured using Academic Achievement in English. ANOVA revealed both cognitive styles and achievement motivation to have both main and interaction effect on academic achievement.

Another finding of the study by Utley (1983) was that cognitive styles were significantly related to reading achievement. One plausible explanation is that FI learners perceive the content analytically and even their learning of social material is motivated intrinsically to achieve self-defined goals. After controlling the effect of intelligence, significant differences were found at grade-level. Fifth-grade students were more FI than third and fourth-grade students. This finding provides support to the belief that with increasing age, one tends to become more FI as they start to draw upon self-references in information processing.

Anxiety in academics is also one of the contributors to low achievement. One possible cause of anxiety is cognitive style. Hadfield (1988) investigated the relationship between cognitive style and mathematics anxiety on 481 secondary school students. They found that FD learners were more prone to mathematics anxiety than FI learners.

Few studies also investigated the influence of teacher's cognitive style of the academic achievement of students and it was found that FI teachers led to greater success in students. FI students taught by FI teachers performed better in Sciences (Homayooni *et al.*, 2006). High achievement in any field requires some amount of field-independence (Srivastava & Asthana, 2014; Geetanjali, 2006). Individuals with more academic achievements were more FI than individuals with lesser accomplishments (Homayooni *et al.*, 2006).

Studies regarding locality of the students, it may be observed that location is a significant variable in determining both cognitive styles. Urban students are generally more FI than their rural counterparts, which may be attributed to the ecological organization as well as the differences in interpersonal relationships among urban and rural people. It was found that FI urban students reported higher academic achievement (Chatterjee *et al.*, 1982; Therakan, 1996). Extensive research spanning over decades shows that cognitive differentiation is more important for academic achievement in science as compared to language and mathematics (Mishra & Berry, 2018).

Contrary to these findings, Rai and Prakash (1989) found neither gender nor cognitive styles influenced academic attainments. Nand, Shrivastava and Venugopal (1994) conducted a study on the cognitive style and achievement of middle-school students using GEFT. The results again showed no relationship between cognitive styles and achievement. The mixed results indicate a gap in research that may be attributed to the sample used, the differences in their need for achievement, and the tests used to assess their achievement. A greater amount of literature still indicates that there is a strong link between cognitive styles and academic achievement.

According to Witkin (1962), the origins of field-dependence-independence cognitive style lie in early socialization experiences. Children who were raised to be more independent and autonomous grew up to be FI, while those who were under strict parental control were relatively more FD. Social conformity and individual and social connectedness are negatively correlated with academic achievement in the domain of science and mathematics. These cultural variables also interact with the development of cognitive differentiation style (Mishra & Berry, 2018). Therefore, children of communities characterized by greater social conformity and individual and social connectedness are likely to display lower levels of academic achievement.

The literature shows that the relationship between cognitive styles and academic achievement has been widely researched in India. This relationship has been studied on different populations ranging from preschoolers to university students, in different countries. A general finding is that there is a significant positive relationship between field-dependence-independence and achievement. FD students make greater use of external social resources in ambiguous situations whereas FI students demonstrate more independence in such situations. One way to explain the high achievement of FI individuals is that they are guided by intrinsic factors and therefore, they set their achievement goals according to their capabilities and needs. They are self-motivated and possess greater problem-solving skills resulting in a better performance in mathematics and science. On the contrary, FD individuals are guided by societal norms in fulfilling their goals. They are more concerned about fulfilling the dreams of others, are more sensitive to criticism and more compliant owing to their cognitive style. As a result, their stress and anxiety due to expectations may lead to lowering the performance and their achievements. However, since they have strong interpersonal skills, they are able to perform better than FI individuals in social sciences.

Impact of Cognitive Styles and Academics on Mental Health

Mental health is not merely the absence of an illness, but rather possessing positive qualities that help in effective day-to-day functioning. It is a concern for all age groups but here we focus on the adolescents who form almost one-fifth of the world population (Bhatia, Vij & Madhura, 2013). An unhealthy mind would not lead to efficiency or achievement.

In most societies, especially in a country like India, where males dominate the society, females tend to be more field-dependent (Hulfish, 1978; Tharakan, 1996). Societal norms expect females to have good interpersonal skills and a conforming nature. As a result, they seek the approval of others leading to an increase in stress. A number of studies have established FDs, especially females to be have greater anxiety and poorer mental health than FI individuals (Witkin, 1962). Ford (1998) found no gender differences in the stress levels of adolescents but their sources of stress varied. While girls were more stressed due to interpersonal situations, boys were stressed due to specific events such as changing schools and poor grades.

The present trend of no rural-urban differences in the anxiety of students (Kumar, Baliya & Bakshi, 2016) shows a significant aspect of academic stress. The urban students are stressed due to the abundance of career options before them. On the contrary, rural students are anxious because of lack of resources and difficulties in finding a course of their choice in their locality. Therefore, there remains no significant difference in anxiety due to academics even though their cognitive styles are different.

Cognitive style comes and goes out of fashion in research but it still remains important in psychology and education. The theory has been criticized for being highly correlated with measures of general mental ability and spatial ability, leading to a doubt whether field-dependence-independence is purely a measure of cognitive style or it rather measures abilities. Field-dependence-independence has been shown to be linked to academic achievement and choice of subjects for college students. Further, the effectiveness of certain instructional techniques also depends on the cognitive styles of both teachers and students (Morgan, 1997). In addition to this, several recent attempts to reformulate the theory indicate that the research on this construct might continue in future despite previous challenges.

Implications for Education

A review of research on these constructs and their interrelationships have several educational implications, which are discussed below.

One drawback of our education system is that it penalizes students whose cognitive styles do not match the instructional methods. Therefore, educationists should consider the results obtained from decades of research in cognitive styles while formulating instructional material so prevent such loss in academic achievement of the students.

Psychological wellbeing of students should be addressed and more attention should be paid to the knowledge of cognitive styles of both the teachers and the students. Failure to understand the teacher's communication creates a kind of cognitive dissonance in the children. This knowledge may lead to the reduction of communication gap between the teacher and the learner.

Schools should encourage a warm and healthy learning environment for students. Support services should be available at school level to prevent serious damage to the child. The mentoring should be in the favour of the child instead of in favour of school or parents, as in the true scenario of most schools at present. If cognitive styles really impact academic achievement and the path of education, it should also be considered during career guidance and counselling to make the correct initial career choice. Since parental overburden is the most prominent cause of poor mental health, it is imperative that parents reduce their expectations and allow adolescents to choose their field according to their own interests and abilities.

Future Directions for Research

Although the research on cognitive styles has been extensive in determining its influence on academic achievement, it is only a part of the theory to explain achievement. It overlaps with other concepts such as cognitive abilities, thinking styles and learning styles, thus, diffusing the impact as a strong predictor of achievement. In this regard, there seem to be three major areas where future research may be directed.

The first concern lies in the validity of cognitive style as a construct. Although there has been significant amount of studies concerning cognitive styles, nevertheless its overlap with other constructs makes its validity questionable. Future research may investigate to find a more definitive understanding of cognitive styles as an autonomous construct or it is in fact, a mix of personality and cognitive ability. Most research has concerned with the cognitive differentiation. Thus, there is a need to integrate the classic theories such as field-dependence-independence with newer theories of thinking styles, assimilation-exploration, and adaptation-innovation to validate the autonomy of the construct.

Secondly, it is necessary to investigate the relationship between cognitive styles with respect to different conceptions of achievement. A number of other factors such as achievement motivation, instructional strategies, and teacher-student interaction guide academic achievement. Future research may study the interactive effects of these variables along with cognitive style on academic achievement.

Thirdly, most studies have assessed the correlation between cognitive style and academic achievement. This limits the understanding of the results and the possibilities of inference causal relationships between style and achievement. One may investigate the underlying mechanism as to why field-independence is essentially leads to better achievement in science. In addition, future studies may also try to identify the strengths of FD students and identify specific areas where their performance is better.

Finally, the use of interventions in improving the competencies of extreme FIs or FDs has been rare. Interventions may provide a way to improve academic performance where poor performance was due to a mismatch between the student's cognitive style and the institution's requirements. Moreover, interventions may also confirm the permanence or impermanence of cognitive styles.

Conclusion

From the above review of literature in the area of cognitive styles, specifically field-dependence-independence and academic achievement, it may be concluded that each style offers significant strengths. FI students tend to be analytic, intrinsically motivated and self-directed in the learning process. On the other hand, FD students who have a holistic approach are passive learners. They draw motivation from external sources, learn social issues better than FI students, and are more receptive to criticisms. However, these differences are not indicative of any cognitive style being better than the other. It simply means that each style has its own advantages and this knowledge of one's cognitive style might be useful for improving performance and overall self-management. By enhancing the areas that they do not use, they can improve their learning and performing power.

For instance, extreme field dependency can be reduced by making use of outlines and timeliness to organize information in the absence of context whereas FI students may work on improving their interpersonal skills to do better in social sciences and humanities. A number of studies have been taken under consideration and several limitations of the studies have been found. Most studies related to cognitive styles were limited to gender-based studies and smaller groups for the sake of generalization. Most importantly, most participants were students of science and technical subjects. Ignoring the students from humanities and social sciences overlooks a large part of the population. With respect to mental health, studies have not assessed the role of cognitive styles on stress and mental health of adolescents. It may be an area of research for future studies.

Investigation of relationships should not be done for the sole purpose of research, but it should have wider applications as well. By incorporating the findings of the research, it might be possible to ensure quality education as well as mental health of students.

References

Adeyemi, M.A. (1992). "Cognitive style and sex as mediators of biology retention-test performance of students exposed to two instructional modes in Benin City, Nigeria", *International Journal of Educational Development*, *12*(1), 3-12.

Agrawal, R.K., and Chahar, S.S. (2007). "Examining role stress among technical students in India", *Social Psychology of Education*, *10*(1), 77-91.

Bal, S. (1988). "Creativity, cognitive style and academic achievement amongst university students", *Psychological Studies*, *33*(1), 10–13.

Banerjee, N., and Chatterjee, I. (2016). "Academic stress, suicidal ideation and mental well-being among 1st semester and 3rd semester medical, engineering and general stream students", *Researchers World*, *7*(3), 73.

Behere, S.P., Yadav, R., and Behere, P.B. (2011). "A comparative study of stress among students of medicine, engineering, and nursing", *Indian Journal of Psychological Medicine*, *33*(2), 145.

Bertini, M., Pizzamiglio, L., and Wapner, S. (1986). "Epilogue: Relation of Witkin's work to future trends in psychology", *Field Dependence in Psychological Theory, Research, and Application*, 5-13.

Bhatia, R., Vij, S., and Madhura, D. (2013). "A Study of Stress Level among Adolescents in Government and Public Schools of Delhi", Addressed to the Academic Editor, *Journal of Indian Education*, Department of Teacher Education, NCERT, New Delhi, 90.

Busari, A.O. (2012). "Evaluating the relationship between gender, age, depression and academic performance among adolescents", *Scholarly Journal of Education*, *1*(1), 6-12.

Chatterjee, R.G. and Paul, B. (1984). "A study of field independence in relation to science achievement, urban-rural habitat and intelligence", *Indian Journal of Psychology*, 59, 1-13.

Chernomas, W.M., and Shapiro, C. (2013). "Stress, depression, and anxiety among undergraduate nursing students", *International Journal of Nursing Education Scholarship*, *10*(1), 255-266.

Chiang, C.X. (1995). "A study of stress reactions among adolescents", *Chinese Journal of School Health*, *26*, 33-37.

Chiang, C.X. (1995). "A study of stress reactions among adolescents", *Chinese Journal of School Health*, *26*, 33-37.

Dasen, P.R., and Mishra, R.C. (2010). *Development of geocentric spatial language and cognition: An eco-cultural perspective* (Vol. 12). Cambridge University Press.

Deb, S., Strodl, E., and Sun, J. (2015). "Academic stress, parental pressure, anxiety and mental health among Indian high school students", *International Journal of Psychology and Behavioural Sciences*, *5*(1), 26-34.

Fawzy, M., and Hamed, S.A. (2017). "Prevalence of psychological stress, depression and anxiety among medical students in Egypt", *Psychiatry Research*, *255*, 186-194.

Frank, B.M. (1986). "Cognitive styles and teacher education: Field dependence and areas of specialization among teacher education majors", *The Journal of Educational Research*, *80*(1), 19-22.

Geetanjali (2006). "A Study of academic achievement in relation to cognitive styles and hemisphericity at secondary stage", M.Ed. dissertation, GNDU, Amritsar.

Hadfield, O.D., and Maddux, C.D. (1988). "Cognitive style and mathematics anxiety among high school students", *Psychology in the Schools*, 25(1), 75-83.

Hall, N.C., Chipperfield, J.G., Perry, R.P., Ruthig, J.C., and Goetz, T. (2006). "Primary and secondary control in academic development: Gender-specific implications for stress and health in college students", *Anxiety, Stress, and Coping, 19*(2), 189-210.

Helen, M., Walt, B. and Clifford, H.A. (1987). "Cognitive learning style and achievement in Mathematics", *Journal of Instructional Psychology*, *14*(1), 26-28.

Homayooni, E., Kadivar, P., and Abdollahi, M. (2006). "The relationship between cognitive styles, learning styles, and deciding fields of study", *Iranian Journal of Psychologists*, 10, 137-144.

Hulfish, S. (1978). "Relationship of role identification, self-esteem, and intelligence to sex differences in field independence", *Perceptual and Motor Skills*, *47*(3), 835-842.

Jayanthi, P., Thirunavukarasu, M., and Rajkumar, R. (2015). "Academic stress and depression among adolescents: A cross-sectional study", *Indian Paediatrics*, *52*(3), 217-219.

Kadapatti, M.G., and Vijayalaxmi, A.H. M. (2012). "Stressors of academic stress: A study on pre-university students", *Indian Journal of Scientific Research*, *3*(1), 171-175.

Kenth, B. (2009). "An investigation of the cognitive styles, learning styles and study skills as predictors of academic achievement of prospective teachers", *Education New Horizon*, *6*(22), 45-50.

Kiranmayi, A., and Vindhya, U. (1996). "Field-dependence-independence as a function of socioeconomic status and academic achievement: A study on adolescent girls", *Journal of Indian Psychology*, 14, 25-35.

Kirk, G.R. (2000). "The relationship of attitudes toward science, cognitive style, and self-concept to achievement in chemistry at the secondary school level. ProQuest Dissertations And Theses; Thesis (Ed.D.)—Florida International University, 2000; Publication Number: AAI9975006; ISBN: 9780599805576.

Kumar R. (2006). "A study of cognitive and learning styles among tribal and non-tribal senior secondary school students of Himachal Pradesh", Ph.D. Thesis, Himachal Pradesh University.

Kumar, M.H. (2014). "Cognitive Styles and Mental Health among College Students in Jammu Division", Department of Educational Studies, Central University of Jammu.

Latiff, L.A., Tajik, E., Ibrahim, N., Abubakar, A.S., and Ali, S.S. B.A. (2016). "Depression and its associated factors among secondary school students in Malaysia", *Southeast Asian Journal of Tropical Medicine and Public Health*, *47*(1), 131.

Malathi, S. and Malini, E. (2006). "Learning style of higher secondary students of Tamil Nadu", *Indian Educational Abstracts*, *6*(2), 16.

Martinetti, R.F. (1994). "Relationship between cognitive processing style and academic achievement", *Perceptual and motor skills*, *78*(3), 813-814.

Masih, P.P., and Gulrez, N.K. (2006). "Age and gender differences on stress", *Recent Trends in Human Stress Management*, 97-104.

Mishra, R.C., and Berry, J.W. (2017). *Ecology, Culture and Human Development: Lessons for Adivasi Education*. SAGE Publishing India.

Morgan, H. (1997). *Cognitive Styles and Classroom Learning*. Praeger Publishers.

Muhammad, A. (2001). "The Role of Cognitive Style in Creative Performance", *Journal of Psychology*, *45*(11), 16-51.

Nand, H., Shrivastava, P., and Venugopal, R. (2014). "Relationship Between Physical Fitness and Well Being", *International Human Research Journal*,{Online Interdisciplinary-Quarterly}, ISSN, 2347-7067.

Ndudi, M.J., and Mkpa, M.A. (2003). "Effects of cognitive styles and instructional strategies on students' achievement in social studies", *The Educational Psychologist*, *1*(1), 172-193.

Noroozi, D. (2003). "Cognitive styles of Students and their relationship with learning", Tehran: Islamic Azad University, the South Branch.

Oltman, P.K., Raskin, E., and Witkin, H.A. (1971). Group embedded figures test.

Onyekuru, B.U. (2015). "Field Dependence: Field Independence Cognitive Style, Gender, Career Choice and Academic Achievement of Secondary School

Students in Emohua Local Government Area of Rivers State", *Journal of Education and Practice*, *6*(10), 76-85.

Panda, S. (1991). Effects of certain organismic variables on cognitive style among pre school children and an analysis of its correlates, Department of Home Science, Utkal University, Bhubaneswar, Odisha. https://shodhganga.inflibnet.ac.in/handle/10603/189804

Rai, P.K., and Prakash, J. (1989). "Cognitive styles and academic achievement among university students", *The Indian Journal of Psychology*, *64*(1-4), 33-40.

Riding, R., and Cheema, I. (1991). "Cognitive styles: An overview and integration", *Educational Psychology*, *11*(3-4), 193-215.

Sharma, H.L., and Priyamvada (2017). "Multimedia: Instructional Strategy to Enhance Achievement of Senior Secondary School Students in Business Studies", *International Journal of Research*, 4(13), 1332-1342.

Srinivas Kumar, D. (2011). *Introduction to Cognitive Styles and Learning Styles*. Kuppam: Prasaranga (Publications Bureau) Dravidian University.

Srivastava, M., and Asthana, M. (2014). "Socio-Cultural Correlates of Cognitive Style: A Study of Primary School Children", *International Journal of Education and Psychological Research* (*IJEPR*), *3*(2), 87-91.

Swanson, L. (1980). "Cognitive style, locus of control, and school achievement in learning disabled females", *Journal of Clinical Psychology*, *36*(4), 964-967.

Tharakan, P.N.O. (1987). "The effect of rural and urban upbringing on cognitive styles", *Psychological Studies*, *12*(7), 119-122.

Tomar, S., Verma, G., David, A., Thakur, M., Ogorchukwu, M.J., Parmar, P., Shriyan, P., and Jaswal, R. (2014). "Study on stress and coping strategies among private and government high school children in Udupi Taluk, Karnataka: A cross-sectional study", *IOSR Journal of Nursing and Health Science, 3(2),* 27-30.

United Nations Development Action Framework 2013–2017 (India UNDAF Report). http://in.one.un.org/img/uploads/India_UNDAF%202013-17_9July2012.

Utley, C.A. (1983). A cross-cultural investigation of field-independent/field-dependent as a psychological variable in Menominees Native American and Euro-American grade school children. Wisconsin Centre for Education and Research.

Venugopal, G. (1994). "Cognitive style and achievement of pupils", *Experiment in Education*, 22.

Verma, S. (2001). "Learning Styles and study skills of two groups of science and arts students", *Prachi Psychocultural Dimension*, 17(2), 113.

Witkin, H.A., Dyk, R.B., Fattuson, H.F., Goodenough, D.R., and Karp, S.A. (1962). *Psychological differentiation: Studies of development*. Wiley.

Witkin, H.A., and Goodenough, D.R. (1981). "Cognitive styles: Essence and origins, *Field dependence and field independence. Psychological Issues*, (51), 1-141.

Witkin, H.A., Oltman, P.K., Raskin, E., and Karp, S.A. (1971). A Manual of the Group Embedded Figures Test. Palo Alto, California: Consulting Psychologists Press.

Yasin, M.A. S.M., and Dzulkifli, M.A. (2011). "Differences in depression, anxiety and stress between low-and high-achieving students", *Journal of Sustainability Science and Management, 6*(1), 169-178.

Yeatts, P.P., and Strag, G.A. (1971). "Flexibility of cognitive style and its relationship to academic achievement in fourth and sixth grades", *The Journal of Educational Research, 64*(8), 345-346.

Zhang, L.F. (2004). "Field-dependence/independence: cognitive style or perceptual ability?: Validating against thinking styles and academic achievement", *Personality and Individual Differences, 37*(6), 1295-1311.

11

Parlous Effect of Loneliness among Adolescents

Shakshi Priya Giri and *Anubhuti Dubey*

Introduction

Imagine one person grew up surrounded by his parents, grandparents and cousins and his entire childhood was spent among the same people. Finally, he had his degree and got a job and his new career requires him to move out to another city. After three months of following various routines he realized that he was not sleeping well. After an unpleasant run-in at the home-office and living alone and a new independent life, he began to feel unwanted and uncared. He was thinking that everyone else is much happier than him.

It does not take a minute to recognize that the person was lonely. Human beings are the social animals that require satisfying social relationships for our better mental and physical well-being. When this relationship gets impaired it can lead to loneliness. It's a painful universal phenomenon that reminds us of the pain and the threat of becoming isolated. Globally, loneliness is a problem that affects not just the elderly, as many would think. Twenty per cent of the population in the United States, that would be sixty million people, are alone and lonely (Steffick, *et al.*, 2000). The Maryland-based National Centre for Biotechnology Information (NCBI), which is a part of the United States National Library of Medicine, stated in an article of 2013 that loneliness is most prevalent during adolescence, with more than 70 per cent of adolescents experiencing recurring loneliness at age 18; this rate declines to 60 per cent by ages 35–40, and 39 per cent for older adults. So, what about India? The National Sample Survey Office reported in 2004 that 4.91 million Indians lived alone. Right now, this number has been increased and most of them feel sufficiently isolated that is a major source of unhappiness in their lives. Consequently, loneliness is taking place and the outcome is health-hazardous (James, 2019).

Like other mental health problems loneliness has no single and common cause that is why its prevention and treatment significantly differs. An adolescent who tries to make a new friend circle needs different tackling strategies; where an older adult who's recently retired from his job needs the different one. To understand this damaging state of mind it is important to have a closer look at exactly what we mean by the term "lonely" as well as what are the various causes, symptoms and its relationship with adolescence stage and also potential intervention plans or treatments for loneliness.

Entering in Loneliness

Everybody feels lonely from time to time, e.g. when we have no one to sit next to at lunch or when we moved to a new city or also when we see nobody has time for us at the weekend. We are living in the most connected time in human history, and yet, an unprecedented number of us feel isolated. Being lonely and being alone is not the same thing. We can be filled bliss by ourselves, and hate every minute when we surrounded by our friends. Loneliness is a purely subjective individual experience. If someone feels lonely, he is lonely. A most common stereotype is that loneliness only happens when someone don't know how to talk to people, or how to behave around others. But when it comes to social connections for adults there is no such difference in terms of social skills. Loneliness can affect anybody and indeed fame, money, good social skills, and a prominent personality—nothing can protect someone against loneliness, because it's a part of our biology (Cattan, White, Bond, & Learmouth, 2005).

Think about hunger and thirst, which make us to pay attention to our physical needs; loneliness makes us to pay attention to our social needs. Therefore, loneliness is a bodily function like other physiological desires (Cacioppo, & Patrick, 2009). Our body cares about our social requirements and connections because prior for our species, it was a great indicator of how likely we were to survive (Theory of Natural Selection, Darwin, 1859). In today's world, people are so busy in their work, social networking sites, dating applications; so, there is not enough time. Therefore, majority of people get stumbled into chronic loneliness by accident. When it becomes chronic an individual cannot escape it merely by 'move out of your shell', or by a makeover, or fixing meetings with somebody.

So, what are the symptoms of being lonely? There are subtle signs that indicate the person is feeling loneliness. Can anyone imagine someone can be lonely without even realizing it? There are N numbers of signs that point towards the lonely individual. Some of the major symptoms are:

- Disruption in sleep pattern, many studies concluded that loneliness is a significant predictor of sleep fragmentation (Kurina, Knutson, Hawkley, Cacioppo, Lauderdale, & Ober, 2011; Cacioppo, Hawkley, Crawford, *et al.,* 2002). Sleep fragmentation is defined as constant awakenings that disrupt the sleep pattern. An individual feels tired constantly.
- Sudden care about material possession, loneliness is likely lead to materialism and in turns materialism contributes to loneliness (Pieters, 2013; Tuttle, 2011). In this, people frequently go out and buy stuffs to alleviate their loneliness. Loneliness causes a sudden change on material possessions and shopping more than normal.
- Feeling hopeless, unwanted, uncared and increased feeling of anxiety and depression, Lonely person feels no one wants him/her and no one cares about his/her feeling. This feeling increases the level of stress and anxiety which could lead to depression (Cacioppo, Hughes, Waite, Hawkley, & Thisted, 2006).
- Spending a lot of time on social media, one study reported that if you are lonely you spend more than two hours of a day on social media in a day and seems to feel more socially isolated (Primack, Shensa, Sidani, *et al.,* 2017).
- Spending time with lone people, if a person is lonely and meets someone it's possible for second person to experience feelings of loneliness too (Cacioppo, Fowler, & Christakis, 2009). In other words loneliness is contagious in social networks.
- Gaining weight, loneliness motivates towards overeating because we tend to compensate for our blues with foodstuff and also gaining weight is a common repercussion of depression. (Shaw, 2018).

Above signs are ratifying the state of loneliness. Studies suggest that the level of loneliness can increase in young adulthood (i.e., 18 to 25) while slowly diminishing throughout middle and afterwards (Cacioppo, & Cacioppo, 2014). Most studies are conducted on millennial group and older group of population but they reported adolescence is quite more vulnerable towards loneliness (e.g. Bernnan, 1982; Larson, 1999; Sullivan, 1953; Ali & Barnagarwala, 2018; James, 2019).

Adolescence and Loneliness

Through various stages human life completes its journey and the most vital stage is adolescence. In the past several decades, it has been suggested that during adolescence loneliness increases (Brennan, 1982; Larson, 1999; Sullivan, 1953; Weiss, 1973; Mahon, Yarcheski, Yarcheski, Cannella, & Hanks, 2006). A global health service company in the United States found that generation Z (18-22 age group) and millennials (generation Y: 23-37 age group) are lonelier than older generations (Cigna, 2018). In 2014, a research project on mental health which was conducted at the university level reveals that students are more vulnerable to mental health related issues like depression, loneliness, social isolation, anxiety, self-harm and suicidal thoughts etc.

Think for a moment you want to pursue higher studies or want to learn some new professional skills or want to switch for a better job for which you need to move out to another city. And what will happen next? One of the prominent newspapers in India published an article, about loneliness, stated that we all know there are so many people in India because we are one of the largest populated countries in the world, but there is no one to connect with (*The Hindu*, 2018). This article shared N numbers of experiences of young adults to show what's going on in modern urban Indian society. A boy, who moved to Bengaluru from Kochi in Kerala for higher education when he was 18, described the feeling of loneliness in the city as exhausting. "It weighs on you unlike anything else," he says. The one girl who is from Mumbai says, "I don't want to see people with other people or people with a sense of purpose because both are elusive to me" (para 2). The idea to share behind these verbatim is to indicate the severity of lonesomeness among adolescents. Urban Indians, particularly the young adults, are sinking into loneliness (James, 2019).

This shows why the familial or social support for youth is important to feel less lonely. However, some studies reported that a lonely young adult may be less competent to sufficiently cope up with stressful situation and also young adults with lesser healthy attachment styles strongly associated with high level of loneliness (Larose & Bernier, 2001). In 2016 the Centre for the study of developing societies conducted a survey on young population (15 to 34 years) of India and found that 12 per cent people feel depressed frequently and 8 per cent reported they felt lonely quite often (Ali & Barnagarwala, 2018). Adolescents may be at greater risk of deleterious mental and physical health outcomes.

Changes during Adolescence that Increase the Risk for Loneliness

Companionship related changes: Over the adolescent years, critical changes occur in the identity of social companionship. There is an articulated move toward age group severance among adolescents: young adults invest less time and energy with their family members and additional time with their peer group (Larson & Richards, 1991). As a result, the reference clusters for social experience changes. By mid-adolescent years, they start enjoying their many evenings with their pals. Hence, an adolescent starts revising his views about what makes him lonesome? Spending time with parents now be seen as social inaccessibility. Moreover, lower level of parental support and regular parental strife can escalate the feeling of loneliness (DeLay, Hafen, Cunha, Weber, & Laursen, 2013).

Identity construction: In adolescent period establishment of identity is a major developmental deed. If a person fails to achieve his identity during adolescence then identity crisis may occur, called identity cohesion vs. role confusion (Erikson, 1968). Crisis results in a loss of ability for self-delineation and obligation to values, goals, or relationships, and a painful sense of inarticulateness (e.g. experience of not fitting in). This can lead to isolation from their cliques and loneliness arises in a consequence (Witvliet, Brendgen, van Lier, Koot & Vitaro, 2010).

Cognitive maturity and changes in social viewpoint: With cognitive maturity a young adult becomes more sophisticated in terms of social exchange ideologies (Laursen & Hartup, 2002). They assess their relationships and they put the interests of the relationship ahead of the interests of the individual. In this cognitive alteration they believe that their close peer relation and their family relation are equal and reciprocal (Smollar, & Youniss, 1985). As a consequence, "demands that parent-child relationships be transformed to resemble peer relationships may meet resistance, which fosters withdrawal and alienation" (para 5, page 5, Laursen, & Hartl, 2013). As a result, sometimes the parent-child relation suffers and loneliness takes place (Laursen & Collins, 1994). Although, the role of cognitive maturity in fostering loneliness, is not well-understood during adolescence yet.

Physical changes: Bodily changes during adolescence i.e. pubertal maturation, affect every aspect of adolescence. Vivid hormonal changes take place that is directly linked to mood vacillation (Susman & Rogol,

2004). Perceptible changes such as changes in body shape in girls and facial hairs in boys and also changes in voice box or larynx for both male and female etc. increases the feeling of 'not fitting in' within an adolescent. This fear can create or escalate social isolation and loneliness (Williams & Currie, 2000).

These changes during adolescence can increase the risk and vulnerability towards loneliness.

Is Social Distancing Due to COVID-19 Increasing Loneliness Among Adolescents?

COVID-19 pandemic presented a series of long term challenges in front of us. Initial lockdown phase and fear of contagion of this disease during unlock phase has prominently up stretched the concern on various mental health issues. Grief and trauma has increased and it's destroying our collective sense of normalcy. Thousands of people committed suicide across the world (Ruiz, 2020). One survey reported adolescents rated high level on loneliness scale due to present isolative deportment from their peer group, teachers and community (Loades *et al.*, 2020). Loneliness, anxiety, depression, PTSD, risk of suicide and other mental health problems are taking place nowadays (King, 2020; Ruiz, 2020; Hoof, 2020). In sum, it's a massive mental health crisis for us. Although, there is a need for additional research to lay down the effect of pandemic and social distancing on adolescent's lonely feeling.

Tackling Strategiés

Looking at the present mental and physical health outcomes that are majorly developed due to loneliness has elevated the interest in intervention to reduce the feeling of loneliness for each group (Rook, 1984; Masi, Chen, Hawkley, and Cacioppo, 2010). We can divide intervention programmes into four major categories to mitigate loneliness, these are: social skills enhancement training, providence of social support related training, increasing opportunities for social interaction programme, and addressing the maladaptive social cognition related training programmes.

Social Skills Enhancement

Good social skills are important to make friends, enjoy yourself in public, and succeed further. Most of the researches identified that feeling of loneliness is first and foremost the result of poor interpersonal skills to maintain and rebuild their relationships (e.g. Rook, 1984; Lea, & Duck, 1982; Masi *et al.*, 2010; Choi, Kong, & Jung, 2012). Healthy relationship or intimacy with others prevent the feeling of emptiness or abandonment state that is directly associated with loneliness (Chernyak, 2020). This kind of intervention involves: teaching people to engage in conversation, how we can take and give compliments, and also how we can communicate our nonverbal communication effectively. The more they practice to be social it will become easy for them (Chernyak, 2020).

Providence of Social Support

Social support is a key component of solid relationship and for our strong mental health. It involves having a net of family and friends or people who care about ourselves that we can turn to in times of exigency. These types of relations play a crucial role for our better functioning in day-to-day life. Many studies identified a solid linkage between social support and loneliness (Santini, Koyanagi, Tyrovolas Haro, & Koushede, 2019; Cattan, White, Bond, & Learmouth, 2005; Austin, 1983). Poor social support indicates the higher level of loneliness and consequently increases the risk of depression, anxiety, suicidal thoughts, drug abuse, cardiovascular illness, and altered brain functioning (Grav, Hellzèn, Romild, & Stordal, 2012). This intervention technique involves—firstly, how we can cast a wide network because it's possible that one person doesn't fit in all, so we have to look for different relationships for different types of support whether it can be personal or professional; how to become proactive in nature, you have to make an effort to get good social relationship; how we can use technology to connect with people; and learn how we can ask for help, asking for help is really important for our better mental peace. And it does not mean you are not valuable or you can't do things alone to seek help and support. It strengthens the relatedness with others (Sturt, & Nordstrom, 2017).

Social Interaction Escalation Programme

Social interaction is a process by which people act and react in relation to others. When you converse, yell, fight, play games this means you are socially interacting. We can form a group of people and do some activity like playing games or sharing own ideas about life or doing some other activities which could help in maximizing our social connection to the outer world (Masi *et al.*, 2010).

Sometimes face-to-face interaction is not easy for someone so in this technique we can teach them or provide them online or social media platform especially to older adults who are living alone and retired. It will help them a lot (Choi *et al.*, 2012).

Addressing Maladaptive Social Cognition

Bandura's reciprocal theory (1978) suggests that our personality is adaptive and can be moulded by social encounters. According to Cacioppo and Cacioppo (2014) a lonely person do not want to become lonely, in fact they find themselves on one extreme of the extent of social connection and feels despondently isolated (Gable & Reis, 2010). This kind of perception increases the level of self-conservation in individual and also it motivates the hyper-vigilance for social threats which activates the attention, memory and confirmatory predispositions. If it's unchecked it can strengthen withdrawal symptoms, negative social interaction and feeling of loneliness ultimately (Cacioppo & Cacioppo, 2014; Cacioppo & Hawkley, 2009). Therefore, in this training individual's attention, memory and confirmatory predisposition could be targeted which can help them to identify their automatic negative thoughts about others and about their social interactions and regarding this it needs to be verify whether these thoughts are real or just their faulty hypotheses. These faulty behavioural confirmation processes could be targeted by training in mindfulness (Cacioppo, Grippo, London, Goossens, & Cacioppo, 2015; Baer, 2003; Creswell, Pacilio, Lindsay, & Brown, 2014) and capitalization e.g. sharing good times with others (Gable & Reis, 2010; Woods, Lambert, Brown, Fincham, & May, 2015).

In sum, these studies empirically suggesting that a wide range of interventions have been developed to envisagement with loneliness. But additional research is required to determine how precisely individual and group level strategies might prove helpful in the treatment.

Conclusion

Loneliness is directly associated with anxiety, depression, maladaptive social cognition, poor social skills and narrow view of social interaction or communication that leads to physical and mental illness for an adolescent. Interventions in these areas can reduce the effect of loneliness in people by providing social support, enhancement in social skill, providing the opportunities for social interaction and by pointing out the maladaptive social cognition to change their faulty assumptions about their social world. As per the researches these are the useful intervention strategies to alleviate the lonely feeling but for advancement in effectiveness of interventions there is a need to focus on individual empowerment as well which allows the individual to manage their own lonesomeness. Another important consideration would be increasing public awareness and also awareness among health care providers that loneliness is a public health issue which can feel by anyone at any moment even popular or higher status people can find themselves lonely and during pandemic period it is really important to consider this feeling as a huge mental health crisis. It can be solved but doing so it needs the full support and engagement of psychological or medical activists.

References

Ali, A., Barnagarwala, T. (2018). *You are not the only one: India stares at a loneliness epidemic.* Retrieved from https://indianexpress.com/article/express-sunday-eye/you-are-not-the-only-one-5154976/

Austin, B.A. (1983). "Factorial structure of the UCLA loneliness scale", *Psychological Reports*, *53*(3), 883–889.

Baer, R.A. (2003). "Mindfulness training as a clinical intervention: A conceptual and empirical review", *Clinical Psychology: Science and Practice*, *10*(2), 125-143.

Brennan, T. (1982). "Loneliness and adolescence", Pulkaisussa: Peplau, Letitia Anne; Perlman, Daniel, (eds.) *Loneliness. A Sourcebook of Current Theory, Research and Therapy*, 260-290.

Cacioppo, J.T., and Cacioppo, S. (2014). "Social relationships and health: The toxic effects of perceived social isolation", *Social and Personality Psychology Compass*, *8*(2), 58-72.

Cacioppo, J.T., Hawkley, L.C., Crawford, L.E., Ernst, J.M., Burleson, M.H., Kowalewski, R.B., ... and Berntson, G.G. (2002). "Loneliness and health: Potential mechanisms", *Psychosomatic Medicine*, *64*(3), 407-417.

Cacioppo, J.T., Hughes, M.E., Waite, L.J., Hawkley, L.C., and Thisted, R.A. (2006). "Loneliness as a specific risk factor for depressive symptoms: Cross-sectional and longitudinal analyses", *Psychology and Aging*, *21*(1), 140.

Cacioppo, J.T., Fowler, J.H., and Christakis, N.A. (2009). "Alone in the crowd: the structure and spread of loneliness in a large social network", *Journal of Personality and Social Psychology*, *97*(6), 977.

Cacioppo, J.T., and Patrick, W. (2009). *Loneliness: Human nature and the need for social connection* (p. 317).

Cattan, M., White, M., Bond, J., and Learmouth, A. (2005). "Preventing social isolation and loneliness among older people: A systematic review of health promotion interventions", *Ageing and Society*, *25*(1), 41-67.

Census of India (2011). Retrieved from https://en.wikipedia.org/wiki/2011_Census_of_India.

Chernyak, P. (2020). *How to Improve Social Skills.* Retrieved from https://www.wikihow.com/Improve-Social-Skills#References.

Choi, M., Kong, S., and Jung, D. (2012). "Computer and internet interventions for loneliness and depression in older adults: A meta-analysis", *Healthcare Informatics Research*, *18*(3), 191-198.

Cigna (2019). Signs and Symptoms of Chronic Loneliness. Retrieved from https://www.cigna.com/individuals-families/health-wellness/chronic-loneliness.

Creswell, J.D., Pacilio, L.E., Lindsay, E.K., and Brown, K.W. (2014). "Brief mindfulness meditation training alters psychological and neuroendocrine responses to social evaluative stress", *Psychoneuroendocrinology*, *44*, 1-12.

Darwin, C. (1859). *The Origin of Species*, ed. JW Burrow.

DeLay, D., Hafen, C.A., Cunha, J.M., Weber, L.N., and Laursen, B. (2013). "Perceptions of parental support buffer against depression for Brazilian youth with interpersonal difficulties", *International Journal of Behavioural Development*, *37*(1), 29-34.

Erikson, E.H. (1968). *Identity: Youth and Crisis* (No. 7). WW Norton & Company.

Gable, S.L., and Reis, H.T. (2010). "Good news! Capitalizing on positive events in an interpersonal context", *Advances in Experimental Social Psychology* (Vol. 42, pp. 195-257). Academic Press.

Grav, S., Hellzèn, O., Romild, U., and Stordal, E. (2012). "Association between social support and depression in the general population: the HUNT study, a cross-sectional survey", *Journal of Clinical Nursing*, 21(1-2), 111-120.

Hoof, V.E. (2020). *Lockdown is the World's Biggest Psychological Experiment- and we will pay the price.* Retrieved from https://www.weforum.org/agenda/2020/04/this-is-the-psychological-side-of-the-covid-19-pandemic-that-were-ignoring/.

James, N. (2019). *Loneliness of a big city dweller.* Retrieved from https://www.thehindubusinessline.com/blink/cover/loneliness-a-universal-problem-among-city-dwellers/article29407877.ece.

King, B.H. (2020). *Loneliness and Mental Health in Young People: Possible Effects of COVID-19 Lockdowns.* Retrieved from https://www.jwatch.org/na51821/2020/06/18/loneliness-and-mental-health-young-people-possible-effects.

Kurina, L.M., Knutson, K.L., Hawkley, L.C., Cacioppo, J.T., Lauderdale, D.S., and Ober, C. (2011). "Loneliness is associated with sleep fragmentation in a communal society", *Sleep*, *34*(11), 1519-1526.

Larose, S., and Bernier, A. (2001). "Social support processes: Mediators of attachment state of mind and adjustment in late adolescence", *Attachment and Human Development*, *3*(1), 96-120.

Larson, R., and Richards, M.H. (1991). "Daily companionship in late childhood and early adolescence: Changing developmental contexts", *Child Development*, *62*(2), 284-300.

Laursen, B., and Collins, W.A. (1994). "Interpersonal conflict during adolescence", *Psychological Bulletin, 115*(2), 197.

Laursen, B., and Hartl, A.C. (2013). "Understanding loneliness during adolescence: Developmental changes that increase the risk of perceived social isolation", *Journal of Adolescence, 36*(6), 1261-1268.

Laursen, B., and Hartup, W.W. (2002). "The origins of reciprocity and social exchange in friendships", *New Directions for Child and Adolescent Development*, 95, 27-40.

Lea, M., and Duck, S. (1982). "A model for the role of similarity of values in friendship development", *British Journal of Social Psychology, 21*(4), 301-310.

Loades, M.E., Chatburn, E., Higson-Sweeney, N., Reynolds, S., Shafran, R., Brigden, A., ... and Crawley, E. (2020). "Rapid Systematic Review: The Impact of Social Isolation and Loneliness on the Mental Health of Children and Adolescents in the Context of COVID-19. *Journal of the American Academy of Child and Adolescent Psychiatry.*

Mahon, N.E., Yarcheski, A., Yarcheski, T.J., Cannella, B.L., and Hanks, M.M. (2006). "A meta-analytic study of predictors for loneliness during adolescence", *Nursing Research, 55*(5), 308-315.

Masi, C.M., Chen, H.Y., Hawkley, L.C., and Cacioppo, J.T. (2011). "A meta-analysis of interventions to reduce loneliness", *Personality and Social Psychology Review, 15*(3), 219-266.

Pieters, R. (2013). "Bidirectional dynamics of materialism and loneliness: Not just a vicious cycle", *Journal of Consumer Research, 40*(4), 615-631.

Primack, B.A., Shensa, A., Sidani, J.E., Whaite, E.O., yi Lin, L., Rosen, D., ... and Miller, E. (2017). "Social media use and perceived social isolation among young adults in the US", *American Journal of Preventive Medicine, 53*(1), 1-8.

Rook, K.S. (1984). "Promoting social bonding: Strategies for helping the lonely and socially isolated", *American Psychologist, 39*(12), 1389.

Ruiz, R. (2020). *Why Suicide Risk May Increase As We Cope With COVID-19.* Retrieved from https://in.mashable.com/social-good/13091/why-suicide-risk-may-increase-as-we-cope-with-covid-19.

Shaw, G. (2018). *9 subtle signs that you're lonely-even if it doesn't feel like it.* Retrieved from https://www.insider.com/signs-of-loneliness-2018-6.

Santini, Z.I., Koyanagi, A., Tyrovolas, S., Haro, J.M., and Koushede, V. (2019). "The association of social support networks and loneliness with negative perceptions of ageing: Evidence from the Irish Longitudinal Study on Ageing (TILDA)". *Ageing and Society, 39*(5), 1070-1090.

Smollar, J., and Youniss, J. (1985). "Adolescent self-concept development", *The Development of Self*, 247-266.

Steffick, D.E., Wallace, R.B., Herzog, A.R., Ofstedal, M.B., Steffick, D., Fonda, S., and Langa, K. (2000). "HRS/AHEAD documentation report: Documentation of affective functioning measures in the Health and Retirement Study", Ann Arbor, MI: Survey Research Centre, University of Michigan.

Sullivan, H.S. (1953). Interpersonal theory of personality. NY Nort.

Susman, E., Rogol, A., Lerner, R.M., and Steinberg, L. (2004). *Handbook of Adolescent Psychology*.

Sturt, D, and Nordstrom, T. (2017). *4 Reasons Why Asking For Help Makes You A Stronger, Not Weaker, Leader*. Retrieved from https://www.forbes.com/sites/davidsturt/2017/11/01/4-reasons-why-asking-for-help-makes-you-a-stronger-not-weaker-leader/#1493c9573c1a.

Tuttle, B. (2011). *The Reason You're in Love With Material Possessions? Loneliness.* Retrieved from https://business.time.com/2011/07/26/the-reason-youre-in-love-with-material-possessions-loneliness/.

UNDP (2020). *United Nations Development Programme*. Retrieved from https://en.wikipedia.org/wiki/United_Nations_Development_Programme.

Weiss, R.S. (1973). *Loneliness: The Experience of Emotional and Social Isolation*.

Williams, J.M., and Currie, C. (2000). "Self-esteem and physical development in early adolescence: Pubertal timing and body image", *The Journal of Early Adolescence*, *20*(2), 129-149.

Witvliet, M., Brendgen, M., Van Lier, P.A., Koot, H.M., and Vitaro, F. (2010). "Early adolescent depressive symptoms: Prediction from clique isolation, loneliness, and perceived social acceptance", *Journal of Abnormal Child Psychology*, *38*(8), 1045-1056.

Woods, S., Lambert, N., Brown, P., Fincham, F., and May, R. (2015). "I'm so excited for you!" How an enthusiastic responding intervention enhances close relationships", *Journal of Social and Personal Relationships*, *32*(1), 24-40.

12

Impact of Cultural Variation, Gender and Chronological Age on Academic Anxiety

Ruchi Tewari and *Aradhana Shukla*

Introduction

Academic anxiety is the fear of studying including not having good study habits and fear of failure among others. It is a physical and psychological state, portrayed by physical, emotional and cognitive changes which can occur in either presence or absence of psychological stress (Afolayan *et al.*, 2013). Academic anxiety is the most prevalent mental health disorder (33.7%) and is a growing worldwide concern, with considerable impact upon cognitive function (Vytal *et al.*, 2013; Bandelow, 2015). Statistics shows that 74 per cent students suffer from anxiety (Aronin *et al.*, 2018), which negatively impacts their learning through influences on working memory leading to poor academic achievement (Hashempour, 2014). For many students "tension" or "pressure" is another word for academic anxiety. Most people think of anxiety as negative but anxiety can also be positively experienced. Academic anxiety has physical and emotional effects on students. It can create positive and negative feelings as per situational demands.

Academic anxiety symptoms are relatively common among children and adolescents and they can interfere their cognitive functioning'. It is a common type of disorder in childhood and symptoms are extremely common in every age and can negatively interfere with general well-being, social life, academic performance and development of social skills. As school education is a very important part in an individual's life and is also a turning point in the academic life. At this stage, the academic performance of a student plays a crucial role in deciding the next stage of his education, which in turn shapes his career. An excess of academic stress during this stage can result in adverse effects that are far-reaching and prolonged.

In today's highly competitive world, students face various academic problems including exam stress, disinterest in attending classes and the inability to understand a subject and academic stress involves mental distress regarding anticipated academic challenges or failure or even the fear of the possibility of academic failure. Academic stressors show themselves in many aspects in the students' environment at school, home, in their peer relations and even in their neighbourhood. Excessive levels of academic stress can result in an increased prevalence of psychological and physical problems like depression, anxiety, nervousness and stress related disorders, which in turn can affect their academic results.

Academic anxiety as a disorder is seen in about 8 per cent of adolescents and children worldwide. Anxiety and stress have a substantial negative effect on their social, emotional and academic success. It is also a reflection of an individual's academic frustration, academic conflict, academic anxiety and academic pressure. The three components of academic anxiety usually identifiable in a student are academic frustration, academic conflicts and academic pressures.

There are a number of reasons why academic anxiety occur to children. Some of these are as follows:

Fear of failure. While the pressure to perform can act as a motivator, it can also be devastating to individuals who tie their self-worth to the outcome of a test.

Lack of preparation. Waiting until the last minute or not studying at all can leave individuals feeling anxious and overwhelmed.

Poor test history. Previous problems or bad experiences with test-taking can lead to a negative mindset and influence performance on future tests.

There are some symptoms that can be seen in students due to academic anxiety:

Physical symptoms. Headache, nausea, diarrhoea, excessive sweating, shortness of breath, rapid heartbeat, light-headedness and feeling faint can all occur. Test anxiety can lead to a panic attack, which is the abrupt onset of intense fear or discomfort in which individuals may feel like they are unable to breathe or having a heart attack.

Emotional symptoms. Feelings of anger, fear, helplessness and disappointment are common emotional responses to test anxiety. Which the students in general feel.

Behavioural/Cognitive symptoms. Difficulty concentrating, thinking negatively and comparing himself to others are common symptoms of test anxiety.

Academic anxiety and its impact is widely studied by Indian and western investigators. Ahamad and Nuna (1987) studied the stress and strains of tribals and suggested a need for education of tribals. They also examined tribals deprivation and suggested uplift of deprived and under-privileged by means of integrated educational development. Agarawal (2005) studied inter-regional part of population in relation to the children attending school. It was concluded that children having higher level of achievement have higher level of academic stress as compared with their low levelled educational and economic attainders. So, it is surely be claimed that academic anxiety interferes with the magnitude of academic achievement and performance as well as social and psychological development among children and adults. (Levine, 2008). Such attempts are very less in Kumaun region of Uttarakhand.

Keeping these views in consideration this study was planned and it was aimed to ascertain the impact of cultural variation, gender and chronological age on academic anxiety. The objectives and hypotheses were as follows:

- The first objective of the study was to find out the impact of cultural variation on academic anxiety. It was hypothesized that variation in culture would cause variation in academic anxiety.
- The second objective of the study was to ascertain the relative efficacy of gender on academic anxiety. It was contended that variation in gender would lay its impact on academic anxiety.
- The third objective of the study was aimed to explore the effect of chronological age on academic anxiety. It was thought that increase in chronological age would cause variation on academic anxiety.
- Fourth objective of this study was to find out the impact of yogic exercises on academic anxiety. It was contended that regular yogic exercises would lay their positive impact and reduce to level of academic anxiety.

Method

Sample—Two hundred forty participants were selected and they were arranged according to the requirements of three-way factorial design with three levels of cultural variation (Tharu, Buxa, General Kumauni), two gender (male, female) and chronological age (10-11 years) i.e., 20 participants in each cell. The experimental design is presented in Table 12.1.

Table 12.1: Schematic presentation of experimental design

	A					
	A1		A2		A3	
	B		B		B	
	B1	B2	B1	B2	B1	B2
C1	20	20	20	20	20	20
C2	20	20	20	20	20	20

Legends:

A – Cultural Variation
A1 - Tharu
A2 - Buxa
A3 - General Kumauni

B – Gender
B1 - Male
B2 - Female

C—Chronological Age
C1 - 10-11 years
C2 - 12-13 years

Measure

In this study only one measure was used it was Academic Anxiety Scale. Abbreviated as A.A.S. this scale is constructed by Paul, Mishra, and Pandey (1975). It is comprised of 35 items in yes/no form and it is a predictor of anxiety faced by students children and/or adolescence during study and examination. Score ranges between 35-70. Low scores indicated high anxiety and high score vice-versa. The reliability of the test is .84. Academic anxiety was assessed by the response of participants.

Procedure: Data collection was done individually and group as per convenience of the participants. Best attempts were made to avoid external distractions.

Results

Obtained data were analysed in three sections. The first section described the impact of cultural variation, gender and chronological age on academic anxiety. The second section discussed the impact of yogic exercises on academic anxiety. And last and third section qualitative analysis of data was made. Findings are presented as follows:

Section I

Impact of culture variation, gender and chronological age on academic anxiety: Obtained data were analyzed by 3 way analysis of variance and interpreted in terms of cultural variation, gender and age as affectors of academic anxiety, findings are reported in Table 12.2.

Table 12.2: Summary table of analysis of variance showing the impact of cultural variation, gender and chronological age on academic anxiety

Sources of Variation	*Ss*	*df*	*MS*	*F*
A	28.50	2	14.125	6.78
B	1.16	1	1.16	0.59
C	3.97	1	3.97	1.91
AB	13.29	2	6.64	3.19
AC	23.70	2	11.85	5.69
BC	12.52	1	12.52	6.01
ABC	24.95	2	12.47	5.99
error within	109.44	228	0.48	
		239		

A close perusal of the table indicates that the main effect of cultural variation was significant (F, 1, 239 = 6.78 P< .01) and it was noted that the magnitude of academic anxiety was shared differently by every cultural segments. Mean values pooled across gender and age were: 67.41, 57.05 and 49.35 and it was noted that general Kumauni participants were least anxious about their academics (X = 49.35) as compared to Buxa (X = 57.05) and Tharu (x = 67.41) participants. Also, it was noted that the magnitude of discrepancy was relatively higher between general Kumauni and Buxa participants while discrepancy between general Kumauni-Tharu and Tharu-Buxa was almost equal. The next main effect of gender was insignificant (F, 1, 239 = 0.59 P>.05) and it was found that males (X = 58.82) and females (X = 57.71) were almost equal in relation to their scores on academic anxiety, but it was clear that females were (X = 57.71) less in academic anxiety than males (X, 58.82). The third main effect of age was also insignificant (F, 1, 239-1.91 P>.05) and it was noted that the 10-11 years old participants were (X = 56.61) less anxious than 12-13 year old participants (X = 59.26).

The two-way interaction of cultural variation and gender was significant (F, 2, 239 = 3.19 P < .05) and it is depicted in Figure 12.1.

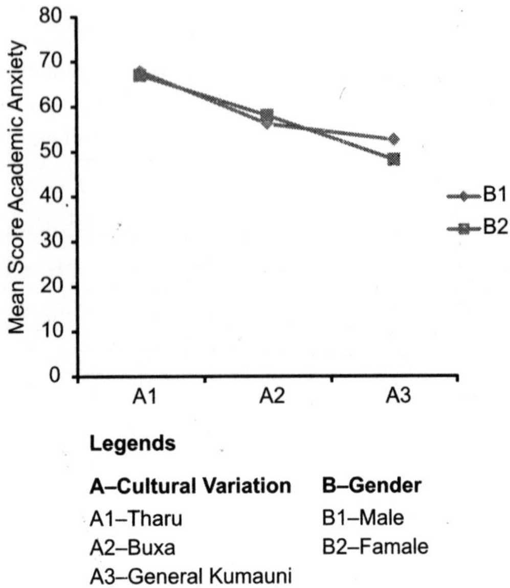

Fig. 12.1: Mean value showing the impact of cultural variation and gender on academic anxiety

Figure reveals that the magnitude of difference related to academic anxiety was higher between Tharus and Buxas. For males and for females the magnitude of discrepancy was almost equal. The magnitude of gender related discrepancy was highly shared by general Kumauni group while in other cultures the magnitude of discrepancy was more or less equal. The next interaction of cultural variation and age was also significant (F, 2, 239 = 5.69 $P < .01$) and it is portrayed in Figure 12.2.

A close perusal of the figure indicated that age related difference is highest in Buxa segment followed by general Kumauni and Tharu segments. Moreover, it was also noticed that culture related gap was almost equal between two groups but the difference between tribal groups was higher as compared to general Kumauni group. Also, it was seen that Tharus were far distinct to general Kumauni population as compared with Buxas and this trend was commonly shared by both age groups.

The gender and age interaction was also significant (F, 1, 239 = 6.01 $P < .01$) and it is reported in Figure 12.3.

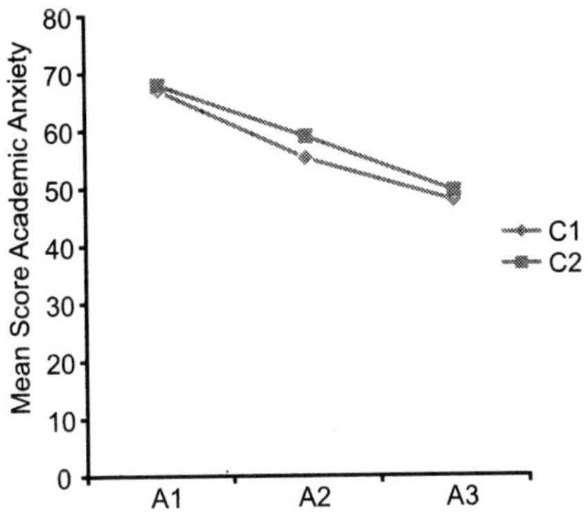

Legends

A–Cultural Variation	**C–Chronological Age**
A1–Tharu	C1–10-11 years
A2–Buxa	C2–12-13 years
A3–General Kumauni	

Fig. 12.2: Mean value showing the impact of cultural variation and chronological age on academic anxiety

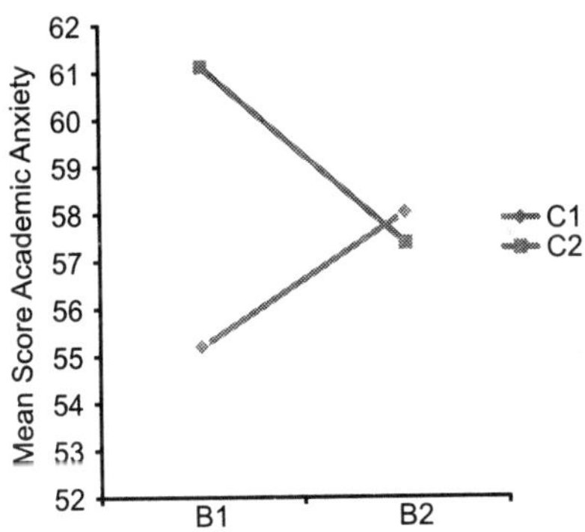

Legends

B–Gender	**C–Chronological Age**
B1–Male	C1–10-11 years
B2–Female	C2–12-13 years

Fig. 12.3: Mean value showing the impact of gender and chronological age on academic anxiety

Figure 12.3 indicates that gender based discrepancy was rather high in 10-11 years old participants (and perhaps it was the cause of significant interaction) as compared to older age group of 13-14 years. Figure also shows that younger aged females were surprisingly high and it is sure to say that the caused significant in the level of interaction.

The three way interaction of cultural variation, gender and age was also insignificant (F, 2, 239 = 5.99 $P < .01$) and it is mentioned in Figure 12.4.

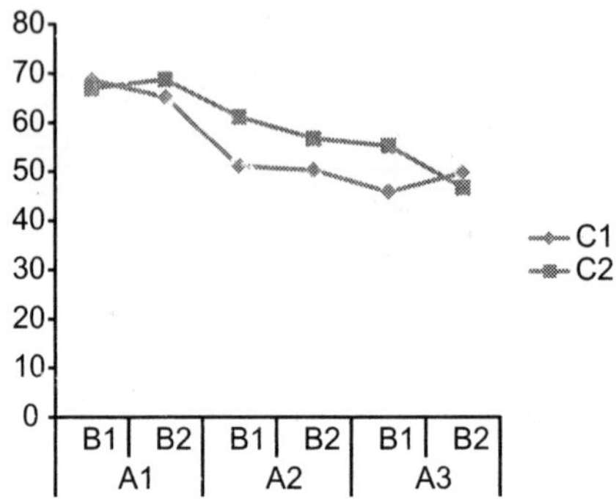

Legends:

A–Cultural Variation **B–Gender**
A1–Male B1–Male
A2–Female B2–Female
A3–General Kumauni
C–Chronological Age
C1–10-11 years
C2–12-13 years

Fig. 12.4: Mean value showing the impact of cultural variation, gender and chronological age on academic anxiety

Figure reveals that all variables laid their impact on academic anxiety.

Section IV

Impact of Yogic Exercise on Academic Anxiety

In this section an attempt was made to find out the impact of Yogic exercises on academic anxiety for this purpose 10 participants from each cell were taken (N = 80) and they were trained on Yognidra for three days. They were, then requested to do it at home for one month and till the time the investigators visited them regularly during this period. Evening time of 5:00-5:30 PM (IST) was prescribed for them and it was convenient for both investigators as well. Participants were also told that they could be cheeked at any time during. After 30 days they were again tested on

Academic Anxiety Scale. Data were analyzed only by mean values and the findings are mentioned in Table 12.3.

Table 12.3: Mean scores of Academic Anxiety as a Function of Gender and Chronological Age

		A1			A				A2	
		B							B	
	B1		B2		B2			B1		B2
C1		60.19			64.57			59.76		60.18
C2		41.38			40.46			46.36		48.54

Legends: **A-Gender**

B-Chronological Age A1–Male

B1-10–1 Years A2–Female

B2-12–13 Years

C-Testing Conditions

C1-Per Yogic condition

C2-Post-Yogic condition

A close perusal of the table indicates that the magnitude of testing condition related was highest in the 12-13 years old male participants.

Section III

Qualitative Analysis of Academic Anxiety

In addition, data of participants was also subjected to qualitative analysis. After filling the Academic Anxiety for some informal observation was made and it was followed by some more inquiries on the basis of which qualitative analysis could by made. As it was a detailed process, so 60 participants (5 from each cell) were taken in consideration and they consisted the framework of the sample.

In this section we had selected only those participants whose data were taken from their homes and they could be contacted again easily. They were those on whom Yog Nidra was also made. The inquiries were related to the individual attention and interest of the child for academic anxiety. Plenty of study materials like books and stationary, disturbance during study, academic care by the parents and other family members, supportive family climate, gender difference for school selection and study, inferiority complex to those studying in better schools and other anxieties related with study. They were presented either in question form or in conversational mode. Apart from the children, parents also took a keen interest and participated actively. The main feature of the findings revealed that in almost families parents showed more anxiety for the academics of their sons. Although they did not reveal any such view but they some time depicted their reluctance with the daughters. As we moved towards the tribal segments we found that the tribal parents were almost very carefree about the education of their children so there was no questions for them to be worried for the academia of their children. Not only for the academics they were not found serious about the physical development and nutritional care of their children. Being studied in the same schools a drastic change in parental behaviour was noticed. The parents who were involved in agriculture showed their interest to involve their children in agriculture also. On the whole, it was noted that the academic anxiety of the participants was based on the climate where they were living.

Findings, in sum, revealed:

1. The variation in academic anxiety was caused by cultural variation.
2. Gender and age were unable to yield their significant impact although the difference existed.
3. All interactions were significant.
4. Qualitative determinants of academic anxiety were also analyzed.

Discussion

Obtained data were analyzed by 3-way analysis of variance and interpreted in terms of culture variation, gender and chronological age as affecters of academic anxiety. It was found that the magnitude of academic anxiety was affected by variation in cultural settings and gender in developmental perspective. Prior to the inception of the study some hypotheses were formulated and the findings will be discussed accordingly.

1. Variation in culture would cause variation in the level of academic anxiety: Our first and foremost hypothesis was related with the impact of cultural variation on academic anxiety. It was noted that variation in cultural setup caused variation in academic anxiety and participants hailing from variant cultures were highly different in relation to their scores on academic anxiety. Culture is a vast phenomena that moves around ourselves and directs our behaviour directly and indirectly. The level and magnitude of academic anxiety revolves around the cultural environment and results accordingly. It was apparently seen in our findings.

In actual sense cultural settings and cultural variation decides all sorts of behaviour. It has underpinned by many factors like, home and school environment, gender and so many other factors. In addition, students own cognitive ability, level of aspiration, past academic scores and peer group also impacts on the magnitude of academic anxiety.

In our study we found that the level of academic anxiety was highest in Tharus followed by Buxas and general Kumauni population. It can be said that general Kumauni participants were found least anxious about their academic anxiety. A close perusal of the environmental observation of general Kumauni sample reveals that they used to study in good and standard public schools and get all sorts of academic amenities that they should have. They have good teaching practices, supportive home and school climate, good academic achievement of siblings, friends and peers. Also, it was noticed that they highly experienced the sense of academic competition with their peers and they work hard for getting good outcomes. Contrarily, the tribal children, although they were worried about their study yet they did not get proper promoting and supporting environment. Moreover, it was also observed that their school climate and peer group psyche was not so supportive. Perhaps, it has caused our findings. Findings are close convenience with Shukla (2012, 2013, 2017, 2018) in which relative superiority of non-tribals over tribals was visited in relation to cognitive, motivational and emotional attributes. Also, our findings are in line of Ahmed and Nuna (1987) and Lee (2009) in which cultural impact on academic anxiety was revealed.

2. Variation in gender would lay its impact on academic anxiety: Our second notion was related with the pattern of gender based discrepancy in academic anxiety. Unfortunately our hypothesis was rejected and we found that boys and girls were almost similar in relation to their scores on academic anxiety. The hair line difference related to gender revealed the fact that girls were less anxious than boys in relation to their scores on academic anxiety.

It is common fact that parents and society expect more with their sons as compared with their daughters. It was our finding and was supported by Pascoe, Hatrik and Parkes (2019). Girls are still supposed to do household chores and maintain the psychophysical balance and health in family. Although, time and temporal demands are changing rapidly and girls are accepting the challenges of life have and occupied higher position in society (the condition has not yet changed in inner world) but the magnitude of change is not so visible. They are more goal-oriented and centred more towards their studies and perhaps, it has caused our findings. In addition, it was also noted that tribal girls were less involved in academic pursuits as compared with nontribal girls. That is why they found less concerned with their academic activities than their non-tribal counterparts because they were deprived of academic amenities (Bhansali & Trivedi, 2017). Findings are in close concern with Barinder (1985), Dev and Walish (2010) and Shukla (2018) in which superiority of non-tribal girls over non-tribal girls is revisited. Our findings are also supported by Gautam (2011) and Yadav (2017) where academic anxiety of female adolescents was observed.

3. Increase in chronological age would cause variation in academic anxiety: Our third hypothesis was related with the impact of developmental changes in academic anxiety. It was found that variation (hairline) in chronological age caused variation in academic anxiety scores age group. Although, the magnitude of discrepancy in both between both age groups was nominal but it recorded its presence. In our common parlance we see that as the chronological age increases the child feels so many academic pursuits in a challenging way and he has to overcome them with increase in academic class. A students has to face many academic responsibilities and burden that develop a sense of anxiety. In this study the participants were the students of VI and VIII classes and the VII graders were found more academically anxious as compared with VI graders. Although there was a nominal difference yet it was noticed that with increase in age and class the load of academic affairs increase and goals are experienced closer. Our findings are in close consonance with Shukla (2012, 2014) in which increasing impact of academic anxiety was appeared with growing age.

Some New Vision Appeared by Qualitative Analysis

It was a new venture for us and we thought that some new aspects and dimensions of academic anxiety would be appeared after qualitative analysis of data. While making an informal observation with the selected participants it was noted that the magnitude of academic anxiety was affected by so many factors like, emotional deformities, health disorders, maladjustment, low self-concept, low aspirational level and intelligence level etc. They were found sheer responsible in the variation in magnitude of academic anxiety. After analyzing the verbal communication with the participants, it was noted that our findings were in consonance with Sri Devi (2013) and Pant *et al.* (2013). Institutional factors were also seen as affectors of academic anxiety and our findings were supported by Mahoto and Jangir (2012), Mattoo and Nabi (2012), Natrajan (2015) and Nadeem *et al.* (2011).

Continuous Yogic Exercises would Deteriorate the Magnitude of Academic Anxiety

Last but not least was the hypothesis in which an attempt was made to find out the impact of yogic exercises on academic anxiety. Participants were selected once they were subjected to yogic exercises following which the measure of academic anxiety was administered again. It was noted that magnitude of academic anxiety decreased after yogic exercises. Therefore, it is surely fair to say that yogic exercises promote positive mental health. Yoga is the control over temperament and *chittvritti*. It is the art of life and impact on knowledge and ways to improve. The basic aim of yoga studies is to shape people exceptional in emotional assumption, desires and planning. Yogis are better than the normal people. The aim of yoga study is:

> "*Yogatsamprapyate gyanam yogarthmasya lakshanam*
> *Yogah param tapogyeyasat dyaktah sambhyasait*"
>
> — *Agni Samhita*

It means that actual knowledge is achieved only by yoga and meditation. Therefore, we should always practice yoga.

In general, yoga aims to:

- develop psychophysical energy
- develop creativity
- reduce tension
- improve and modify life style against nature
- provide mental peace
- develop positive energy
- make the body free from diseases
- make the body drug free
- maintain world unity and world peace.

All these aim, if followed carefully develop a person in psychophysical perspective. Dealing with the impact of yogic exercise on academic anxiety, it was noted that not only the magnitude of academic anxiety was decreased changes in behaviour was also visited.

Here are some valuable strategies that will help, manage and overcome the causes and effects of academic anxiety:

Make a to Do Lists
Time management
Make a reward system
Ask for help and move on
Take breaks to breathe
Eat healthy
Take a restful sleep
Do exercise daily
Have some days to relax
Seek help if necessary
Take time for self-care
Learn to change your thinking
Take assignment one baby step at a time
Deeding the goals as per capacity and capabilities
Stay balanced during study.

Findings, sum reveal, the relative efficacy of cultural variation, gender and chronological age on academic anxiety. Parental support positive home and school climate and teachers willingness to reduce academic anxiety are the need of hour and they should be followed strictly.

References

Afolayan, J., Donald, B., Onasoga, O., A,. A. and A., A. (2013). "Relationship between anxiety and academic Performance of nursing students", Niger Delta University, Bayelsa State, Nigeria. *Advances in Applied Science Research*, *4*(5), pp. 25-33.

Agrawal, A. (2005). Pattern of well-being in police man, *Paper presented at NAOP* XV held at K.S. Saket Mahavidyalaya, Ayodhya, Faizabad.

Ahmad, A. and Nuna, S.C. (1987). "Stress and Strain of tribals", *Journal of Educational Planning and Administration.*

Alam, M.J.F. (2017). "Relation between academic anxiety and academic achievement among school students of Murshidabad district," *International Journal of Advanced Research and Innovative Ideas in Education*, *3*(3), 3354-3357.

Bandelow, B., and Michaelis, S. (2015). "Epidemiology of anxiety disorders in the 21st century", *Dialogues in Clinical Neuroscience, 17*(3): 327-335.

Bhansali, R. and Trivedi, R. (2017). "Is academic anxiety gender specific: A comparative study", *Journal of Social Science,* 17, 1-3.

Barinder, M. (1985). "A Study of general anxiety and list anxiety with reference to the environmental factors and extraversion-intraversion of Delhi students", Unpublished Doctoral Dissertation, Department of Psychology, Delhi University, in M.B. Busch (1988-1992). *Fifth Survey of Educational Research,* New Delhi, NCERT, 2, (337).

Gautam, S. (2011). "Academic anxiety of urban and rural adolescents girls in relation to their socioeconomic status", *International Referred Journal, 3*(33), 27-31.

Hashempour, S. and Mehrad, A. (2014). "The Effect of Anxiety and Emotional Intelligence on Students' Learning Process", *Journal of Education and Social Policy, 1*(2), pp. 115-119.

Levin, G. (2008). "A favocaltian approach of Academic anxiety", *Journal of American Educational Studies Association, 44*(1), 62-76.

Mahato, B. and Jangir, S. (2012). "A study on the academic anxiety among adolescents of Minicoy Island", *International Journal of Science and Research, 1*(3), 12-14.

Matto, N.H. and Nabi, R. (2012). "A study on academic anxiety among adolescents (14-16 years)", *International Journal of Social Science Tomorrow, 1*(3), 37-42.

Nadeem, M. *et al.,* (2011). "Impact of anxiety on the academic achievement of students having different mental abilities at university level in Bahawalpur, (Southern Punjab)", *Pakistan's International Online Journal of Educational Sciences, 4*(3), 519-528.

Natrajan, G. (2015). "Study on anxiety level among school students undergoing higher secondary examination", *International Journal of Student Research in Technology and Management, 3*(03), 302-304.

Pascoe, M., Hetrick, S.E. and Parker, A.G. (2019). "The impact of stress on students in secondary schools and higher education", *International Journal of Adolescents and Youths*, 104-112.

Paul, S.K., Mishra, K.S. and Pandey, K. (1975). *Academic Anxiety Scale,* Varanasi Rupa.

Shukla, A. (2012). "Psychological Consequences of Environmental stress in Kumaun Region of Uttarakhand", *Unpublished Report,* University Grants Commission, New Delhi, Published by LAP, Germany (2015).

Shukla, A. (2013). *Psychosocial Pattern of Children in Kumaun Region of Uttarakhand.* Indian Council of Social Science Research, New Delhi.

Shukla, A. and Joshi, R. (2017). "Academic stress among professional and non-professional students", *The International Journal of Indian Psychology, 4*(4), 182-188.

Shukla, A. (2018). "Culture, Climate and Psyche of children in Uttarakhand: A Developmental Approach", *Unpublished Report*, University Grants Commission, New Delhi.

Vytal, K., Cornwell, B., Letkiewicz, A., Arkin, N. and Grillon, (2013). "The complex interaction between anxiety and cognition: Insight from spatial and verbal working memory", *Frontiers in Human Neuroscience*, 7.

13

Styles of Parenting and Perceived Social Support as Predictors of Social Anxiety in Adolescent Boys and Girls

Turfa Ahmed and *Tilottama Mukherjee*

Introduction

The period of development from the onset of puberty to the attainment of adulthood is called adolescence which usually begins between 11 and 13 years of age and terminates legally at the age of usually 18 years (Coleman, 2025). Social development influenced by families, parenting styles and peer support most often explains behavioural problems during adolescence. Parents and peers are both crucial sources of social support for adolescents because they obtain different provisions of social support from these relationships and when one relationship is lacking in social provisions, other relationships become increasingly important provisional resources (Gaertner, Fite & Colder, 2010).

Parenting can be defined as activities of parents aimed at helping their child to bring forth. There are two main dimensions underlying parental behaviour (Maccoby & Martin, 1983): parental responsiveness and parental demanding behaviour. Parental responsiveness refers to the extent parents are warm, responsive, supportive, and sensitive to children's personal requirements for fostering individuality, self-regulation, and self-assertion of their child (Baumrind, 1971). Parental demanding behaviour or parental control refers to the firm demands, discipline and supervision entailed by parents for becoming integrated into the family, and willingness to accost the child who defies (Baumrind, 1991). Perception of social support is defined as the phenomena when an individual perceives that his or her social network is ready to provide aid and assistance if needed (Wethington & Kessler, 1986), which influences their appraisal of and response to the stressful situation. People with high perceived support believe that they can count on their family and friends to offer quality assistance during times of stress and has been associated with both physical and mental health outcomes (Wilks, 2008). Social anxiety as a state of emotional distress and avoiding behaviour in real or imagined social interactions has infrequently been a subject of research during adolescence. Relationships with peers become increasingly important during adolescence. At the same time, self-consciousness develops among adolescents due to their self-awareness, which stirs them up. Not coincidentally, this is the stage at which *excessive* social anxiety typically starts developing. They are preoccupied by persistent doubts and worries, and their excruciating distress may lead them to start avoiding any situation that might provoke it. Eventually, this avoidance begins to interfere with their ability to function at home or school (Foa & Andrews, 2006). Indeed, adolescents could have difficulties to cope this period which is characterized by a stressful shift, including behavioural, cognitive, environmental and social challenges (Collins, 2001). Psychological health is a major element contributing to the overall well-being of an adolescent and multiple factors influence that at any one time. Factors that may contribute to stress during adolescence include a desire for greater autonomy, the pressure to conform to peers, quality of their home life and their relationships with their peers and gender norms. Withdrawal or avoidance of family, peers or the community can exacerbate isolation and loneliness, perpetuating emotional problems, excessive irritability or frustration in addition to depression or anxiety (World Health Organization, 2018).

Keeping in view the foregoing discussions, the aim of the present study is to investigate in a non-clinical sample, whether there exists a significant difference among the two groups, namely, morbid and non-morbid groups and boys and girls with respect to styles of parenting, perceived social support and social anxiety; and to determine the relative contributions of styles of parenting and perceived social support in predicting social anxiety.

Material and Method

For the purpose of the study, the sample consisted of 200 adolescents aged between 12 and 17 years. The General Health Questionnaire-12 (GHQ-12) is a screening tool that has been used in the present study and the non-morbid group and the morbid group have been defined on the basis of the scores obtained in the tool. Non-morbid group comprised of individuals who scored 12 and below (here, considered as absence of psychological morbidity) and morbid group comprised of individuals who scored above 12 (here, considered as presence of psychological morbidity) in GHQ-12. Both groups consisted of 50 boys and 50 girls each on the basis of their scores in GHQ-12.

At first, the participants were approached in schools with the assistance of school authorities and they were explained about the purpose of the present study. This was followed by obtaining consent from parents of all the participants to be included in the study. The participants were assured complete confidentiality regarding the data obtained from them. The questionnaires were filled in the presence of the assessor so that any clarification could be done immediately and that no item was omitted or left incomplete. The administration of the questionnaires followed a pre-determined sequence as: Information Schedule, General Health Questionnaire-12 (GHQ-12), Scale of Parenting Style, Multidimensional Scale of Perceived Social Support (MSPSS) and Liebowitz Social Anxiety Scale for Children and Adolescents-Self Report (LSAS-CA-SR).

The information schedule was used for collecting socio-demographic information such as name, age, gender, nationality and education, information about whether parents are living or deceased, marital status of parents, monthly family income, information about any history of major physical or psychiatric illness in the family or in the individual.

General Health Questionnaire-12 (GHQ-12) (Goldberg, 1972) is a brief, self-administered screening test designed to detect current mental disturbances and disorders. The GHQ-12 comprises 12 items describing mood states, six of which are positively phrased and six negatively phrased. Each item of the GHQ-12 has four possible response options. For the assessment of psychological distress, Likert Scoring System (0-1-2-3) was used, with a score range of 0–36 (Goldberg, *et al.,* 1997). The cut-off point for psychological morbidity was considered 12, that is, scores upto 12 were considered normal and a score more than 12 was considered as an evidence of psychological distress.

Scale of Parenting Style (Gafoor & Kurukkan, 2014) measures perceived parenting styles of adolescents. Items measure the responsiveness and control of parents as perceived by their adolescent wards. The participants are required to respond on the five-point scale ranging from 1 (Very wrong) to 5 (Very right). There are no negative items. Half of the items in scale are responsiveness items and half of them are control items. The total score of control and total score of responsiveness were found out by the sum of scores of each parent, taken for overall score of an item.

The Multidimensional Scale of Perceived Social Support (MSPSS)

(Zimet, Dahlem, Zimet & Farley, 1988) is a self-administered test. It is a 12-item scale that is specifically designed to assess perceptions of social support adequacy from three specific sources which form three separate subscales: Significant Other, Family and Friends. The items are rated ranging from 1 (Very Strongly Disagree) to 7 (Very Strongly Agree). The scale consists of a total score and three subscale scores.

The Liebowitz Social Anxiety Scale for Children and Adolescents-Self Report (LSAS-CA-SR) (Masia-Warner, Storch, Pincus, Klein, Heimberg & Liebowitz, 2003) assesses both fear and avoidance across a number of social situations. It contains 24 items: 12 items are social interaction situations, and the other 12 are performance situations. Each item assesses the fear level and the avoidance level on a Likert type scale: ratings of anxiety (0 = none; 1 = mild; 2 = moderate; 3 = severe) and avoidance (0 = never; 1 = occasionally; 2 = often; 3 = usually). It provides scores of total anxiety, total avoidance and a total score of social anxiety.

Following data collection, responses were scored according to the standard procedures given in the manuals and appropriate statistical treatment was used upon the obtained scores. Statistical analysis was done by computing the means, standard deviations (SD) and Pearson's product moment correlation for the scores. Following this, obtained data was analyzed by means of independent samples t-test and Two-Way Analysis of Variance (2×2 ANOVA). Finally, to find out the relative contributing variables for social anxiety multiple regression analysis was done. For analysis, 0.05 and 0.01 levels of significance were accepted.

Results

The mean age of the sample was 15 (SD-1.59) years, for boys was 14.97 (SD-1.48) years, for girls was 15 (SD-1.7) years, for non-morbid group was 14.82 (SD-1.62) years and for morbid group was 15.18 (SD-1.54) years.

Table 13.1 shows the means and standard deviations (SD) of the non-morbid and morbid subgroup among boys and girls respectively. The significance of differences between the mean scores with respect to each of the dimensions considered in the study were tested with the help of independent samples t-test are also tabulated. Table 13.1 shows that among boys, there was a significant difference of mean scores on Parental Responsiveness ($t_{(98)} = 2.517$, $P < 0.05$), Family subscale ($t_{(98)} = 2.859$, $P < 0.01$), Total Anxiety ($t_{(98)} = -4.368$, $P < 0.01$), Total Avoidance ($t_{(98)} = -3.451$, $P < 0.01$) and Total score of Social Anxiety ($t_{(98)} = -4.528$, $P < 0.01$) between the non-morbid group and the morbid group.

Among girls, there was a significant difference of mean scores on Parental Responsiveness ($t_{(98)}$ = 2.167, P<0.05), Family subscale ($t_{(98)}$ =

Table 13.1: Comparison between the male and female group with respect to the level of morbidity (Non-morbid and Morbid) for Styles of Parenting, Perceived Social Support and its three sub-scales, and Social Anxiety and its two sub-scales

Groups Dimensions	*Boys*			*Girls*		
	Non-Morbid (N = 50)	*Morbid (N = 50)*	*$t_{(98)}$*	*Non-Morbid (N = 50)*	*Morbid (N = 50)*	*$t_{(98)}$*
	Mean (SD)	*Mean (SD)*		*Mean (SD)*	*Mean (SD)*	
Styles of Parenting						
Parental Responsiveness	155.42 (17.27)	146.12 (19.61)	2.517*	151.20 (18.10)	142.04 (23.78)	2.167*
Parental Control	155.56 (21.02)	152.56 (17.72)	.772	151.14 (19.72)	142.40 (25.98)	1.895
Perceived Social Support						
Significant Other	5.52 (1.42)	5.36 (1.36)	.558	5.25 (1.59)	5.20 (1.43)	.165
Family	6.27 (0.97)	5.68 (1.11)	2.859**	5.54 (1.30)	4.70 (1.44)	3.061**
Friends	5.48 (1.38)	5.26 (1.25)	.799	5.66 (1.17)	5.22 (1.58)	1.600
Total Perceived Social Support Index	5.76 (0.93)	5.43 (0.95)	1.706	5.48 (1.09)	5.04 (1.00)	2.123*
Social Anxiety						
Total Anxiety	10.74 (7.93)	19.84 (12.42)	-4.368**	15.48 (9.84)	26.48 (12.11)	-4.984**
Total Avoidance	15.46 (10.51)	22.66 (10.35)	-3.451**	17.32 (11.55)	27.74 (11.18)	-4.583**
Total Score of Social Anxiety	26.20 (16.17)	42.50 (19.66)	-4.528**	32.80 (19.49)	54.22 (21.58)	-5.208**

*P < 0.05, **P < 0.01. N = number of individuals; $t_{(98)}$ = t statistic at 98 degrees of freedom.

3.061, P < 0.01) and the total perceived social support index ($t_{(98)}$ = 2.123, P < 0.05), Total Anxiety ($t_{(98)}$ = –4.984, P < 0.01), Total Avoidance ($t_{(98)}$ = –4.583, P < 0.01) and Total score of Social Anxiety ($t_{(98)}$ = –5.208, P < 0.01) between the non-morbid group and the morbid group.

Table 13.2 shows that there was a significant main effect of morbidity on Parental Responsiveness ($F_{(1,196)} = 10.811, P < 0.01$), Total Perceived Social Support Index ($F_{(1,196)} = 7.400, P < 0.01$) and Family subscale ($F_{(1,196)} = 17.357, P < 0.01$), and in Total Anxiety ($F_{(1,196)} = 43.865, P < 0.01$), Total Avoidance ($F_{(1,196)} = 32.609, P < 0.01$) and Total Score of Social Anxiety ($F_{(1,196)} = 47.623, P < 0.01$). There was a significant main effect of gender on Parental Control ($F_{(1,196)} = 5.841, P < 0.05$), Total Perceived Social Support Index ($F_{(1,196)} = 5.761, P < 0.05$) and Family subscale ($F_{(1,196)} = 24.791, P < 0.01$), and Total Anxiety ($F_{(1,196)} = 14.061, P < 0.01$), Total Avoidance ($F_{(1,196)} = 5.059, P < 0.05$) and Total Score of Social Anxiety ($F_{(1,196)} = 11.234, P < 0.01$). There was no interaction effect between morbidity and gender in neither of the dimensions.

Table 13.2: Means (M), Standard Deviations (SD) and F ratios (at df = 1,196) for the main effects of morbidity and gender and their interaction effects on Styles of Parenting, Perceived Social Support and its three subscales, Social Anxiety and its two sub-scales

GROUPS DIMENSIONS	Morbidity		Gender		Main effects (F values)		Interaction effect (F values)
	Non-Morbid	Morbid	Male	Female	Morbidity	Gender	Morbidity* Gender
	M (SD)	M (SD)	M (SD)	M (SD)			
Styles of Parenting							
Parental Responsiveness	153.31 (17.73)	144.08 (21.78)	150.77 (18.97)	146.62 (21.52)	10.811**	2.186	.001
Parental Control	153.35 (20.40)	147.48 (22.71)	154.06 (19.40)	146.77 (23.37)	3.787	5.841*	.905
Perceived Social Support							
Significant Other	5.38 (1.51)	5.28 (1.39)	5.44 (1.38)	5.22 (1.51)	.249	1.174	.065
Family	5.90 (1.20)	5.19 (1.37)	5.97 (1.08)	5.11 (1.43)	17.357**	24.791**	.506
Friends	5.57 (1.27)	5.24 (1.42)	5.37 (1.31)	5.43 (1.40)	2.929	.124	.377
Total Perceived Social Support Index	5.62 (1.02)	5.23 (0.99)	5.60 (0.95)	5.26 (1.07)	7.400**	5.761*	.198
Social Anxiety							
Total Anxiety	13.11 (9.20)	23.16 (12.65)	15.29 (11.33)	20.98 (12.29)	43.865**	14.061**	.532
Total Avoidance	16.39 (11.03)	25.20 (11.02)	19.06 (10.99)	22.53 (12.46)	32.609**	5.059*	.298
Total Score of Social Anxiety	29.50 (18.12)	48.36 (21.37)	34.35 (19.69)	43.51 (23.12)	47.623**	11.234**	.350

*P < 0.05, **P < 0.01.

Table 13.3: Pearson's Product Moment Correlation (r) between Social Anxiety and its two sub-scales, and the two Styles of Parenting and Perceived social support and its three subscales

Dimensions	*Styles of Parenting*		*Perceived Social Support*			
Social anxiety	Parental responsiveness	Parental control	Significant other	Family	Friends	Total perceived social support index
Total Anxiety	–.065	–.082	–.136	–.234**	–.096	–.208**
Total Avoidance	–.081	–.100	–.119	–.205**	–.203**	–.236**
Total Score of Social Anxiety	–.080	–.100	–.139*	–.240**	–.163*	–.243**

*P < 0.05, **P < 0.01.

Table 13.3 shows that there was a significant negative correlation between the sub-scale of total anxiety and the subscale of family and total perceived social support index. Significant negative correlation was found between the sub-scale of total avoidance and the sub-scales of family and friends, and total perceived social support index. There was a significant negative correlation between the total score of social anxiety and the sub-scales of significant other, family and friends, and total perceived social support index.

Table 13.4: Linear Regression Analysis showing Criterion Variable and Predictor Variables in the Sample

Criterion	F ratios	R^2	Predictors	β	T values
Total Anxiety	$F_{(2, 197)}$ = 6.042**	.058	Family	–.174	–1.737
			Total Perceived Social Support Index	–.082	–.818
Total Avoidance	$F_{(3, 196)}$ = 4.592**	.066	Family	–.149	–1.274
			Friends	–.146	–1.260
			Total Perceived Social Support Index	–.023	–.141
Total score of Social Anxiety	$F_{(3, 196)}$ = 4.850**	.069	Family	–.168	–1.441
			Friends	–.062	–.537
			Total Perceived Social support Index	–.076	–.473

**P < 0.01.

Table 13.4 shows the values of multiple regression analysis for the respective dimensions. Overall perceived social support with support from both family and friends were found to be predictors of social anxiety and its two sub-scales of total anxiety and total avoidance.

Discussion

Differences in the Psychological Profiles of Non-Morbid and Morbid Groups

Parental responsiveness, parental control, and perceived social support from family, friends and significant other were higher within the non-morbid group than in the morbid group and the non-morbid group had lower social anxiety scores compared to the morbid group. Hence, this suggests that parenting behaviours characterized by warmth, responsiveness, autonomy granting, and firmness are considered important contributors to healthy development with a positive impact on mental health in adolescents (Steinberg, 2001). The quality of family relationships is additionally a crucial protective factor influencing an individual's social and emotional well-being (Rees, Bradshaw, Goswami & Keung, 2010); and perceived social support from family is negatively related to behavioural problems that makes a major contribution to the adolescents' perceived social support levels and accepted as moderate to strongly related to many personal, health, and social indicators adolescents (Ikiz & Savi Çakar, 2012). When parental support is higher, generally measured as support from family at times, it has consistently been associated with less general psychological distress and emotional problems (Demaray, *et al.*, 2005). Moreover, compared to those having weak social support systems and lower global functioning, the symptoms of anxiety and behavioural problems are less in adolescents whose level of social support are high in view of the stressful life events—thus supporting the buffer theory (Rockhill, Stoep, McCauley & Katon, 2008). A study (Rubin & Burgess, 2001) found that limited social relationships are a causal factor of social anxiety among individuals, as the individual with social anxiety experiences physiological and psychological discomfort due to limited social network leading to maladjustment in social situations. In general, the adolescents' close friendships and the qualities associated with it (i.e., intimacy, support) have been associated with lower levels of social anxiety (La Greca & Lopez, 1998), suggesting that friendships may serve a protective mental health function and promote psychological well-being, as has been found in the present study. However, the actual behaviour of peers should also be considered. The effect of being negatively treated and being rejected by peers (Verduin & Kendall, 2008) should not be underestimated. Adolescents who are socially anxious develop a lack of social skills and hence when they are rejected by peers they will presumably react with further avoidance of social situations.

Adolescents with social anxiety often overlook positive feedback from highly valued peers that could have affected them positively (Jarcho, *et al.,* 2015). This successively will decrease their opportunity to improve their social skills resulting in a vicious cycle of social anxiety, poor social skills and peer rejection. The conditioning theory (Mowrer, 1939, 1960) might explain the presence of high scores of anxiety and avoidance in the morbid group in the present study. Fear persists because avoidance of the conditioned stimulus (CS) prevents the extinction that normally occurs through repeated non-reinforced exposures. From a cognitive perspective, avoidance behaviour prevents the gathering of information that disconfirms catastrophic misappraisals and over-prediction of fear, motivating avoidance behaviour that prevents dis-confirmation opportunities, and consequently such appraisal and their resultant fear and anxiety are maintained (Clark, 1988; Rachman, 1994). Hence it explains the prevalence of higher avoidance score in the morbid group when compared to non-morbid group, with an adolescent in the morbid group avoiding anxiety-provoking situations more.

Differences in the Psychosocial Profiles among Boys and Girls

Parental responsiveness and parental control, and overall perceived social support from family are greater in the boys than in the girls. From the early years, girls and boys may be educated with different gender roles. It is also probable that the social behaviour of females is more strictly controlled by parents and society than in the male's case, tolerating fewer mistakes and explaining their higher anxiety score on the subscales (Caballo, 2014). Hence these explanations support the finding in the present study where girls have scored higher anxiety and avoidance scores. Consistent with gender schema theories (Bem, 1981) parents' gender-differentiated use of controlling and autonomy-supportive strategies is perhaps influenced by parents' gender-role stereotypes (such as more harsh discipline of boys than girls, more gentle control and guidance of girls than of boys). When parents develop non-stereotypical ideas about the gender roles, they might practice gender-differentiated parenting more often that reinforces behaviour that is inconsistent with gender roles (e.g., more gentle control and guidance of boys than of girls, more harsh or physical control of girls than of boys). Additionally, the total score of Social Anxiety is greater among girls than in boys. However, the girls witnessed greater support from their friends than the boys. Social support might be more important to girls because stressors having interpersonal significance are stronger predictors of negative psychological outcomes in girls relative to boys, hence adolescent girls typically report more intimacy and support in their friendships than boys (Urberg, 1995; Rose & Rudolph, 2006) and when these needs are thwarted adolescent girls are more likely to report more symptoms of social anxiety than adolescent boys (La Greca & Lopez, 1998). Hence, problems in close friendships may be more strongly linked to feelings of social anxiety for girls than for boys. Additionally, feelings of social anxiety-particularly generalized social avoidance and distress may lead to disengagement from peer interactions (La Greca & Lopez, 1998), and interfere with the development of close and supportive ties. Generally, girls are more emotional as compared to boys; thus, they might be able to communicate more openly with friends. By doing so, the girls perceive having someone to talk to as having adequate social support. On the other hand, boys are expected to adhere to certain social gender role expectations that have been set and that if they were to share their feelings, it would be considered as their vulnerability. Hence, boys tend to perceive lower social support from friends because they are more likely to feel that they have no one to express their feelings. In case of the present study, however, boys experience more social support from their family which might be explained by the cultural differences in socialization practices of the family. Moreover, this finding can be corroborated by a study (Walen & Lachman, 2000) which found that family support was predictive of well-being measures and supportive networks were found to buffer the detrimental effects of stressful interactions.

There was no significant interaction effect between morbidity and gender concerning the variables considered in the present study which can be explained by the fact that inadequate parenting styles and lack of perceived support from the social circle are equally distressful to any adolescent irrespective of gender which further exacerbates their anxiety and avoidance in social contexts when they have underlying psychological morbidity. Moreover, despite styles of parenting and perceived social support having a significant correlation with anxiety and avoidance, neither single sub-domain from any of the variables were predictors of anxiety and avoidance among adolescents because there are additional factors such as life experiences, conditioning, trauma, biological determinants and/or other psychological factors which add to the risks of developing social anxiety; and neither responsiveness nor control under parenting styles nor perceived social support from family nor friends in isolation leads to the development anxiety and avoidance among adolescents.

A limitation of this study is that since data were collected from a specific geographical area, the sample could have been more representative of the population and generalizability of the findings could have been increased by taking a larger sample size. Predictive statistical analysis could have been done for the groups—non-morbid and morbid groups, and boys and girls and a more detailed analysis of the sample could have been observed. Additionally, if the contributions of life experiences, trauma, coping strategies, parental psychopathology, or stressful home environment could have been specifically measured, then the study would have been qualitatively enriched because several factors interact for the development of social anxiety as a disorder. Nevertheless, the findings of the present study will help to design various management programmes where adolescents in the non-clinical population can be screened for any manifestation and trained to deal with their crises and prevent the development of social anxiety.

Conclusion

Since adolescence is a period when they undergo significant internal turbulence with regard to issues of identity and other challenges pertaining to transition to adulthood, it's imperative for those around these adolescents to be more tolerant and patient in understanding the reasons of their behaviour in order to reduce the interpersonal conflict, and the resultant anxiety. Presence of psychological morbidity is associated with a low perception of support and warmth from parents and family and with development of social anxiety. Thus, the value of familial as well as extra-familial relationships in serving as buffer against the socially anxious adolescents is highlighted in the present study.

References

Baumrind, D. (1971). "Current patterns of parental authority", *Developmental Psychology Monograph*, *4* (1, Pt. 2), 1-103.

Baumrind, D. (1991). "The influence of parenting style on adolescent competence and substance use", *Journal of Early Adolescence*, *11*, 56-95.

Bem, S.L. (1981). "Gender schema theory: A cognitive account of sex typing", *Psychological Review*, *88*(4), 354–364.

Caballo, V.E., Salazar, I.C., Irurtia, M.J., Arias, B., Hofmann, S.G., and CISO-A Research Team (2014). "Differences in social anxiety between men and women across 18 countries", *Personality and Individual Differences*, *64*, 35–40.

Clark, D.M. (1988). "A cognitive model of panic attacks", In: Rachman, S., Maser, J.D., Rachman, S., Maser, J.D. (Eds.), *Panic: Psychological Perspectives,* pp. 71-89. Hillsdale, NJ, US: Lawrence Erlbaum Associates Inc.

Collins, M.E. (2001). "Transition to adulthood for vulnerable youths: A review of research and implications for policy", *75*(2), 271–291.

Colman, A.M. (2015). *Oxford Dictionary of Psychology* (4th ed.). New York, NY: Oxford University Press.

Demaray, M.K., Malecki, C.K., Davidson, L.M., Hodgson, K.K., and Rebus, P.J. (2005). "The relationship between social support and student adjustment: A longitudinal analysis", *Psychology in the Schools, 42*(7), 691–706.

Foa, E.B., and Andrews, L.W. (2006). *If Your Adolescent has an Anxiety Disorder: An Essential Resource for Parents*, New York, NY: Oxford University Press.

Gaertner, A.E., Fite, P.J., and Colder, C.R. (2010). "Parenting and friendship quality as predictors of internalizing and externalizing symptoms in early adolescence", *Journal of Child Family Studies, 19*, 101–108.

Gafoor, A.K., and Kurukkan, A. (2014). "Construction and Validation of Scale of Parenting Style", *Guru Journal of Behavioural and Social Sciences, 2*(4), 315-323.

Goldberg, D. (1972). "The detection of psychiatric illness by questionnaire: A technique for the identification and assessment of non-psychotic psychiatric illness", London, New York: Oxford University Press.

Goldberg, D.P., Gater, R., Sartorius, N., Ustun, T.B., Piccinelli, M., Gureje, O., and Rutter, C. (1997). "The validity of two versions of the GHQ in the WHO study of mental illness in general health care", *Psychological Medicine, 27*(1), 191–197.

Ikiz, F.E., and Savi Çakar, F. (2012). "Behaviour problems in relation with perceived social support", In: L. Barış, and Ö. Uzun (Eds.), *Psychology of Adolescence* (pp. 1-48). New York: Nova Science Publisher. Inc.

La Greca, A.M., and Lopez, N. (1998). "Social anxiety among adolescents: Linkages with peer relations and friendships", *Journal of Abnormal Child Psychology, 26*, 83–94.

Maccoby, E.E., and Martin, J.A. (1983). "Socialization in the context of the family: Parent-child interaction", In: P. Mussen and E.M. Hetherington, (Eds.) *Handbook of Child Psychology, Volume IV: Socialization, Personality, and Social Development,* pp. 1-102. New York: Wiley.

Masia-Warner, C., Storch, E., Pincus, D., Klein, R., Heimberg R.G., and Liebowitz, M.R. (2003). "The Liebowitz Social Anxiety Scale for Children and Adolescents: An initial psychometric investigation", *Journal of the American Academic of Child and Adolescent Psychiatry, 42*, 1076-1108.

Mowrer, O.H. (1939). "A stimulus-response analysis of anxiety and its role as a reinforcing agent", *Psychological Review, 46*(6), 553–565.

Mowrer, O H. (1960). 'Sin': The lesser of two evils", *American Psychologist, 15*(5), 301–304.

Rachman, S.J. (1994). "The over-prediction of fear: A review", *Behaviour Research and Therapy, 32*(7), 683–690.

Rees, G., Bradshaw, J., Goswami, H., and Keung, A. (2010). *Understanding Children's Wellbeing: A National Survey of Young People's Well-Being*, London: The Children's Society.

Rockhill, C.M., Stoep, A.V., McCauley, E., and Katon, W.J. (2008). "Social competence and social support as mediators between comorbid depressive and conduct problems and functional outcomes in middle school children", *Journal of Adolescence*, *32*(3), 535–553.

Rose, A.J., and Rudolph, K.D. (2006). "A review of sex differences in peer relationship processes: Potential trade-offs for the emotional and behavioural development of girls and boys", *Psychological Bulletin*, *132*, 98–131.

Rubin, K.H., and Burgess, K.B. (2001). "Social withdrawal and anxiety", In: M.W. Vasey and M.R. Dadds (Eds.), *The developmental psychopathology of Anxiety* (pp. 407–434). New York: Oxford University Press.

Steinberg, L. (2001). "We know some things: Adolescent-parent relationships in retrospect and prospect", *Journal of Research on Adolescence*, *11*(1), 1–19.

Urberg, K.A., Degirmencioglu, S.M., Tolson, J.M., and Halliday-Scher, K. (1995). "The structure of adolescent peer networks", *Developmental Psychology*, *31*, 540–547.

Verduin, T.L., and Kendall, P.C. (2008). "Peer perceptions and liking of children with anxiety disorders", *Journal of Abnormal Child Psychology*, *36*, 459–469.

Walen, H.R., and Lachman, M.E. (2000). "Social support and strain from partner, family, and friends: Costs and benefits for men and women in adulthood", *Journal of Social and Personal Relationships*, *17*, 5-3.

Wethington, E., and Kessler, R.C. (1986). "Perceived Support, Received Support and Adjustment to Stressful Life Events", *Journal of Health and Social Behaviour*, *27*(1), 78-89.

Wilks, S.E. (2008). "Resilience amid Academic Stress: The Moderating Impact of Social Support among Social Work Students", *Advances in Social Work*, *9*(2), 106-125.

World Health Organisation (WHO) (2018); Adolescent mental health. Retrieved from https://www.who.int/news-room/fact-sheets/detail/adolescent-mental-health

Zimet, G.D., Dahlem, N.W., Zimet, S.G., and Farley, G.K. (1988). "The Multidimensional Scale of Perceived Social Support", *Journal of Personality Assessment*, *52*, 30-41.

14

COVID-19 and Mental Health of Children and Adolescents

Challenges and Coping Strategies

Manish Kumar Jaisawal, Rajbala Kumari and *Dhananjay Kumar*

Introduction

COVID-19 is a highly infectious disease with no proper treatment so far. The cases of corona virus infection first came in China and gradually it became a global disease. Patients of this disease (COVID-19) continue to rapidly increase day by day. So far millions of people have been affected by Corona and thousands of lives have been lost. Corona has shaken the economy of the whole world. This devastating and prevalent virus has caused damage all over the world. World Health Organization has declared it a pandemic. Along with all these, the one thing that makes this situation even more worse is that, so far no medicine has been found for the treatment of COVID-19.

People all around the world are struggling to fight and cope with Corona virus. There is an uncertainty about life and future (Guo *et al.*, 2020). In absence of any treatment, as an effort to control the surge of this disease, social restrictions have been enforced. It lead billions of people globally, to remain locked in their homes. It means in a way people are lacking their social support and connection (Cao, Fang, Hou, Han, Xu, Dang, & Zheng, 2020). Many people may be very worried and scared, confused, distraught or upset with the current situation. Physiological symptoms are very apparent and getting enough attention. But in this whole chaos, sometimes the psychological health is being left behind or somehow neglected (Huang & Zhao, 2020; Rajkumar, 2020). Symptoms like depression and anxiety often go unnoticed, but it should not be accounted for less (Wang *et al.*, 2020). In a study Wang *et al.* (2020) reported that approximately 16-28 per cent of the participants experienced anxiety and depressive symptoms, while eight per cent reported moderate to severe stress due to COVID-19. All the age group is deeply affected by this abrupt change due to corona but, children and adolescents are the age group who needs special care and consideration (WHO, 2020). Children and adolescents are that age group who are considered as highly vulnerable for COVID-19 and are taken care for their physiological symptoms (Dong, Mo, Hu, Qi, Jiang, Jiang, 2020). Perhaps a more important but easily neglected issue is the psychological impact on children and adolescents (Dalton, Rapa, & Stein, 2020). Mental health care is very important because it is deeply rooted in this phase of life, making it essential that mental health needs are identified early and treated during this sensitive time in child development (Golberstein, Wen, & Miller, 2020). The pain, wounds and traumatic experiences of corona can affect children's mental health to a great extent, especially children who come from lower unprivileged society (Mukherjee, Bandopadhyay, & Chatterjee, 2020). This problem associated with COVID-19 is an unprecedented problem for us. The sudden emergence of this virus has forced us to change many aspects of how we live our lives.

The lock-down may have changed people's habits but a large section is living in the midst of stress. This stress is about illness and future anxiety (Wang, Zhang, Zhao, Zhang, & Jiang, 2020). Children whose caregivers are infected with COVID-19 or who have died from the disease might be more susceptible to mental health problems because of their higher risk of infection, and the grief and fear caused by parental loss or separation. Stressors such as prolonged school closure, fears of infection and death, frustration and boredom, inadequate information, lack of in-person contact with classmates, friends, and teachers, lack of personal space at home, and family financial loss can have even more problematic and enduring effects on children and adolescents (Wang, Zhang, Zhao, Zhang, & Jiang, 2020). Mental health is an issue, if not given proper intervention can lead to many negative health and social outcomes in adulthood. Hence, it is crucial to pay fine attention on the psychological challenges faced by children in this pandemic situation and empower them to effectively cope with it. Medical Association is working tirelessly to deal with the spread of this virus. And in ensuring medical care to those infected with COVID-19 who has physical symptoms are employed. But at this time it is also important that mental health of the people should also be given priority. The issue of mental health due to corona virus has also emerged in the country rapidly. As it is very well known that psychological health of a person is connected to the various aspects of his/her life (Luo & Wang,

2009; Meng *et al.*, 2011; Low *et al.*, 2012), the researchers feel the need to understand the different challenges of children's life in this scenario to get a better picture of their mental health. In this review paper authors will discuss the challenges faced by the children during this pandemic with a special focus on the psychological health. Also, rather than just focusing on the challenges this review provides insights on some possible interventions to effectively cope and overcome this situation.

Childhood and Mental Health

Childhood is a formative period of an individual's life. Childhood memories, traumas, anxieties etc. remains in a person's mind throughout his/her life (Venter, Demyttenaere, & Bruffaerts, 2013). Studies have found a significant impact of childhood mental health on the overall functioning in later life (John, Leon, & McCulloch, 2005). Hence, it is very important to take good care of this foundation phase. In this crisis situation the focus should be given to the identification of vulnerabilities among children and to protect them from adversities.

Physical Challenges

Physical challenges of COVID-19 are something that is very apparent. COVID-19 has very high spread rate, absence of medicine for it make it very fatal in nature (Kar *et al.*, 2020; Fegert *et al.*, 2020). Only way to control the disease is massive lock-down and social distancing. That causes people to have very limited amount of interaction with others and prohibited to go outside from the home. Evidence suggest that now that children are out of school since march, they are physically less active, have much longer screen time, irregular sleep patterns, and less favourable eating habits (Fegert *et al.*, 2020). Children are in the phase of early physical development and they need healthy and proper diet and life style. However, fewer workouts can cause the problem of obesity, cardio-respiratory disease, and early age diabetes in them (Fegert *et al.*, 2020). Additionally, expanded use of mobiles and laptops can harm their eyesights and cause nausea, dizziness, and headaches as some children are sensitive to flickering lights.

Educational Challenges

COVID-19 has substantially affected the educational system all around the world. Among the various actions taken to endorse social distancing, many schools have been closed and online classes are started on home-based distance-learning models. School closures is an important step to control the outbreak of COVID-19, however it has substantially disrupted the lives of students and their families (Viner *et al.*, 2020; Lanker & Parolin, 2020). The Ministry of Education estimates that more than 247 million children are confined to their homes; this includes 180 million primary and secondary students and 47 million preschool children.

Schools have been closed since March and there is still no certainty about their reopening. Children are taking these classes via video call on mobile or laptop. Online classes have given children an opportunity to learn and right now it seems the only way to stop wasting precious time of children and to continue their studies. However, it also calls for a lot of effort from governments as most of the countries have unequal educational system which can disproportionately affects the poor and marginalized children (Ahmed, Pissarides, & Stiglitz, 2020). Many children do not have proper equipment such as internet connectivity, mobile phone or laptop at home (Viner *et al.*, 2020). In some cases family members are not supportive to continue the child's education in this crisis situation. Poor families struggle a lot to support their children in education. However, these COVID-19 induced economic crisis, job and income losses are forcing people into a dilemma to choose between education, health care or food. Hence, there is a significant chance of so many children from poor families to stop their education (Ahmed *et al.*, 2020). It means the drop-out rates can be increased. In this situation children can experience various reasons for stress and anxiety like loss of learning, deprivation or lack of opportunities. These conditions are amplified for children who are already vulnerable or unprivileged such as girls, migrant children, or children with disabilities (Lancker & Parolin, 2020; Vieira, Franco, Restrepo, & Abel, 2020).

Apart from these, schools are not just the place to provide education, but an important source of nutritious meals for children especially in developing countries. In this closure situation children are missing out on a main source of their meal (Lancker *et al.*, 2020).

Therefore, we must consider the potential association school closures have with children's well-being and what can be done to mitigate them.

Behavioural Challenges

The abrupt outbreak of COVID-19 has resulted in so many behavioural changes among children and adolescents. Apart from being less physically active due to closure of public places including stadiums, parks, dance classes and playgrounds it has created several other issues. Also, there is a lack of daily routine or schedule because children do not have to go to their schools or outside home. It has severely affected the sleeping patterns and eating habits of children. Apart from these, COVID-19 has abruptly pushed many children's daily lives online.

Irritability: Nowadays, especially teenagers like to spend some time alone in their home as they wish. Some like to play, fight or gossip with their friends. But due to the lock-down, the parents are always in the house. Everything is closed and most of the parents unnecessarily keep an eye on the children and interrupt in everything. This is especially increasing pressure on adolescent boys and girls. As a result, irritability is occurring in them and appearing in the form of needless resentment.

Also, children are facing such a situation for the first time in their life when they are locked in homes for so long. Most of them are unable to adjust with the situation. The ability to mould them according to the situation is not well developed in this early stage of life. By continuously staying in one place, they start feeling suffocated. All these factors combined and create irritability in them.

Longer screen times: COVID-19 has abruptly pushed many children's daily lives online, and they are spending even more hours online than before. Online solutions provide huge opportunities for continuing learning, socializing and playing. Excessive gaming can lead to "gaming disorder" that leads to reduced sleep or day-night reversal, loss of appetite, aggression, headaches, and attention problems. Another thing is that, it has become harder for parents to keep eye on what their child is doing online, which has sometimes risky consequences. It can lead to child access to inappropriate websites showing violence and pornographies. Easy internet access among children can raise the cases of cyber bullying.

***Disrupted sleep-wake and eating* cycles:** Another prevalent issue that is seen during corona infection is a lack of routine in children's life. Due to being in the house round the clock, there has been a lot of upheaval in their routine. On the one hand, where some adolescents are troubled by the problem of not sleeping at night, on the other hand some people get excessive sleep. Both types of problems are harmful to their physical and mental health.

Psychological Challenges

The corona epidemic has also affected people's mental health, in this situation it is not difficult to see the faces with anxiety around; and children are no exception. While keeping them locked at home government is making good efforts to protect them from virus, but in this environment of social distancing and longingness from friends their mental health is being affected.

According to UNICEF, the current corona virus epidemic also causes anxiety, stress and uncertainty among children. Protecting children from corona virus infection is a major concern. This time of lock-down is such that children in this situation need more love and care.

We can classify the psychological challenges faced by children in following ways:

Anxiety: Suspected or diagnosed COVID-19 children have fears about severe infectiousness and malfeasance to severe high levels (Wang *et al.*, 2020). Physical symptoms of COVID-19 such as fever, hypoxia, and cough, as well as adverse effects of prescribed medications (corticosteroids), may lead to greater anxiety and mental distress (Wang *et al.*, 2020). A recent study of 1210 participants from 194 cities in China reported that 53.8 per cent had moderate or severe psychological effects, 36.4 per cent had some type of anxiety and 32.4 per cent had some type of stress (Liu *et al.*, 2020).

Depression: Due to lock-down, children's social relationships are strongly restricted to close family members; contact with peers is severely limited or restricted. This can damage children's privacy, often children share their thoughts with their peers and in this situation children and/or adolescents may feel loneliness that may lead them to depression. Quarantined people typically experience boredom, loneliness, anger, depression, anxiety, denial, hopelessness, insomnia, harmful substance use, suicide, and suicidal feelings (Wang *et al.*, 2020; Dong & Bu, 2020; Li *et al.*, 2020). In the same study Li *et al.* (2020) found 31.3 per cent of 1210 COVID-19 cases had some type of depression.

Self-harm and Suicidality: Several psychosocial and environmental factors of current situation such as prolonged social isolation, feeling of emptiness, and death of family members etc. have promoted self-harm behaviour during this epidemic crisis. There are reports of suicides in India due to extreme fear of being affected by COVID-19 (Goyal *et al.*, 2020).

Post-traumatic Stress Disorder: Many families are facing financial constraints due to lock-down, and their socio-economic status has become very weak. That in turn leads to substance abuse among parents that affects a child's relationship with parents (Fegert *et al.*, 2020). Younger age attachment to parents is considered relevant to psychological development.

Due to COVID-19 separation and/or loss parents that occurred in the early years of childhood may disrupt current attachment processes, which may be associated with adverse mental health outcomes like mood disorder, psychosis, and death from suicide later in adulthood (Fegert *et al.*, 2020). Sprang *et al.* (2013) reported that children who were isolated during the epidemic were more likely to have acute stress disorder, adjustment disorder, and grief. 30 per cent of the children who were isolated met the diagnostic criteria of Post-traumatic stress disorder (Sprang & Silman, 2013). Survivors with COVID-19 are also at significant risk for developing several mental disorders such as depression, anxiety, and PTSD (World Health Organization, 2020).

Obsessive-Compulsive Disorder: The COVID-19 epidemic may increase the risk of pre-existing mental disorders due to fear, anxiety, and even panic situation. Perhaps no groups of individuals with other mental illness are as affected by the worsening outbreak of COVID-19 as those with obsessive-compulsive disorder (OCD). An adolescent with pre-existing OCD may face strong obsessive fears about contamination, and may lead to harmful compulsive behaviour. For these adolescents, corona-virus may be the only thing to think about. In continuation of safety behaviour with repetitive patterns, children may develop obsessive-compulsive disorder (Li *et al.*, 2020).

Intervention Strategies

There are several steps that can be taken to effectively cope with this pandemic situation.

Parental Support and Care

Parents and caregivers are the closest and reliable persons when it comes to the responsibility of a child (Wang *et al.*, 2020; Singh & Singh, 2020). This is even true in the present scenario of COVID-19 and home confinement. They are the best resource for children to ask for any help. Parents are the role models for their children. This implies that parents can help their children to cope up with this hectic situation by maintaining a good physical and psychological health. It is evident that children and adolescents can be fearful and anxious in present situation. However, a calm and attitude of parents provides a sense of control and predictability in children which in turn help to reduce their negative effects (WHO, 2020).

Open communication is another key aspect of parenting during this pandemic (Dalton, Rapa, & Stein, 2020). It becomes particularly crucial when children are away from their friends and have nobody to share their emotions. Good communication with their parents can help them to share their psychological and physical issues. It has a comforting impact on children in prolonged isolation. Parents need to monitor their child's behaviour and performance while respecting his/her identity and needs.

Apart from so many negative impacts home confinement is an opportunity for children and family members to enhance their interaction and relationship. It is a good time to involve children into family activities and strengthen the togetherness of family members.

Besides monitoring child performance and behaviour, parents also need to respect their identity and needs, and they need to help children develop self-discipline skills. Children are constantly exposed to epidemic-related news, so having direct conversations with children about these issues could alleviate their anxiety and avoid panic. Home confinement could offer a good opportunity to enhance the interaction between parents and children, involve children in family activities, and improve their self-sufficiency skills. With the right parenting approaches, family bonds can be strengthened, and child psychological needs met (Cluver *et al.*, 2020).

Physical Activities and Exercises

Home confinement has reduced the physical activity of children and its negative consequences are very well-known. However, to overcome this virus, it is very important to be physically fit (Jiménez-Pavón, Carbonell-Baeza, & Lavie, 2020). For this, stay at home and exercise and keep your immunity strong. WHO has recommended 150 minutes of moderate-intensity or 75 minutes of vigorous-intensity physical activity per week, or a combination of both to maintain good fitness. These commendations can be attained at home, with no extraordinary equipment and even in limited space. This can be in the courtyard, terrace, veranda and balcony of the house. Exercises can include spot running, jumping, stretching, shaking of hands, legs and waist, sit ups and push-ups. While exercising we breathe deeply, it provides the brain more oxygen. It also has a positive effect on your blood pressure, pulse speed, heart rate and other body parts.

Staying locked at home for a long time can be boring, but do something which requires physical activity (i.e. exercises, yoga, dancing, household chores etc.) can be enjoyable and healthy, both physical and mental.

Daily Routine and Schedule

It is very important to have a daily routine. It is not possible for a child to mirror the school curriculum and classes at home, but effort should be given in the direction to keep a daily routine for game, study and sleeping.

Also, long-term distance from books will affect their study habit. It is important for the children up to the early grades to take care of the study habits; so that the tendency of reading is maintained in children. Special attention should be paid to homework by determining the time of reading. Along with this, there is a need to motivate them about the rehearsal of the previous class as well as the upcoming class. For this, the alertness of the parents is necessary. In such a situation, motivating children to follow the rehearsal and homework would be a better medium.

Their routines are changing due to long-term school closures and children staying in their homes. Parents should take care of this and motivate the children for regular reading, along with this they can connect them to study by motivating them for homework and practice. Regular education along with entertainment is quite necessary.

Enhancing control, predictability and moderation at home can be addressed through balancing structure and flexibility in daily routines. Some caregivers have found it difficult to implement a routine while juggling their responsibilities.

Indoor Recreational Activities

Recreational activities can play important role to help children fight with boredom and learn new things. This could be reading a book, painting, dancing or listening to music. It is important to stay connected with close friends and family members by communicating through phone or internet.

Apart from this, children can watch films or television shows. However, it is advised to not watch news related to COVID-19 so many times in a day; as it can create unnecessary anxiety and fear in child. Repeatedly listening to and watching negative news can bring negative thoughts in mind and children can start falling prey to despair and negativity.

During this home confinement, there are a lot of activities to do with the family in which they can be busy and this time will not be too boring for them. Also, children can learn something new through these activities and can develop a skill that was not there before.

Community Health Services

Communities can serve as valuable resources in managing difficulties of this crisis. Family matters. Community members can work together to bridge the needs of children. An increased number of violence against children, adolescents, and women have been reported during this period of lock-down. Community members can help in identifying children and adolescents suffering from abuse and violence and provide them support. A group of trusted individuals can be identified within the community who can keep communication and support children facing situations such as domestic conflicts, tension with parents, and anxiety of becoming infected.

Finally, owing to a shortage of professionals, the establishment of psychological intervention teams in many areas is not feasible. Teams might consist of psychological counsellors, nurses, volunteers, or teachers majoring in psychology and other related fields, with no professional and experienced psychologists and psychiatrists. One individual often has multiple responsibilities, which can reduce the effectiveness of interventions.

Online Mental Health Services

Online counselling process of children can be effective to solve the concerns of a child. Not all children need this online counselling, but when possible, it can help in the short term. Government should start twenty four hours online counselling hotline. Online mental health app can also be helpful and more works should be done in this direction. Children's access to mental health services can be enhanced by joint online systems comprising psychiatrists, psychotherapists, researchers, and community volunteers.

There is already a shortage of professionals working in mental health care. This situation can be resolved by strengthening personnel training, optimising organisational policies, and constantly reviewing experiences in practice.

Policies

The whole world is fighting against this pandemic in every possible way. However, in this process the governments and legislators need to pay keen attention that these policies must take care of the unprivileged and marginalized children. Children from lower socioeconomic background are struggling hard to meet the psychological and educational needs in this crisis situation. There are inequalities and difference of resources. Policies should be made and implemented with such a concern that these gaps and inequalities are not amplified in a long run.

Acceptance-based Strategies

During this scenario there is an environment of substantial and persistent stress and anxiety. These types of situations sometimes require acceptance-based coping strategies. It involves being aware of the present feelings so that one can accept his/her affect, thought and feelings as reasonable and fair. Any anxious and threatening situation can cause a series of unpleasant thoughts and fear in children. Most of the time children and adolescents try to run away from their thoughts; which often lead to more negative consequences. Parents or caregivers should encourage their child to accept their fears and anxieties and not controlling them.

Accepting our emotions helps to inhibit these emotions from taking over. During this pandemic there will be phases when a child can experience overwhelming and intense negative emotions. Trying too hard to get rid of these feelings is sometimes difficult. Parents on the other hand can remind children that human beings are made for resilience, to survive and that happiness comes after every adversity.

Resilience

Resilience can be understood as the ability of a person to withstand adversity (Jackson, Firtko, & Edenborough, 2007). A resilient person can cope with hardship effectively. Resilience can help children manage stress, anxiety and feelings of uncertainty. Resilience skills can be learned and parents/caregivers can help children to develop it. Building a strong family connection, structuring daily routine, proper exercise, diet and rest, positive self-image etc. are considered very helpful for resilience. Finally, encouraging kids to look beyond present i.e. helping them recognise things outside the current adversity and that the future can be good. An optimistic attitude empowers child to see good things and keep going even in the toughest phases of life (APA, 2011).

Conclusion

The outbreak of COVID-19 embodies a vigorous, significant and actual hazard to the health and well-being of children and adolescents. Keen consideration and efforts are essential to tackle these challenges effectively so that any long-term consequences can be avoided. Furthermore, the interaction between lifestyle changes and psychosocial stress caused by home confinement could further aggravate the detrimental effects on child's physical and mental health, which could cause a vicious circle. To mitigate the consequences of home confinement, the government, non-governmental organisations (NGOs), the community, school, and parents need to be aware of the downside of the situation and do more to effectively address these issues immediately.

References

Ahmed, F., Ahmed, N.E., Pissarides, C., and Stiglitz, J. (2020). "Why inequality could spread COVID-19", *The Lancet Public Health*, *5*(5), e240.

American Psychological Association (2011). "Resilience guide for parents and teachers", *No pages. Online: http://www.apa.org/helpcentre/resilience.aspx*.

Cao, W., Fang, Z., Hou, G., Han, M., Xu, X., Dong, J., and Zheng, J. (2020). "The psychological impact of the COVID-19 epidemic on college students in China", *Psychiatry Research*, 112934.

Cluver, L., Lachman, J.M., Sherr, L., Wessels, I., Krug, E., Rakotomalala, S., … and Butchart, A. (2020). *Parenting in a time of COVID-19.*

Dalton, L., Rapa, E., and Stein, A. (2020). "Protecting the psychological health of children through effective communication about COVID-19", *The Lancet Child and Adolescent Health*, *4*(5), 346-347.

De Venter, M., Demyttenaere, K., and Bruffaerts, R. (2013). "The relationship between adverse childhood experiences and mental health in adulthood: A systematic literature review", *Tijdschrift Voor Psychiatrie*, *55*(4), 259-268.

Dong, Y., Mo, X., Hu, Y., Qi, X., Jiang, F., Jiang, Z., and Tong, S. (2020). "Epidemiology of COVID-19 among children in China", *Pediatrics*, *145*(6).

Fegert, J.M., Vitiello, B., Plener, P.L., and Clemens, V. (2020). "Challenges and burden of the Coronavirus 2019 (COVID-19) pandemic for child and adolescent mental health: a narrative review to highlight clinical and research needs in the acute phase and the long return to normality", *Child and Adolescent Psychiatry and Mental Health*, *14*, 1-11.

Golberstein, E., Wen, H., and Miller, B.F. (2020). "Coronavirus disease 2019 (COVID-19) and mental health for children and adolescents", *JAMA Pediatrics*.

Goyal, K., Chauhan, P., Chhikara, K., Gupta, P., and Singh, M.P. (2020). "Fear of COVID 2019: First suicidal case in India!", *Asian Journal of Psychiatry*, *49*, 101989.

Guo, J., Feng, X.L., Wang, X.H., and van IJzendoorn, M.H. (2020). "Coping with

COVID-19: Exposure to COVID-19 and Negative Impact on Livelihood Predict Elevated Mental Health Problems in Chinese Adults", *International Journal of Environmental Research and Public Health*, *17*(11), 3857.

Huang, Y., and Zhao, N. (2020). "Generalized anxiety disorder, depressive symptoms and sleep quality during COVID-19 outbreak in China: A web-based cross-sectional survey", *Psychiatry Research*, 112954.

Inter-Agency Standing Committee. Interim Briefing Note Addressing Mental Health and Psychosocial Aspects of COVID-19 Outbreak (developed by the IASC's Reference Group on Mental Health and Psychosocial Support)| IASC [Internet]. 2020 [cited 2020 Apr 20].

Jiménez-Pavón, D., Carbonell-Baeza, A., and Lavie, C.J. (2020). "Physical exercise as therapy to fight against the mental and physical consequences of COVID-19 quarantine: Special focus in older people", *Progress in Cardiovascular Diseases*.

Kar, S.K., Arafat, S.Y., Kabir, R., Sharma, P., and Saxena, S.K. (2020). "Coping with mental health challenges during COVID-19", In *Coronavirus Disease 2019 (COVID-19)* (pp. 199-213). Springer, Singapore.

Klomek, A.B. (2020). "Suicide prevention during the COVID-19 outbreak", *The Lancet Psychiatry*, *7*(5), 390.

Li, H.O. Y., and Huynh, D. (2020). "Long-term social distancing during COVID-19: A social isolation crisis among seniors?" *CMAJ*, *192*(21), E588-E588.

Low, N.C., Dugas, E., O'Loughlin, E., Rodriguez, D., Contreras, G., Chaiton, M., and O'Loughlin, J. (2012). "Common stressful life events and difficulties are associated with mental health symptoms and substance use in young adolescents", *BMC Psychiatry*, *12*(1), 1-10.

Luo, Y., and Wang, H. (2009). "Correlation research on psychological health impact on nursing students against stress, coping way and social support", *Nurse Education Today, 29*(1), 5-8.

Meng, X.H., Tao, F.B., Wan, Y.H., Yan, H.U., and Wang, R.X. (2011). "Coping as a mechanism linking stressful life events and mental health problems in adolescents", *Biomedical and Environmental Sciences*, *24*(6), 649-655.

Mukherjee, A., Bandopadhyay, G., and Chatterjee, S.S. (2020). "COVID-19 pandemic: Mental health and beyond: The Indian perspective", *Irish Journal of Psychological Medicine*, 1-11.

Patrick, K., Stanbrook, M.B., and Laupacis, A. (2020). "Social distancing to combat COVID-19: We are all on the front line".

Rajkumar, R.P. (2020). "COVID-19 and mental health: A review of the existing literature". *Asian Journal of Psychiatry*, 102066.

Singh, Jaspreet and Singh, Jagandeep. "COVID-19 and Its Impact on Society" (April 3, 2020). *Electronic Research Journal of Social Sciences and Humanities*, Vol. 2: Issue I, 2020. Available at SSRN: https://ssrn.com/abstract = 3567837

Sprang, G., and Silman, M. (2013). "Posttraumatic stress disorder in parents and youth after health-related disasters", *Disaster Medicine and Public Health Preparedness*, *7*(1), 105-110.

St. John, T., Leon, L., and McCulloch, A. (2005). "Lifetime Impacts: Childhood and Adolescent Mental Health-Understanding the Lifetime Impacts." Report of a Seminar Organised by the Office of Health Economics and the Mental Health Foundation, April 2004. Mental Health Foundation.

Van Lancker, W., and Parolin, Z. (2020). "COVID-19, school closures, and child poverty: A social crisis in the making", *The Lancet Public Health*, *5*(5), e243-e244.

Vieira, C.M., Franco, O.H., Restrepo, C.G., and Abel, T. (2020). "COVID-19: The forgotten priorities of the pandemic", *Maturitas*.

Viner, R.M., Russell, S.J., Croker, H., Packer, J., Ward, J., Stansfield, C., ... and Booy, R. (2020). "School closure and management practices during coronavirus outbreaks including COVID-19: A rapid systematic review", *The Lancet Child and Adolescent Health*.

Wang, C., Pan, R., Wan, X., Tan, Y., Xu, L., McIntyre, R.S., ... and Ho, C. (2020). "A longitudinal study on the mental health of general population during the COVID-19 epidemic in China", *Brain, Behaviour, and Immunity*.

Wang, G., Zhang, Y., Zhao, J., Zhang, J., and Jiang, F. (2020). "Mitigate the effects of home confinement on children during the COVID-19 outbreak", *The Lancet*, *395* (10228), 945-947.

WHO (2020). Coronavirus disease (COVID-19) advice for the public.

World Health Organization. (2020). *Mental health and psychosocial considerations during the COVID-19 outbreak, 18 March 2020* (No. WHO/2019-nCoV/MentalHealth/2020.1). World Health Organization.

15

Adolescent Orphans: "A Socially Excluded Group"

Psychological Problems and Challenges

Adil Azeez and *Anubhuti Dubey*

Introduction

Major proportion of the world's population is covered by children and adolescents. In 2019, it was estimated that 26 per cent of the total population of the world is below 15 years of age. And India leads this table with the highest number of the child population in the world. About 41 per cent of the total population of India is under 18 years of age or belongs to children and adolescents group. Adolescence can be defined as a transitional period of development and growth between childhood to adulthood and generally its age range is considered between 13-19 years. The WHO defines adolescent as "any individual as adolescence who ages between 10-19 years of age". Adolescent term is taken from the Latin word "Adolescere" which means to grow up. In its simplest form it is a period between children to adulthood.

The term adult is conceptualized differently in different societies and cultures; right to vote, minimum marriage age are some common criteria for conceptualizing adults or who has completed adolescence. In India, most community define adult to those, who start earning of its own. But biologically and theoretically, adolescence is the age between 13-19 years, the age group we known as "teen age". It can be sub-divided into three parts: (i) Early adolescents, (ii) Middle adolescents, (iii) Late adolescents.

This is stressful period for adolescents because many biological changes occur during this period like growth spurt, development of primary sex organs, maturity of other sex characteristic, maturity in reproduction etc. These biological changes occurred due to hormonal changes that lead naturally towards anxiety and stress. Adolescents also encountered many psychological problems during this period like identity confusion, undeveloped self-esteem, search of autonomy; unstable relationships, mood swings, risk taking behaviour and aggression are the common reported problems of adolescents.

Adolescent period is also crucial for the healthy development of cognitive processing. Piaget (1983) stated in his theory of cognitive development, that "Formal Operational stage" is the final stage of cognitive development is in which abstract and hypothetical thinking develops and this stage is from 12 years of age to adulthood which we normally known as adolescence period.

Vygotsky (1987) also stated in his theory of socio-cultural theory of cognitive development about the importance of childhood and adolescence. According to Vygotsky, for the healthy cognitive development, social and cultural interaction is necessary for the child and he also emphasized about the role of highly skilled persons who can support child to resolve the daily life's obstacles.

This stage is also very important for the development of personality. Erickson (1997) in his theory of psychosocial stages of development defines this stage as a period between 13-20 year of age, in which major problem faces by the adolescents are "identity vs. role confusion" in which adolescents search for their identity, their role in the society and their usefulness for the society. If adolescents resolve this confusion then they can enter healthily in the next stage of development, i.e. adulthood.

Sometimes because of some unusual consequences they are deprived and excluded from the main stream society and this can be done directly or indirectly. Because they have not developed enough coping and reasoning abilities and they are still not in autonomy, they are forced to face its impact in its full strength. In simple words, social exclusion disturbs the psychological, social and often biological development of adolescents.

Social Exclusion

The term 'Social exclusion' was first used in France and related to social disadvantage. It is a social phenomenon is which majority group removes minority group from mainstream because of either they are of no use or because of the problems, threats, disease, and stigma etc. from them to the society. Social exclusion is also known as 'Marginalization'. This is the process in which not only dominant put the weaker out of periphery but also abundant them from getting their basic and fundamental essentials and block them from participating and contributing in the society. According to Saksena (2014), marginalization can be done on the basis of religion, disease, race, ethnicity, culture, gender etc. According to WHO (2015) social exclusion is a multidimensional process in which unequal power relationship interacts, in different level from individual to global and result in unequal access to the resources and rights which leads to health consequences. Social exclusion can be enforced to an individual or to a group (Baskin, 2003; Tamara, 2006).

Psychological problems of marginalized were not accessed for years but affect the life in adverse form. Excluded one's has little or no control over the resources available. Social exclusion is an overt action of human societies in which unreliable are excluded out of the existing system of safety, health and opportunities but it can also be implemented indirectly.

One of the major groups of social exclusion is orphans. Orphans are defined differently in different context. UNAIDS (2004), define orphan as a child less than 18 years of age and who has lost his/her both parents. Orphans face many psychological problems like loss of social support, depression, low self-esteem, stigma, cognitive distortion, isolation etc. and if the cause of orphan-hood is due to HIV/AIDS then the impact of stigma and isolation is severe and intensified.

Orphan

In common, an orphan does not have any surviving parent to care. According to Merriam-Webster Dictionary (2012), the term orphan is derived from Greek word "Orphanos" which means, "a child whose parents is dead or abandoned them permanently". One of the legal definitions for orphan in US is "death or disappearance of, abandonment or desertion by, or separation or loss from, both parents" (UCSIS definition for immigration purposes). Some other groups like UNICEF, Joint United Nations Programme on HIV and AIDS (UNAIDS) label any children who lost one parent as an orphan. In this view any child who lost his/her mother is called maternal orphan, child who has lost his father is termed as paternal orphan and double orphan who has lost both parents (UNAIDS Global Report, 2008). UNAIDS (2004) define orphan as a child less than 18 years of age and who has lost his/her both parents.

International Children Charity (2018) found that approx 20 million of Indian child population is orphan, which is equal to 47 per cent of total child population. It is estimated that India has the largest child population in the world which is approximately 41 per cent of the population is below 18 years of age.

The one of the leading cause of orphan-hood is AIDS. This disease caused large increase in the mortality rate of adults during their reproductive age (Porter & Zaba, 1986; Blacker, 2004) and as a consequence the increased number of children is orphaned by HIV/ AIDS (Monasch & Boerma, 2004). Many orphans forced to drop school because of financial reasons and blocks their economic growths and future opportunities. These children are always at increased risk of malnutrition, physical and mental problems, sexual exploitation and stigmatization (Brown & Sittitrai, 2005; UNICEF, 2006).

People who have reached adulthood when they lost their one or both parents are not considered as orphan, but sometimes they are also called as adult orphan. Basically, the term orphan has been reserved for children who lost his/her parents before adulthood while they were too young to support themselves. In simple words, orphans are children who lost one or both parents before adulthood, means until adolescence period.

Children who have no one to look after or no one is willing to look after are shifted to residential institutions made up for the care and welfare of orphans. These institutions are called Orphanage. Mostly the process of shifting was done forcefully. Children remain in complete blank and often become hopeless about the future. In simple words, they were excluded from the main stream society and their participation in the welfare of society has been stopped, their reach to the basic resources were blocked, their potentials has been then neglected and they had no or little control on their own lives.

In India and most of the other countries the orphans were released from orphanage or deinstitutionalized when they reach adulthood. Orphans were provided education according to their interest and cognitive capabilities and other occupational trainings during their stay in orphanage that will help them to survive outside of the orphanage.

Orphanage

It is a residential institution for the care of orphans or for those children whose parents were unable to rear their children. In simple terms, it is a resident for those children who has no one to look after. Orphanage is an only way which provides education, food and safety to the orphans. Orphanages can be governmental or private.

Orphanage has been facing criticism because it is often found that they do not fulfill the essential and basic needs of the orphans which are necessary for complete development of the adolescents. The findings of many researches on nutrition showed that orphans of orphanage suffer from malnutrition (Chowdhury *et al.*, 2017) and are compatibly below the non-orphans on physical health dimensions (Braitstein *et al.*, 2013).

Problems and Consequences of Orphans

There can be a long list of problems faced by the orphans in their life span and specially, during their stay in orphanage. The orphans faced malnutrition that can lead to delayed intellectual development (UNICEF, 2006), loss in opportunities, loneliness, little or no social support and other several social and psychological problems. Death of the parents interrupt the emotional intelligence, skills, communication and other cognitive processing (Fredriksan & Kandous, 2004), they manifest lack of hope, negative perception of future and low self-esteem (Kedija, 2006). Orphans are deprived from social context that's why they show more emotional distress, hopelessness and frustration than non-orphans (Mbozi, Debit, & Munyati, 2006).

Profound and lifelong impact on self-esteem and psychological well-being on orphans can be seen after the death of parents. Adolescents can engaged in unresolved bereavement because of their developmental vulnerability and emotional dependency and being an AIDS orphan place them at heightened risk of prolonged mental problems (Hiwot *et al.*, 2011).

The beginning of orphan-hood imposes many new changes and challenges to orphans. This involves moving from home place to other, separation from siblings which is mostly done arbitrarily and division of orphaned brothers and sisters in relatives without due considerations of their needs. This can be very stressful and poses new demands and constraints to life of adolescents or orphans (Sengendo & Nambi, 1997).

With the death of the parents, orphans experience profound loss, grief, hopelessness etc. with long-term consequences such as chronic depression, low self-esteem, disturbed social behaviour and other major psychological problems. This can take the form of "self-stigma" in which children start blaming themselves for their parents' death and for the family's misfortune (Smart, 2003).

Here, we will discuss about some current and major issues related to the orphans of orphanage.

Orphans and Self-Esteem

Self-esteem is broader term and gained the focus of both academic and other popular circles (Mruk, 1999). There has been a lack of agreeableness on the concept of self-esteem. Many psychologists define self-esteem as a domain specific variable while some other defines self-esteem as a whole. After going through several definitions, one most straight forward definition can be "an evaluation of oneself" (Zeigler-Hill & Jordan, 2010, p. 392). One of the most renowned persons who has greatly contributed in conceptualizing self-esteem is Martin Rosenberg (1960) who defines self-esteem as "a feeling of self worth".

Other issues related in conceptualizing is whether self-esteem is a state or trait, or it should be used as an affective or cognitive process and whether implicit and explicit self-esteem are different from one another (Mruk, 1999, Zeigler-Hill & Jordan, 2010).

Rogers (1959) analyzed the self-esteem and find that the self-esteem has three components:

The view we had of ourselves (self image):

- How much value we place on ourselves (self worth).
- What we wish we were really like (ideal self).

Rogers also stated that high self-esteem is related to positive view of ourselves and it improves confidence, build our beliefs in our capabilities and lead to optimism and self-acceptance (Rogers, 1959).

The first psychological term was traced back from the work of William James (1890) generally called as "father of modern psychology" has defined self-esteem as "success divided by pretension". According to James, "the more success we have and the lower our expectations or pretensions then the higher our self-esteem". He defines two options to boost our self-esteem:

- Lower our expectations of ourselves.
- Increase our achievements.

James also identified two level of "self" processing; process of knowing called I-self and resulting knowledge from the I-self is called Me-self and these two processing create three types of knowledge which collectively account for Me-self:

- Matcrial self,
- Social self,
- Spiritual self.

Self-esteem was found to be associated with confidence and optimism (Rogers, 1959) and it also has positive association with social adjustments and happiness. Self-esteem is strongly related with happiness and people who has high self-esteem is more likeable, and can make strong relationship with others and can have a better impact on others than people with low self-esteem (Twenge & Campbell, 2009). Many studies showed that orphans show significantly lower level of self-esteem than non-orphans. This lead orphans toward negative self-image and negative self-evaluation.

Shifting from biological parents to adoptee caretakers is a stressful process and separation from siblings or friends from orphanage imposes extreme emotional impact on orphans, and create maladjustment in their environment. Assessing maladjustment and self-esteem in orphans, Farooqi and Intezar (2010) investigated about the level of self-esteem in orphans living in orphanage and non-orphans living with their parents. Their finding reveals that orphans show lower level of self-esteem than non-orphans and their findings also reveals that, children who were adopted from other cities or countries show significantly lower level of self-esteem and increased risk of developing mental problems as well as social maladjustment.

He and Ji (2007) conducted a study to assess the influence of AIDS related orphan-hood on nutrition status, well being and quality of life in Henan in China. Their findings reveal that there was no significant difference in nutrition status, both orphan and non-orphan getting poor nutrition, while low self-esteem, more depression and poor quality of life was found in orphans. Finding also revealed that low self-esteem mediates the association between orphan-hood and low quality of life.

Uma and Thomas (1991) conducted a study in Thiruvanathapuram, India to examine the personality of orphans and non-orphans. The dimensions were alienation, locus of control, hostility and self-derogation. The findings reveal that all the dimensions were significantly different in orphan and non-orphan. Self-derogation was higher in orphan than non--orphan, hostility was found higher in orphan and orphans assume that their locus of control is from external source.

Arsalan (2009) conducted a study to find the association between self-esteem, perceived social support and trait anger on 499 adolescents and the findings reveal that there were significant negative relationship between self-esteem and trait anger. The findings also reveal that self-esteem is significantly positive correlated with anger control and with the social support received from teachers and family.

Orphans and Perceived Social Support

Social support is a kind of help that we will get from our surroundings, social context or by significant others when we need it to overcome from any physical and mental obstacles of life and also when our coping resources are not enough. It can be tangible, in the form of any physical or concrete things like money, or it can be in a non-tangible form, which do not have any physical form like sympathy.

Social support means having people with us during the times of crisis to broaden our focus and attention and to create more positive self-image. It can enhance our quality of life and provide a buffer against adversities of life. Social support can be categorized in two categories:

- ***Actual/Received social support***: It can be defined as the help and support we actually receive in the times of adversity and crisis from our social context and important one's in our life.
- ***Perceived social support***: It can be defined as the hope, wish or desire about the kind and amount of support that we will get during the times of adversities from our social context and from the significant others.

Perceived social support can be broadly divided in four different types. These four types are:

- ***Emotional support***: It is also called as non-tangible support and it is related to the emotional back-up provided by others and gives a sense of care.
- ***Instrumental support***: It is also called as tangible support and related to worldly things that help someone to overcome from any difficult situation. Like providing money to someone in economical crisis.
- ***Informational support***: This is a kind of support that is delivered by providing any information related to the problem that can minimize the problem or provide new and innovative ways to look at any problem and find a solution and it can be any information that can be useful for other person.
- ***Appraisal or Companionship***: It is closely related to the emotional support and provides sense of belongingness or self-evaluation.

It has been seen that social support helps adolescents to make a clear sense of self and cope better in their life. Orphans does not get social support as much as they needed or in the time of crisis when they need it most. AIDS related orphans severely lack this because of the stigma associated with this disease.

In one study by Elamurugu and Indiramma (2015) on orphans of Tamil Nadu, India, found that orphans get less social support when others are aware of the cause of the orphan-hood is HIV/AIDS. The finding also reveals that scheduled caste (socially excluded) get less support than the other caste.

Social support was also found to be positively associated with many social aspects like the sense of cohesiveness, school grades, interpersonal relationship, etc. and negatively associated with many psychological aspects, such as, distress, anger, cognitive distortions etc.

In one study conducted by Caserta *et al.* (2016) was planned to assess how social support varies from context to context in orphan related characteristics in South Africa. It was also designed to investigate the relationship with emotional well-being and emotional distress. The finding reveals that orphans of orphanage shows higher level of perceived social support than non-orphans. The finding reveals that emotional and companionship support was associated for higher emotional well-being and lower emotional distress.

It was seen that support group interventions positively associated with performance and healthy emotional behaviour. It was seen that support, whether in form of peer group or significant other improved performances. In one such study by Osuji *et al.* (2018) was conducted to examine the role of social support by different sources on AIDS orphans in Uganda. The finding reveals that social support from caregivers, teachers, and classmates has positive impact on school outcome. This finding highlight the role of extended relationship beyond family is also crucial. Kumakech et al. (2004), conducted a study on AIDS orphans in Uganda. The findings reveal that school based peer support can significantly improve the school grades.

Orphans and Cognitive Distortions

Aron T. Beck in his book "Depression; causes and treatment" (1972), first conceptualized about the model of depression in which he mentioned about the thought processing by depressed patients. He showed about the false beliefs including self-blaming, negative self-evaluation and self-criticism by the depressed person. And these thought processing was then termed as "cognitive distortions".

Cognitive distortions are inaccurate thoughts that usually reinforce both negative thinking and emotions and convince us for something to be true which is actually irrational. Cognitive distortions make us feel to look at any event in a distorted way. Turkcapar (2009) define it as Going beyond content, negatively biased thought processes are called "Cognitive Distortion" or "Thinking Mistakes".

Cognitive distortions are basically irrational, biased and distorted form of our thought processing that leads to perceived things inaccurately. It creates an unending cycle of self-defeating thoughts from which escape looks impossible and it is also closely related with many psychological disorders specially depression and anxiety. Cognitive distortions are at the focus of many cognitive therapies in which psychotherapist try to change the irrational thought pattern and processes by the more rational one.

The cognitive distortions were conceptualized by Beck, but David Burns was known for popularizing its common names and examples in his book "Feeling Good: The New Mood Therapy (1980)". Some of the main cognitive distortions are:

- ***Filtering:*** In which we take negative details and filter the positive information of any event.
- ***Polarized Thinking/Black or White Thinking***: In this type of distortion, in which individual construct two extreme poles of evaluation of his performance. For example, being perfect or he will be a complete failure.
- ***Overgeneralization***: In this type of distortions individual use a single event or information to make generalization.
- ***Jumping to the conclusion***: In this type of distortions people assume that they know how others think for them and why they are acted like this.
- ***Personalization***: In this type of distortion people relate every bad event and failure with them. They feel that they were the reason for this failure. People also compare themselves with other and demoralize themselves.
- ***Catastrophizing***: In this type of distortion people feel that any disaster will happen no matter why and when but they continuously fell that, what if that happens?

Basically IQ (Intelligence Quotient) is the measure of intellectual functioning and high IQ is associated with good in cognitive functioning. IQ of an individual is associated with environment, surroundings, socio-economic status, nutrition, family background and other factors. The cognitive functioning of ex-institutionalized orphans varies according to the time spent in orphanage, post-orphanage placement and also the age at the time of adaptations (Maclean, 2003).

Barriga *et al.* (2000) conducted a study in Ohio to assess the self-serving and self-debasing cognitive distortions and their relationship with internalizing and externalizing problematic behaviour. Self-serving cognitive distortions specifically related to externalizing behaviours, whereas self-debasing cognitive distortions specifically related to internalizing behaviours.

According to Beck's theory of depression, negative thinking about self, future and world is due to depression and that is the other way for looking at the cognitive distortions. So, if we look at some of the previous researches conducted to study the level of depression in orphans, we will find that orphans show higher level of depression than non-orphans specially those orphans residing in orphanage.

In one study by Ramagopala *et al.* (2016) was conducted to assess the level of depression among orphans and non-orphans of Tamil Nadu. The finding of his research reveals that female orphans were more depressed than non-female participants (53%) and 48 per cent male orphans were found depressed and all of them were between age group of 15-17 years.

Cognitive distortions block the real view of the psychological environment that inhibits the full potentials of the orphans and as a result it blocks the paths of achievements and happiness and leads toward depression and hopelessness.

Discussion

Adolescence period is considered as a crucial stage because it plays an important role in healthy development of the individual as an adult because it works as a bridge between children to adulthood. The negative psychological impacts during this period which were not seen for year can ruin the healthy development. Erikson (1997) also stated about the importance of this transitional period; defining goals, creating self-identity and accepting duties and roles will move adolescence as a healthy adult.

Social exclusion is a multidimensional and social phenomenon (Saksena, 2014) and can be implemented on individual or group (Baskin, 2003; Tamara, 2006). When marginalization is implemented on a whole community or group, it causes little bit less negative impact because the whole marginalized community can stand for one another and provide some sort of support for each other. When it is implemented individually it enforces many psychological, social and development problems which cannot be tackled or resolved without the interference and proper planned interventions.

Marginalization can be indirect, like in the cases of orphans, during the age of rapid biological, psychological and social development they were excluded from society and institutionalized and this process blocks their opportunity and affect their overall development. 20 million of Indian child population is orphan *(*International Children Charity, 2018*)*. Collectively this is a very large number and sharing 47 per cent of total Indian child population. This large number of population is neglected and put out of the periphery. Their potentials can be used for the development and welfare of the society and nation.

The self-esteem plays an important role in using our capabilities in full strength and for a better self-image and self-evaluation but it is found that orphans often show low self-esteem as compared to non-orphans. Self-esteem was also found to be associated with maladjustment, happiness, quality of life, well-being etc. and this is found to be true with several findings.

Such as, Farooqi and Intezar (2010) found that orphans of orphanage show lower level of self-esteem than non-orphans and adopted orphans show lower level of self-esteem that cause mental problems and maladjustments. Self-esteem also found to be associated with happiness and has important role in quality of life. Twenge (2009) found that self-esteem is associated with happiness and those who has high self-esteem is more likable and can make log term relationships. He & Ji (2007) found that orphans show low self-esteem and poor quality of life and also found that self-esteem mediates between orphan-hood and quality of life. Self-esteem is also highly positively correlated with anger control (Arsalan, 2009).

Social support is needed by everyone, even normal people in their normal times needs emotional support that can provide a feeling of care, belongingness and affection. It was found that orphans perceived, social support more than non-orphans. It means that they expect more from us, from society and from their surroundings. It is also helpful in building coping strategies and improved performances. Many researcher uses social support as an intervention to improve academic grades and performance.

Caserta *et al.* (2016) found that orphans of orphanage show higher level of perceived social support than non-orphans and also found that emotional support is associated with high emotional wellbeing and lower emotional distress. Osuji *et al.* (2018) and Kumakech *et al.* (2004) found that peer based intervention programmes improve school grades and these findings draw the attention on importance of relationship beyond family. AIDS is perceived as stigma in our society and it inhibits the AIDS related orphans to get accurate social support from the society and significant others. Elamurugu and Indiramma (2015) found that orphans receive less social support by significant others when they are aware that AIDS is the cause of orphan-hood.

Cognitive distortions distort our thinking and perception and create an irrational belief about self, future and environment and this concept was taken from the thinking process of depressed patient. Cognitive distortions make orphans self-handicapped, hopeless and did not allow them to use their potentials in full strength and to cope properly and effectively.

In such study focusing on the negative effect of cognitive distortions, Maclean (2003) found that cognitive functioning of orphans depend on the time they spent in orphanage, age at the time of adoptation and surrounding where they have been adopted. Ramagopala and associates (2016) found that 53 per cent female and 48 per cent male orphans were depressed and all aged between 15-17 years of age. Barriga et al. (2000) found that self-serving cognitive distortions are related with externalizing behaviour problems and self-debasing cognitive distortions are related with internalizing behaviour problems.

Conclusion

It was found that orphans has many psychological problems and are at heightened risk-mental problems. Government and policy-makers are working for orphans and launches several schemes and policies for the development and welfare of the orphans in India. For example; Platinum jubilee orphan children education scheme by Indian Air Force which provide monthly grants from KG up to XII, scheme of assistance to voluntary organization for homes (Shishu Grih) for infants and young children for promoting in country adoption, for destitute and orphans of age 0-6 (by CARA under the ministry of social justice and empowerment), The 'Education for All' campaign the government is addresses a large number of male and female children in which 60 per cent are girls of age group between 6-14 years (Indian women welfare, orphan welfare) etc. but these policies are not providing the up to the mark improvement and result because of the failure in implementing it properly. And without proper supervision, follow-up and feedback government cannot extract the desired results from these policies. The failure of these policies did not help the orphans to overcome from psychological and social problems and are unable to merge in the main stream.

Implications

In India the main focus of government and policy-makers were previously on physical health and nutrition of orphans, now it is shifted on the education of orphans but they should also focus their attention on psychological aspects for overall development of orphans. Without the planned and empirically supported results, schemes and policies will not give a better or desired outcome. Good intervention plans are required to provide psychological help and this required knowledgeable and skilled counsellor and psychologist develop interventions and implement it to resolves the maximum psychological problems. For this government should recruit good and skilled counsellors and psychologist in every orphanage and NGO to understand the cause and consequences of the problems and to resolve it. The quality and standard of government owned orphanage should also be improved and private orphanage should be under the supervision of government. Policies for the welfare and development of orphans should be followed and observed critically for maximum result and should be updated time by time and those policies which were not providing effective outcome should be change. Adoption is also under the government schemes and it should be promoted on large level because the rate of adoption in our country is very low (approx 6,000 per year).

Some intervention programmes can be effective some area but not for others because every orphan has some unique demands and problems and it is impossible to resolve it but if we look at any specific region we will find that a general pattern of problems emerge and that will be almost same for all of the orphans of that region and that would be easy to handle and resolve by providing special treatment, intervention, policy, counselling and psychotherapy related to that general pattern of problem.

References

Andrews, G., Skinner, D., and Zuma, K. (2006). "Epidemiology of health and vulnerability among children orphaned and made vulnerable by HIV/AIDS in sub-Saharan Africa", *AIDS Care, 18*, 269-276.

Arsalan, C. (2009). "Anger, Self-esteem and Perceived Social Support among Adolescence", *Social Behaviour and Personality, 37*(4), 555-564. https://doi.org/10.2224/sbp.2009.37.4.555.

Barriga, A., Q., Landau, J., R., Stinson, B., L., and Liau, A., K. (2000). "Cognitive distortions and problem behaviours among adolescents", *Criminal Justice and Behaviour, 27*(1), 36-56. https://doi.org/10.1177/0093854800027001003.

Baskin, C. (2003). "Structural social work as seen from an Aboriginal Perspective", In: W. Shera (Ed.), *Emerging Perspectives on Anti-oppressive Practice,* pp. 65–78, Toronto: Canadian Scholar's Press.

Beck, A., T. (1972). *Depression; Causes and Treatment*, Philadelphia: University of Pennsylvania Press.

Burns, D. D. (1980). *Feeling Good: The New Mood Therapy*, New York: Morrow.

Braitstein, P., *et al.* (2013). "Nutritional Status of Orphaned and Separated Children and Adolescents Living in Community and Institutional Environments in Uasin Gishu County, Kenya", *PLoS One, 8*(7), https://doi.org/10.1371/journal.pone.0070054.

Caserta, T. A., Punamaki, L-R., Pirttila-Backman, M-A. (2016). "The Buffering Role of Social Support on the Psychosocial Wellbeing of Orphans in Rwanda", *Wiley Online Library,* https://onlinelibrary.wiley.com/doi/abs/10.1111/sode.12190.

Chawdhury, A.B. M.A., Wasiullah, S., Haque, Md.I., and Muhammad, F. (2017). "Nutritional status of orphans living in orphanage of Dhaka, Bangladesh", *Malaysian Journal of Nutrition, 23*(2).

Csikszentmihalyi, M. (2020). *Adolescence*, Encyclopaedia Britannica https://www.britannica.com/science/adolescence.

Duffin, E. (2019, September 20). "Proportion of selected age groups of world population in 2019, by region", Statista. https://www.statista.com/statistics/265759/world-population-by-age-and-region/.

Elamurugu, M., Indiramma, V. (2015). "Perceived Social Support among children orphaned by HIV/AIDS in Trichy, India: A cross-sectional study", *Journal of School of Social Work, 12*(2).

Erikson.E. H., and Erikson J.M. (1997). *The Life Cycle Completed,* New York: Norton.

Farooqi, N., and Intezar, M. (2009). "Differences in self-esteem of orphan children and children living with their parents", Department of Applied Psychology. University of Punjab, Lahore, Pakistan, vol. *46*(2).

He, Z., and Ji, C. (2007). "Nutritional status, psychological well-being and the quality of life of AIDS orphans in rural Henan Province, China", *Trop Med International Health, 12*(10), 1180-1190. https://doi.org/10.1111/j.1365-3156.2007.01900.x.

Hilary, S. (1994). Social Exclusion and Social Solidarity: Three Paradigms, *International Labour Review, 133* (5–6), 531–78.

Hiwot, G., Fentie, A., Lakew, A., and Wondoesn, K. (2011). "Psychological distress and its predictors in AIDS orphan adolescents in Addis Ababa city:

A comparative survey: *Ethiopia Journal of Health Development, 25*, 135-14.

https://www.who.int/social_determinants/themes/socialexclusion/en/

http://www.lawctopus.com/academike/problems-marginalized-groups-india/

https://www.merriam-webster.com/dictionary/orphan

http://files.unaids.org/en/media/unaids/contentassets/documents/unaidspublication/2004/GAR2004_en.pdf

http://data.unaids.org/pub/globalreport/2008/jc1510_2008_global_report_pp11_28_en.pdf

https://www.soschildrensvillages.ca/india-now-home-20-million-orphans-study-finds

https://web.archive.org/web/20120527084514/http://www.ashlyns.herts.sch.uk/about/history.htm

https://indianairforce.nic.in/content/platinum-jubilee-orphan-children-education-scheme-0.

https://www.womenwelfare.org/Orphan%20Welfare.html

https://www.google.com/search?q = indian+government+schemes+for+orphans & oq = in & aqs = chrome.0.69i59j69i57j69i60l3j69i65l3.3946j0j7 & sourceid = chrome & ie = UTF-8

James, W. (1890). "The Self and Its Selves", In: C. Lemert (Eds.) (2010) *Social Theory: The Multicultural Readings* (pp. 161-166). Philadelphia: Westview Press.

John, M. (2017). "An Investigation of Factors Affecting the Academic Performance of Orphaned Children: A Case of Selected Upper Primary Schools in Nchelenge District, ZAMBIA", *The International Journal of Multi-Disciplinary Research*, Information and Communications University School of Education.

Kumakech, E., Crantor-Graae, E., Maling, S., and Bajunirwe, E. (2009). "Peer-group support intervention improves the psychosocial well-being of AIDS orphans: cluster randomized trial", *Soc Sci Med*, 68(6), 1038-1043. https://doi:10.1016/j.socscimed.2008.10.033.

MacLean, K. (2003). "The impact of institutionalization on child development", *Development and Psychopathology, 15*, 853–884.

Manuel, P. (2002). "Assessment of orphans and their caregivers' psychological well-being in a rural community in central Mozambique", *Institute of Child Health*, London.

Maqbool, A. and Ganai, M.Y. (2016). "A Study of Self-Concept, Mental Health and Academic Achievement of Orphan and Non-Orphan Adolescents", Anchor Academic Publishing.

Mbozi, P.S., Debit, M.B., and Munyati, S. (Eds), (2006). "Psychosocial conditions of orphans and vulnerable children in two Zimbabwean Districts", HSRC Press, Cape Town, South Africa.

Osuji, H., L., Nabunya, P., Byansi, W., Parchment, T., M., Ssewamala, F., McKay, M., M., Haung, K-N. (2018). "Social support and school outcomes of adolescents orphaned and made vulnerable by HIV/AIDS living in South

Western Uganda", *Vulnerable Child Youth Stud., 13*(3), 228-238. https://doi.10.1080/17450128.2018.1439211.

Piaget, J. (1983). "Piaget's Theory", In: W. Kessen (Eds.), *Handbook of Child Psychology, 1, Theoretical model of human development,* 103-128. New York: Wiley.

Ramapogal, G., Narasimhan, S., Uma Devi, L. (2016). "Prevalence of depression among children living in orphanage", *International Journal of Contemporary Pediatrics, 3*(4), 1326-1328. doi: http://dx.doi.org/10.18203/2349-3291.ijcp20163670

Rogers, C.R. (1959). "A Theory of Therapy, Personality, and Interpersonal Relationships: As Developed in the Client-Centred Framework", In: S. Koch (Ed.), *Psychology: A Study of a Science. Formulations of the Person and the Social Context* (Vol. 3, pp. 184-256). New York: McGraw Hill.

Sengendo, J., and Nambi, J. (1997). "The psychological effect of orphanhood: a study of orphans in Rakai district", *Health Transition Review, 7*, 105-24.

Smart, R. (2003). "Policies for Orphans and Vulnerable Children: A Framework for Moving Ahead", Washington, DC.

Tamara, W. (2006). "A right to inclusion? Homelessness, human rights and social exclusion" (PDF). *Australian Journal of Human Rights*. 12, 185–204. https://doi.org/10.1080/1323238X.2006.11910818.

Twenge, J.M., and Campbell, W.K. (2009). *The Narcissism Epidemic: Living in the Age of Entitlement*. New York: Free Press.

Uma J., and Thomas, I. (1991). "Personality differences between orphans and non-orphans", *The Creative Psychologist, 3*(1), 31-38.

Voux, A. (1988). *Social Support: Theory, Research and Intervention*, New York, N.Y.: Praeger.

Vygotsky, L.S. (1987). "Thoughts and words", In R.W. Riebe and A.S. Carton (Eds.), *The Collected Works of L.S. Vygotsky, 1, Problems of general psychology,* 243-288. New York: Plenum.

Wills, T.A. (1985). "Supportive functions of interpersonal relationships". In S. Cohen; L. Syme (eds.). *Social Support and Health*. Orlando, FL: Academic Press. 61–82.

Zeigler-Hill, V., and Jordan, C.H. (2010). "Two faces of self-esteem: Implicit and explicit forms of self-esteem", In B. Gawronski and B.K. Payne (Eds.), *Handbook of Implicit Social Cognition: Measurement, Theory, and Applications* (pp. 392-407). New York, NY: Guilford Press.

16

Role of Self-disclosure and Emotion Regulation in Parent-Adolescent Relationship

Sweta Pathak, Mithilesh Kumar Tiwari and *Shubhra Sinha*

Introduction

Good health both physical and mental is of paramount importance for human existence. It is often conceived as an outcome of interaction between individual and environment, mutually affecting each other. Good health helps in building strong relationship, better adaptation to change and in dealing effectively with life's challenges. During adolescence, adolescents face countless physical, cognitive, emotional, social and behavioural changes due to various factors including biological, social, psychological etc. Psychological changes of adolescence include autonomy demands, identity development, development of knowledge and skills, changes in emotional understanding about oneself as well as others and also several abilities of abstract thinking, introspection and practice of moral values in behaviour (Myers, Laurent & Hodges, 2014).

In this phase of development, many times a rift may develop between parents and their children, because it is a time of rapid physical/ psychological development and deep emotional changes, which are often confusing and uncomfortable for adolescents and parents alike. Identifying accurate emotional cues from outside as well as from inside, differentiating between different emotional states, using appropriate behavioural strategies in different emotional situations etc., which are collectively referred as emotional intelligence, significantly affect the emotional experience and ultimately mental health of individuals (Underwood, Moore & Rosenhan, 1973).

Emotion regulation is another important aspect of emotional development which is aimed at modifying emotional experiences through using various strategies, to make emotional experiences congruent to the individual's adaptation (Aldao, Nolen-Hoeksema, & Schweizer, 2010; Gross, 2015; McLaughlin, Hatzenbuehler, Mennin, & Nolen-Hoeksema, 2011).

Emotion regulation is conceived as "the extrinsic and intrinsic processes responsible for monitoring, evaluating, and modifying emotional reactions, especially their intensive and temporal features, to accomplish one's goals" (Thompson, 1994). Gross (1998) identified various strategies which further divided into two broader categories—Cognitive reappraisal and expressive suppression. Each strategy has different short-term as well as long-term health consequences.

Conventionally adolescence has been characterized as a stage of storm and stress. Due to a lot of changes in hormonal, maturational and expanded network of relationship as well as globalization, adolescent's expectations from their immediate family environment change. Adolescents demand more autonomy in their decisions related to various aspects of their life, at the same time, parents become more vigilant about their whereabouts, their activities and friend circle. Parents and adolescent's behaviour are contingent upon each other. Parents adopt different strategies and to control, monitor and supervise their adolescent's behaviour, which collectively referred to as parenting styles (Barnhart *et al.*, 2013). Parenting style is basically a type of interaction between parents and adolescents through which both share their expectations and demands with each other. The quality of interaction between them is a very crucial factor in determining the overall development of adolescents. There is plethora of studies related to different type of parenting styles and their impact on different aspects of adolescents' development (Bornstein & Putnick, 2012; Pomeranz & Wang, 2009).

Self-disclosure is a type of communication in interpersonal relationships which have significant contribution in the quality of relationship and ultimately on the mental health and well-being of the participants involved in it. Self-disclosure is a process of voluntarily divulging something personal with some significant other in the relationship. Content of the self-disclosure may be of personal, emotional, conceptual or both and may be related to any issue, of the outer world (Ignatius & Marja, 2007). Thus, the quality of self-disclosure in terms of quantity, frequency, accuracy, truthfulness and content have significant impact upon the quality of interpersonal relationship. Self-disclosure is not having to be all or nothing. Disclosing one's mental health is a very personal and subjective matter and while disclosing something personal, it is also important to accept negative responses from others.

Self-disclosure: The Conceptual Framework

Self-disclosure is a form of interpersonal communication which plays an important role in the management of the parent-adolescent relationship. Self-disclosure is defined as "an act of revealing information to others" (Archer, 1980) and has been regarded as a major factor in influencing the course of development, maintenance, and deterioration of a relationship (Derlega *et al.,* 1993; Laurenceau & Barret, 1998). The context of self-disclosure includes one's personal thoughts, feelings, and experiences (Derlega *et al.*, 1993). Self-disclosure involves an implicit or explicit understanding that the personal information revealed to the other party will not be relayed further (Yovetich and Drigotas, 1999). Through self-disclosure, an individual lets himself or herself be known to the other person, in a way it, "reduces the mystery" between people (Jourard, 1971). Self-disclosure is one of the most important mechanisms in the development of intimacy (Lauer *et al.,* 2000).

Dolgin and Kim (1994) reported that adolescence is characterized by increased peer pressure and the tendency to disclose more to their peers while concurrently decreasing disclosure to parents. It represents a significant change from the disclosure patterns of childhood where parents serve as primary confidants for their children. This situation presents two major challenges before parents. First is to protect the emotional bond between parents and adolescents which is naturally at stake because of the heightened autonomy demands and second is to exert control on the ideas and behaviour of adolescents to prevent them from potentially risky situations and from getting them culturally uprooted. The whole venture of parenting is directed towards these two goals. Now, it is important to understand self-disclosure though the lenses of two major theoretical substrates dealing with it.

The social exchange theory (Homans, 1958) examine the relationship choices that individuals made on the basis of costs and benefits associated with the relationship. Theory suggests that when the rewards exceed the costs, there is equity in the relationship and the partners are motivated to stay in it. But when the costs exceed the rewards, the partners are likely to consider other alternatives, such as leaving the relationship entirely or initiating relationships with others. Applying same principle, Altman & Taylor (1973 & 1987) concluded that every self-disclosure has certain costs as well as certain rewards or payoffs. Rewards include developing trust and liking for each other, finding solutions to their problems by talking to reliable others and getting a chance to release one's pent up emotions.

On the other hand, the cost may be putting one's image at stake, getting socially stigmatized, experiencing rejection, social isolation and threats to personal well-being. Besides this, another feature of disclosure is that it creates an obligation for the listener to return the disclosure with the same amount of breadth and intimacy, which may not be achieved at all times. So the decision of disclosing or not disclosing oneself to others depends upon careful consideration of these possibilities.

The Social penetration theory was given by Altman and Taylor (1987) to provide an insight to the development of interpersonal relationships. They proposed that as relationships grow, interpersonal communication moves from relatively shallow, non-intimate levels to deeper levels and finally reaches to more personal ones. Altman and Taylor (1987) suggested that this closeness in relationship occurs through a gradual process of self-disclosure, which proceeds from superficial to intimate levels of exchange as a function of both immediate and final outcomes. The term "social penetration" is used to refer to both overt interpersonal behaviours that take place in social interaction and internal subjective processes that precede, accompany and follow overt exchange. This theory is perhaps best known for its onion analogy. It claims that our relationships progress through four stages before reaching stability where communication is open and partners are highly intimate.

- Orientation stage
- Exploratory affective stage
- Affective stage
- Stable stage.

When the relationship starts breaking down and costs exceed benefits, there is a gradual withdrawal of disclosure which leads to termination of the relationships. This process is called de-penetration. Both theories explain the notion, function and process of self-disclosure in interpersonal relationships but with respect to parent-child relationship the Social exchange theory appears more suitable, as this relationship is biological and extremely intimate from the beginning.

Self-disclosure: Types and Dimensions

Depending upon its nature and content self-disclosure is categorized into different types. For example, Waring (1987) suggested two types of disclosure namely *Personal self-disclosure* which means disclosure about oneself and *Relational self-disclosure* which focuses on disclosing one's relationship with another person. Pathak & Sinha (2018) also found similar factor structure in their study where they developed a scale measuring self-disclosure in parent-adolescent relationship, as suggested by Waring (1987).

Zur (2009) identified four types of self-disclosure used in clinical settings, described as follows:

1. **Unavoidable Self-Disclosure:** As the name implies, unavoidable self-disclosure encompasses those attributes/mannerisms that are obvious in someone. It might include the gender, age and physical characteristics of the person disclosing the information. Unavoidable self-disclosure is uncontrollable. There is nothing that people can do about it. It covers disclosure through place of practice, tone of voice, pregnancy, foreign or any accent, stuttering, visible tattoos, obesity and many forms of disability, such as paralysis, blindness, deafness or an apparent limp (Zur, 2007, 2009). Counsellors reveal themselves also by their manner of dress, hairstyle, use of make-up, jewellery, perfume or aftershave, facial hair, wedding or engagement rings, or the wearing of a cross, or any other symbol (Barnett, 1998; Zur, 2007). Body language can include any non-reflexive or reflexive movements of parts of the body. Clients, are often more attuned to non-verbal cues, such as body language and touch, than to verbal communication (Knapp & Hall, 1997).
2. **Accidental Self-Disclosure:** Accidental self-disclosure occurs when there are incidental (unplanned) encounters outside the office, spontaneous verbal or non-verbal reactions, or other planned and unplanned occurrences that happen to reveal counsellors' personal information to their clients. (Knox, Hess, Petersen, & Hill, 1997; Strieker & Fisher, 1990).
3. **Deliberate Self-Disclosure:** This refers to the counsellor's intentional, verbal or non-verbal disclosure of personal information, information about who the counsellor really is which is not commonly known. A deliberate self-disclosure may occur when the counsellor exposes some personal and family photographs in his/her office which will go a long way in providing background information about the counsellor. (Barnett, 1998; Mahalik, Van Ormer & Simi, 2000; Zur, 2007). Two types of deliberate self-disclosures are identified by Knox,

Hess, Petersen, & Hill, (1997). These are self-revealing (the disclosure of information by counsellors about themselves) and self-involving (counsellors' personal reactions to clients).

4. **Clients' Deliberate Actions:** These are also potential sources that can reveal personal information about the counsellor. Inquiries can be initiated by clients about their counsellor by conducting a simple Web search. Such searches can reveal a wide range of professional and personal information, such as family history, criminal records, family tree, volunteer activity, community and recreational involvement, political affiliations and much more. Counsellors do not always have control over what is posted online about them, which means they may not have control or even knowledge of what clients may know about them. A client's deliberate tracking, spying or stalking their therapist can reveal a significant amount of private and personal information (Zur, 2007, 2008).

Above mentioned four types of self-disclosure suggested by Zur (2007, 2008) were specifically for clinical settings, which are applied in other settings as well i.e.—peer group, parent-child relationship etc.

Three different dimensions of self-disclosure were also identified by Omarzu (2000) as **breadth, duration** and **intimacy**, where breadth refers to the diversity of contexts and topics during self-disclosure, durations means amount of time people utilizes in sharing information with others and intimacy means that how much importance individual places on the topic they discuss with others.

Self-disclosure serves two important functions which are important within every network of relationship (Ando, 1990; Derlega *et al.*, 1993). First is personal function (emotional expression, self-clarification, social validation) and second is interpersonal function (relationship development, social control and intimacy maintenance). Both of these are very vital for the successful development as well as maintenance of the relationship. Self-disclosure may be either unplanned or planned. People may prefer planned disclosure about potentially stigmatizing information because it maximizes privacy regulation.

The term "reciprocity" is an important and thoroughly investigated aspect of self-disclosing behaviour (Barack & Gluck-Ofri, 2007). Various authors have referred to this process as the "dyadic effect" or the "mutual effect" (Jourard, 1991). This concept refers to the process of mutual exposure by communicating partners, in which a disclosure by one partner is followed by disclosure by the other (Barack & Gluck-Ofri, 2007).

The self-disclosure of children to their parents is the dominant source of information for parents to gain knowledge about their children and their daily lives. Parental knowledge of their children's whereabouts and daily lives has been linked to several positive outcomes. The more parents know about their kids, the lower the rate of behaviour problems among children, and the higher the children's well-being.

Self-disclosure can be strongly influenced by the culture we live in. There are cultures in the world that are much more intimate and are less reserved when it comes to personal space. Some studies have suggested that it is not only parenting style or child's personality that determines the level of disclosure, the nature of issues and cultural norms about discussing such issues with parents also play a crucial role in controlling the width, depth and intensity of child's disclosure to parents. For example, Youniss and Smollar (1985) found that adolescents tend to discuss their school work, future plans, and social issues with their parents, but they do not communicate much about issues like dating (although they disclose more to mothers than fathers.

Mental Health and Well-being of Adolescents: Role of Self-disclosure and Emotion Regulation

Emotion regulation is an important aspect of individuals wellbeing, it focuses on how effectively people manage their and others emotional experiences, expressions and reactions in day to day life. Previous studies suggest, inadequate emotion regulation leads to several psychological problems, interpersonal difficulties and poor resilience to stressful situations (Aldao *et al.*, 2010, 2015; Gross, 2015; Moore, Zoellner, & Mollenholt, 2008; Webb, Miles, & Sheeran, 2012).

Gross (1998) proposed a model of emotion regulation, known **as Process model of emotion regulation** and reported five essential points of emotion regulation which are *situation collection, situation alteration, attentional disposition, cognitive variation* and *response adjustment.* There are two types of strategy which people adapt during the process of emotion regulation, i.e.—*Cognitive reappraisal (CR) and Emotion expressive suppression (ES).*

Cognitive reappraisal strategy is antecedent focused, which acts before the completion of emotional response and useful when the stressful situation cannot be changed (Gross & John, 2003). It decreases the emotional impact of stressful situation by reframing the present perception of stressful situation. It is an effective and frequently used strategy in modifying the impact of emotional experiences. Expressive suppression (ES) is a response-focused strategy, which includes reduction of facial expression and regulation of positive and negative emotions. It may have negative emotional and psychological effects on individuals as it reduces expressive behaviour knowingly. Previous studies support cognitive reappraisal strategy more than expressive suppression strategy because, rather than disturbing emotional response cognitive reappraisal focuses on provoking stimulus and leads to greater life satisfaction, positive emotions, high self-esteem and good social relationship (Webb *et al.,* 2012; Haga, Kraft, & Corby, 2009; Balzarotti, John, & Gross, 2010; Cabello, Salguero, Fernández-Berrocal, & Gross, 2013; John & Gross, 2004; Lougheed & Hollenstein, 2012; Moore *et al.*, 2008).

Pennebaker and O'Heeron (1984) concluded in their study that talk with confidant was the important factor contributing to health and psychopathology of spouses of victims of suicide and other accidental death. Those who talked with confidant experienced less intrusive and unwanted thoughts related to death of their spouse. Several mechanisms were proposed to explain why and how self-disclosure is contributing to the health and well-being of individuals.

From inhibition/disinhibition perspective, self-disclosure leads to disinhibition of thoughts and feelings related to various aspects of life which in turn lead better health & well-being, whereas non-disclosure related with the psychological inhibition of thoughts and feelings and these thoughts/feelings becomes intrusive, ruminating in nature and in turn affect their mental health. Cole & colleagues (1996) in their study on psychological inhibition among men having HIV found that those who were classified as "closeted" i.e. concealed about their identity and homosexuality with others, have higher risk of developing diseases as compared to those individuals who were classified as "open" i.e. disclosed about their identity and homosexuality with others. Preoccupation model of secrecy (Lane & Wegner, 1995) maintained that secret thoughts and feelings are associated with the obsessive preoccupied other cognitive thoughts. These obsessive thoughts/ feelings associated with secrecy, are self-sustaining in nature and lead to various kinds of mental health issues. In contrast to self-disclosure, non-disclosure in the form of maintaining secrecy have negative consequences upon the health of individuals.

Expressing own thoughts and feelings in any form (talking, writing etc.) lead to less stressful experiences. Expression of cognitive processing in writing or talking allow individuals to accept their own psychological state as well as being acceptable in their network of relationship with whom they share their thoughts/feelings. Constructing narratives to express their feelings help people in exploring meaning in their experiences, alternatives and validate their experiences (Lepor, Ragan & Jones, 2000).

Pathak and Sinha (2018) conducted their study specifically on parent-adolescents relationship exploring relationship between self-disclosure of adolescents and emotion regulation strategies. Researchers found that those who disclosed more on personal issues, use emotion suppression technique more as compared to those who disclose less, whereas no significant difference appeared on the dimension of cognitive reappraisal. Emotion expression provides information to observers about a person's social intentions and his/her feelings regarding the current relationship. Expressive suppression is quite common during social interactions (Gross & John, 2003) and several evidences suggest important links between emotion expression, social relationships and health (House, Landis, & Umberson, 1988; Schwarzer & Leppin, 1991; Seeman, 2001; Uchino, Cacioppo, & Kiekolt-Glaser, 1996).

Conclusion

Although research into self-disclosure and emotion regulation in parent-adolescent context is in its relative infancy, there is sufficient evidence which suggest that self-disclosure helps adolescents to communicate and express their positive and negative emotions to their parents easily, so that they suffer less from emotional chaos and bond positive relations with their parents. Sufficient evidence suggests that adolescent should use strategies that influence their appraisal of the situation to create the most appropriate emotional climate to respond. Research suggests that this approach is likely more effective than the suppression of emotions that have already happened. In short, where dysfunctional emotions are concerned, prevention might be better than cure. Further study should focus on cultural criteria that influence self-disclosure. Although there is widespread study on gender differences in self-disclosure, more research is needed on the psychological and social sustaining of these effects.

References

Aldao A., Nolen-Hoeksema S., and Schweizer S. (2010). "Emotion-regulation strategies across psychopathology: A meta-analytic review", *Clinical Psychology Review*, *30,* 217–237.

Aldao, A., and Tull, M.T. (2015). "Putting emotion regulation in context", *Current Opinion in Psychology, 3*, 100–107.

Altman, I., and Taylor, D.A. (1973). *Social Penetration: The Development of Interpersonal Relationships.* New York: Holt, Rinehart & Winston.

Altman, I., and Taylor, D. (1987). "Communication in interpersonal relationships: Social penetration theory", *Interpersonal Processes: New Directions in Communication Research*, 257-277.

Ando, K. (1990). "Jiko no sugata no hyoshutsu no dankai, the step of—disclosure of self", In Y. Nakamura (Ed.),—Jikokatei no shinrigaku [Psychology on —the process of self-] (148 198). "Tokyo: Tokyo daigakushuppan-kai".

Archer, R.L. (1979). "Role of personality and the social situation", In G.J. Chelune (ed.), *Self-disclosure: Origins, Patterns, and Implications of Openness in Interpersonal Relationships*, London: Jossey-Bass.

Balzarotti, S., John, O.P., and Gross, J.J. (2010). "An Italian adaptation of the emotion regulation questionnaire", *European Journal of Psychological Assessment, 26,* 61–67.

Barnett, C. (1998). "The cultural turn: Fashion or progress in human geography", *Antipode, 30,* (4), 379-394.

Barnhart, C., Raval, V., Jansari, A., and Raval, P. (2013). "Perception of Parenting style among college students in India and the United States", *Journal of Child Family Studies, 22* (5), 684-693.

Bornstein, M. and Putnick, D. (2012). "Cognitive and socioemotional caregiving in developing countries", *Child Development, 83* (1), 46-61.

Cabello, R., Salguero, J.M., Fernández-Berrocal, P., and Gross, J.J. (2013). "A Spanish adaptation of the emotion regulation questionnaire", *European Journal of Psychological Assessment, 29*, 234–240.

Cole, S.W., Kemeny, M.E., Taylor, S.E., Visscher, B.R. and Fahey, J.L. (1996). "Accelerated course of human immunodeficiency virus infection in gay men who conceal their homosexual identity", *Psychosomatic Medicine, 58* (3), 219-231.

Derlega, V.J., Metts, S., Petronio, S., and Margulis, S.T. (1993). *Self-disclosure.* Newbury Park, CA: Sage.

Gross, J.J. (1998). "The emerging field of emotion regulation: An integrative review", *Review of General Psychology, 2*(3), 271-299.

Gross, J.J. (2007). *Handbook of Emotion Regulation*. New York, NY: Guilford Press.

Gross J.J. (2015). "The extended process model of emotion regulation: Elaborations, applications, and future directions", *Psychological Inquiry, 26*, 130–137.

Gross, J.J., and John, O.P. (2003). "Individual differences in two emotion regulation processes: Implications for affect, relationships, and well-being", *Journal of Personality and Social Psychology, 85,* 348–362.

Haga, M.H., Kraft, P., and Corby, E. (2009). "Emotion regulation: Antecedents and well-being outcomes of cognitive reappraisal and expressive suppression in cross-cultural samples", *Journal of Happiness Studies, 10*, 271–291.

Homans, G.C. (1958). "Social Behaviour as Exchange", *American Journal of Sociology, 63* (6), 597-606.

House, J.S., Landis, K.R., and Umberson, D. (1988). "Social relationships and health", *Science, 241,* 540—545.

Ignatius, Emmi; Marja Kokkonen (2007). "Factors Contributing to Verbal Self-disclosure", *Nordic Psychology*. *59* (4), 362-391.

Jaurard, J.M. (1971). *Self-disclosure: An Experimental Analysis of the Transparent Self.* New York: Wiley-Interscience.

John, O.P., and Gross, J.J. (2004). "Healthy and unhealthy emotion regulation: Personality processes, individual differences, and life span development", *Journal of Personality, 72(6),* 1301-1334.

Knapp, M.L., and Hall, J.A. (1997). *Nonverbal Communication in Human Interaction* (4th Ed.). New York: Harcourt Brace.

Knox, S., Hess, S., Petersen, D., and Hill, C.E. (1997). "A qualitative analysis of client perceptions of the effects of helpful therapist self-disclosure in long term therapy", *Journal of Counselling Psychology, 44*, 274-283.

Lane J. and Wegner D. (1995). "The cognitive consequences of secrecy", *Journal of Personality and Social Psychology, 69,* 237–253.

Lauer, Robert H. and Jeanette C. Lauer. (2000). *Marriage and Family: The Quest for Intimacy. (4).* Boston: McGraw Hill.

Lougheed, J.P., and Hollenstein, T. (2012). "A limited repertoire of emotion regulation strategies is associated with internalizing problems in adolescence", *Social Development, 21*, 704–721.

Lepor, S.J., Ragan, J. and Scott, J. (2000). "Talking facilitates Cognitive-emotional processes of adaptation to an acute stressor", *Journal of Personality and Social Psychology, 78* (3), 499-508.

Mahalik, J.R., Van Ormer, E.A., and Simi, N.L. (2000). "Ethical issues in using self-disclosure in feminist therapy", In M.M. Brabeck (Ed.), *Practicing Feminist Ethics in Psychology* (189-201). Washington DC: American Psychological Association.

McLaughlin, K.A., Hatzenbuehler, M.L., Mennin, D.S., and Nolen-Hoeksema, S. (2011). "Emotion dysregulation and adolescent psychopathology: A prospective study", *Behaviour Research and Therapy*, *49*(9), 544-554.

Moore, S.A., Zoellner, L.A., and Mollenholt, N. (2008). "Are expressive suppression and cognitive reappraisal associated with stress-related symptoms?", *Behaviour Research and Therapy, 46*, 993–1000.

Myers M.W., Laurent S.M. and Hodges S.D. (2014). "Perspective taking instructions and self-other overlap: Different motives for helping", *Motivation and Emotion, 38,* 224–234.

Omarzu, J. (2000). "A disclosure decision model: Determining how and when individuals will self-disclose", *Personality and Social Psychology Review, 4*, 174-185.

Pennebaker, J.W., and O'Heeron, R.C. (1984). "Confiding in others and illness rate among spouses of suicide and accidental death victims", *Journal of Abnormal Psychology, 93*, 473-476.

Pomeranz, E.; Wang, Q. (2009). "The Role of parental Control in Children's Development in Western and East Asia Countries". *Current Directions in Psychological Science, 18* (5), 285-289.

Schwarzer, R., and Leppin, A. (1991). "Social support and health: A theoretical and empirical overview", *Journal of Social and Personal Relationships, 8*, 99–127.

Seeman, T. (2001). "How do others get under our skin? In C.D. Ryff and B.H. Singer (Eds.), *Emotion, Social Relationships, and Health,* 189–210. New York: Oxford University Press.

Stricker, G., and Fisher, M., (Eds.). (1990). *Self-disclosure in the Therapeutic Relationship*. New York: Springer Science Business Media.

Thompson, R.A. (1994). "Emotion regulation: A theme in search of definition", *Monographs of the Society for Research in Child Development, 59*, 250–283.

Uchino, B., Cacioppo, J.T., and Kiekolt-Glaser, J.K. (1996). "The relationship between social support and physiological processes: A review with emphasis in underlying mechanisms and implications for health", *Psychological Bulletin, 119,* 488–531.

Underwood, B., Moore, B.S. and Rosenhan, D.L. (1973). "Affect and self-gratification", *Developmental Psychology, 8*, 209–214.

Waring, E.M. (1987). "Self-disclosure in cognitive marital therapy", In V.J. Derlega and J.H. Berg (Eds.), *Self-disclosure: Theory, Research and Therapy* (285-305) New York: Plenum.

Webb, T.L., Miles, E., and Sheeran, P. (2012). "Dealing with feeling: A meta-analysis of the effectiveness of strategies derived from the process model of emotion regulation", *Psychological Bulletin, 138*, 775–808.

Yovetich, N.A., and Drigotas, S.M. (1999). "Secret transmission: A relative intimacy hypothesis", *Personality and Social Psychology Bulletin, 25*, 1135-1146.

Zur, O. (2007). *Boundaries in Psychotherapy: Ethical and Clinical Explorations*, Washington, DC: American Psychological Association.

Zur, O., Williams, M.H., Lehavot, K., and Knapp, S. (2009). "Psychotherapist Self-Disclosure and Transparency in the Internet Age", *Professional Psychology: Research and Practice, 40(1)*, 22-30.

17

The Role of Empowerment in a School-based Community Service Programme

Kalpana Sahoo

In today's globalized era, personal intellectual advancement must go hand in hand with broader goals of sustainable development, poverty reduction, peace and human rights. The recent economic crisis has highlighted societal commitment to education, underscored by the decision of some of the leading economic powers to spend massively on education as a sound investment for economic recovery and growth. But it has also highlighted the fact that society has endowed its educational institutions with greater social responsibilities and the expectations are high. It must start its journey from the grassroot level. Social responsibility might mean, as it relates to education, so that it must be creating a more "socially responsible education" can be better understood. Education is the sector which is the most eligible and socially rewarding effort to be looked upon to discharge its social responsibility. Supporting education at any level will mean, re-energized education sector which can transform our country into a true knowledge power and realize a future of prosperity and sustainable growth. We now look to education not just to educate our children and youth, but to bring us out of poverty and set us on the path to peace and sustainable development. It is the food for thought to analysis whether institutions of higher education carry through on their growing responsibilities in the domain of socio-economic development. For that reason, these responsibilities require a radical re-shaping of the dominant higher educational system and philosophy. Producing the leaders of tomorrow and instilling in them the values and knowledge, it is necessary to building a more sustainable future, that it is also the social responsibility of institutions of higher education to take on an anticipatory role—to foresee and alert society to emerging trends and, ideally, to help prevent major crises before they happen.

Education has a strategic importance in the current era; meanwhile it can be viewed as a systematic strategy which is used to create desired changes in individual behaviour in society. One large advantage is present in students is that Indian maximum youth falls in the age range of 18-25. This group is the so-called Gen Y, the Net Generation. This group is the most tech-savvy within the general population. These youth power should be properly used in understanding the social action of organizations. Young people are concerned about their world and want to have a voice and feel that they have power to make a difference. Community Service-learning is unique in that it brings together all students who are at all different levels. It starts with the students as focal point and each student is valuable to contribute. Bhaerman, Cordell and Gomez (1998) believe that service learning is not only as programme, but rather than as instructional strategy, a philosophy and a process. Community engagement pedagogies, often called "service learning," are ones that combine learning goals and community service in ways that can enhance both student growth and the common good.

The article highlights a community service learning assignment as a means of promoting students empowerment. It may result towards better teacher and student's engagement through their community service. In general, the school does not have any specific curricular for community service projects which may be integrated with academic calendar. If we talk about the public a government based educational system, there is no policy and regulation for community learning service. It is the responsibility for the teacher and the leader of the school to initiate in their academic curriculum. The student must be exposed to the ground reality of the social issues. In this process the teacher will create more social leaders for the society from the very beginning. This platform injects more leadership qualities among students. Students themselves feel more empowered. The activity will construct more autonomy and independence among the students. Research also formed that the cooperating teachers appears to be more influential person in the development of the student teacher (Coulon, 1994; Gonzalez and Carter, 1996).

One of the studies of teacher's stages of development, a number of researchers have noted that student teacher begins their experience with a concern for self, followed by a concern with feeling and then followed by student learning behaviour (Campbell & Wherthly, 1983).

Student Empowerment

The middle school years are challenging for many students (Simmons &

Bluth, 1987). Issues such as a lack of self-confidence, social problems such as bullying, and disengagement increases during early adolescents are pervasive (Goldring & Rosen, 2004). How do school environments, pedagogy, and curricular practices impact these learners? Service learning is a teaching and learned tool that shows promise in engaging, motivating, and empowering early adolescents. Service learning can benefit student's personal development and can enhance empowerment. Through this service-learning project, the students notice a notably more clear understanding of class content. It bridges the gap between theory and practice. **Student's empowerment** is any attitudinal, structural, and cultural activity, process or outcome where students of any age gain the ability, authority and agency to make decisions and implement changes in their own schools, learning and education, and in the education of other people, including fellow students of any age and adults throughout education. There are countless ways this can happen as well as many potential outcomes, all of which feature learning, teaching and leadership. *Student empowerment happens in schools child and students' empowerment happen outside of schools.* Student empowerment generally happens through *student authorization* and *student action.* Student authorization, which is part of the cycle of engagement, happens when students acquire the knowledge and positions they need to affect schools.

Children are the future of the society. They are the architecture of the community. During this time, greater independence from parents and on increase in peer influence combined with changes in physical, social and psychological sphere in the minds of the children. Specifically, the school children must be vulnerable to maximum opportunity where they have the chance to begin to develop a sense of self-empowerment and social orientation toward others. However, the students must successfully integrate their increased need of autonomy with their drive for affection.

Service learning is a social progress where more students can be engaged. They will be exposed to service opportunities. There are many benefits for students, schools and the community. It is about courage, compassion, change, challenge, creativity, and connections. Students learn to decipher and understand complex social issues in our society. Service learning is about teaching for social responsibility.

Service-learning can nurture a lifelong commitment to civic participation and social justice. Quality service-learning is linked to the curriculum—student-centred and student-driven. Students have ownership of their own learning. It is applied, hands-on, and experiential learning. This can empower students for meaningful social change. Learning takes on new meaning because it is authentic, holistic and constructive learning.

Experience is the best teacher. The Chinese proverb says "I hear, and I forget, I see, and I remember. I act and I understand. Our educational process is a one-way learning process. Education must be continually changing experiment and learning as a continuous learning process.

It also indicates students serving in community-based helping organization. For example, hospital, nursing homes, handicapped and retired centre, old age home and connected with some NGO. A community service programme can be designed in two ways. One, is formally planned where community service is considered part of the school's official academic requirements. Second, is more spontaneous alternative tendency to serve for society.

Levinson (1994) indicates three broad theoretical rationales for community service:

1. Community service as experimental education.
2. Community service as means to promote adolescent psychological development.
3. Community service to foster active and informed citizenship.

Working with youth who have experienced serious personal trauma necessitates a programme rooted in social work that offers a resilience-oriented form of intervention. Addressing low self-esteem, poor self-confidence, and other harmful self-perception issues is integral in ultimately targeting positive health outcomes. Bridges programming gives youth new avenues of communication. Additionally, it equips them with new ways of coping with the tensions they experience as a result of the trauma they have faced, building confidence. "We stress the development of confidence as an antidote to this worldview that tells them the world is unsafe and dangerous," says Dr. Abramovitz. "But not only that, it helps decrease any sense of shame they might have, which is an important part of dealing with traumatized youth, and essential for their healing."

The model can be proposed by author (see Fig. on next page).

Rationale of the Study on Community Service Learning

Why school and other educational institutes will promote community service learning? There are several reasons which supports community service programmes can be an effective strategy for enhancing the student's empowerment. **First**, students' academic curriculum is completely a

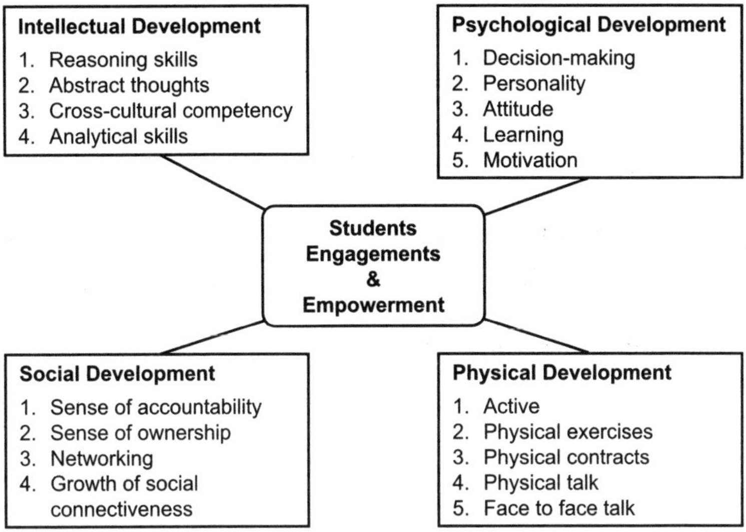

theoretical in nature. Most of the learning pedagogy is based on lecture model. There is no effective interaction between teacher and student for understanding and assimilating the concept.

In lecture mode learning, teachers vomit all the jargons to the students even if they are given life time examples. But sometimes the students are unable to reconnect them. Hence there is a huge gap between the theory and practice. Our education system never encourages the end way feedback or multiple feedback (360-degree feedback) from different stakeholders. So, students gain knowledge for the examination point of view. They are unable to connect with the social relevance and its significance in our day to day life.

Second, their community service activities promote the students to practice reflection. Poland and Anglin (1993) have noted that their ability to reflect on one's teaching can enhance teachers' stage development. It gives student teacher opportunities to extend their visions of the teaching role to encompass that of community liaison.

Third, with respect to the engagement of service learning project, teachers need to take more risk and will take the new path for teaching pedagogy. The learning outcomes include development of leadership and problem-solving skills, connecting the theoretical with the practical, and educating students for citizenship.

Fourth, students transition from the role of student-only to a sense of adulthood where they take on a challenge facing the community and used their knowledge to offer expert advice. This intangible benefit pays dividends to students as they transition from the classroom to their careers.

Fifth, it improves inter-personal and human relations skills which are increasingly viewed as the most important skills in achieving success in professional and personal spheres. It provides guidance and experience for future career choice.

Community service learning really gives a lifetime experience for the students. It boosts their self-efficacy and their passion can be integrated with their purpose. Students can perform better when their confidence level is high. They derive more joy and happiness being involved in that activity. High self-efficacy leads to effort and persistence in dealing with issues and obtain higher goals. While low self-efficacy led to hopeless and stop working. (Bandura, 1999). People with high self-efficacy look at issues as a challenge to learn more, not a treat that they should avoid it. They spread their interests in the area where they do things and they feel severe commitment to do it. Students' aim is to gain new things with fun and joy. This community learning programme really boosts their self-efficacy as well as happiness.

Self-Efficacy and Happiness

The expectancy for classroom success, or self-efficacy, involves beliefs about how well one can successfully perform academic activities and enhance cognitive skills. It is directly associated with behavioural, cognitive, and motivational engagement in academic practices. Self-efficacy influences the learning strategies and intrinsic motivation, (Bandura, 1997). If students have all of the above, and perceive it important, higher cognitive achievement is attained. At this point, students should be aware of self-efficacy in terms of its value and it being positively linked to teaching and learning. Cone studied the effect of service learning on enhancing self-efficacy beliefs of pre-service elementary teachers. The findings indicated that service learning significantly influenced pre-service teachers and their expectancy in achieving equitable teaching and learning outcomes (Cone, 2009a). Bandura explained the role of self-efficacy and how it is linked to educational outcomes 'as a situation-specific construct concerned with how an individual judges his/her ability to organize and successfully performed in prospective situations. Not only is self-efficacy enhanced in the context of service learning, but civic engagement.

Many research points to inclusive classroom environments, with greater parental involvement, and student empowerment. Additionally, student engagement must not be viewed in isolation, but must include school, teacher, and cultural contexts. The above-mentioned contexts for learning (school, teacher, culture) are also very important in building strong service learning environments. Student leadership, voice and community involvement is linked to increased engagement, and these are fundamental aspects of service learning (Billig, 2011). Newman's concepts of school belonging and authentic work are linked directly to service learning. By involving students in all aspects of school and community functioning and building an inclusive community, this research on engagement supports a direct connection to the authentic, place based work of service learning.

For Vanderbilt University's Janet S. Eyler (winner of the 2003 Thomas Ehrlich Faculty Award for Service Learning) and Dwight E. Giles, Jr., it is:

> "a form of experiential education where learning occurs through a cycle of action and reflection as students. seek to achieve real objectives for the community and deeper understanding and skills for themselves. In the process, students link personal and social development with academic and cognitive development, experience enhances understanding; understanding leads to more effective action."

Carlisle (2011) focused on students who built positive relationships with teachers, other students and school staff in service learning experiences. Researchers recognize that adolescence is a period when students tend to disregard adult role models and focus on their peers instead (Carlisle, 2011; Becker & Luthar, 2002). These happen primarily during unstructured times such as locker and lunch breaks. Researchers have studied how developing healthy relationships between teachers, schools staff and students, through participation in service learning projects, can combat some of these problems. Key findings include improvements in student behaviour in terms of lessening bullying and office referrals, and an increase in students expressing a need for healthy relationships (Carlisle, 2011). By synthesizing theory and practice, this educational method provides a distinctive, meaningful, and influential life experience. Students build relationships, solve problems, value a sense of community, and gain self-awareness. Service-learning is beyond memorable; it can influence one's career path and enhance civic responsibility. Service-learning extends learning beyond the academic term; it lays the foundation for continual personal growth throughout the student's academic experience and beyond. According Jane Kendall service-learning is a philosophy of "human growth and purpose, a social vision, an approach to community, and way of knowing." (Kendall, 1990).

The implications for this literature review include a deep understanding of how service learning can impact students. This understanding can be applied at the school, district, state and national level. In addition, this review lays the groundwork for further study in the experiences of early adolescent students engaged in service learning. Service learning is served to engage learners in developmentally appropriate pedagogy and this can in turn lead to greater personal development in students.

References

Bhaerman, R. and Cordell, K., and Gomez B. (1998). *The role of service-learning in educational reform*, Raleigh, North Carolina: National Society for Experiential Education, Simon Schuster Custom Publishing.

Bandura, A. (1997). "Exercise of personal and collective efficacy in changing societies", In: Bandura, A. (editor). *Self-efficacy in the Changing Societies*, Cambridge: Cambridge University Press, pp. 1-45.

Billig, S. (2011). "Making the most of your time: Implementing the K-12 Service-Learning standards for quality practice", *Prevention Researcher*, *18*(1) 8-13.

Cone, N. (2009a). "A bridge to developing efficacious science teachers of all students: Community-based service-learning supplemented with explicit discussions and activities about diversity", *Journal of Science Teacher Education*, *20*, 265-383.

Cone, N. (2009b). "Community-based service-learning as a source of personal self-efficacy: Preparing preservice elementary teachers to teach science for diversity", *School Science and Mathematics*, *109*(1): 20-30.

Cone, N. (2009c). "Preservice elementary teachers' self-efficacy beliefs about equitable science teaching: Does service learning make a difference", *Journal of Elementary Science Education*, *21*(2): 25-34.

Carlisle, M. (2011). "Healthy relationships and building developmental assets in middle school students", *Canadian Journal of Education*, *34*(3), 18-32.

Campbell, P., and Wheatley, G. (1983). "A model for helping student teachers", *Mathematics Teacher*, *76*(1), 60-63.

Coulon, S.C. (1994). The Effect of post-teaching conferences on instructional behaviour of students teachers. Papers presented at the annual meeting of the American Educational Reasearch Association, San Francisco.

Simmons, R.G., and Blyth, D.A. (1987). *Moving into adolescence: The impact of pubertal change and school context.* Hawthorne, NY: Aldine de Gruyter.

https://www.marquette.edu/youth-empowerment-program/program_social_work_model.shtml assessed on 3.2.2020.

18

Development of Sustainable Intervention Programme in Autism Spectrum Disorder

A Case Study

Garima Gupta, Anushka Singh, Monika Shukla, and
Usha Verma Srivastava

Autism Spectrum Disorder

Autism Spectrum Disorders (ASD) is a neuro-developmental disorder. It is characterized by lack of interest, impairment in communication and social interaction with restricted and repeated behaviour (Zwaigenbaum, 2001). According to Diagnostic Statistical Manual of Mental Disorders-Text Revision (DSM-IV-TR), three types of disorders are categorized under ASD: Autistic disorder, Asperser's disorder and Pervasive Developmental Disorder Not Otherwise Specified (PPD-NOS). Additionally, it is also classified according to its severity i.e. mild, moderate, and severe. The Centre for Disease Control and Prevention (CDC) reported that about 1 in 88 children had been identified with ASD in the United States (CDC, 2012). The terms Autism and Autism Spectrum Disorders (ASDs) are used interchangeably in this paper.

People with ASD reflect many symptomatic manifestations in terms of positive and negative behaviours such as hand flapping, emotional meltdowns, avoidance of eye contact. They are skilled at perceiving details as opposed to whole gestalts. They perform better than their peers. This was proved in a study where ASD children demonstrated better performance on WISC-IV by matching a pattern by taking blocks that are all white, all red, or mixtures of red and white and putting them together (Shah & Frith, 1993). They were found better on EFT than neuro-typical children (Baron-Cohen, 1998; Shan & Frith, 1993).

The estimated prevalence of ASD in U.K. is 1 per cent and 1.5 per cent in the US (Taylor, Jick, & MacLaughlin, 2013) but the recent data based on the surveys showed an increase in the prevalence of ASD worldwide. The prevalence was estimated to be 61.9/10,000 globally in 2012 (RCI, India). The estimated prevalence in India is more than 2 million (Rudra, Belmonte, Soni, Banerjee, Mukerji, & Chakrobarti, 2014). However, the reported studies on ASD are largely from hospital-based data and therefore the prevalence estimates of this disorder lacks information in India (Kumar, Juneja, & Mishra, 2016; Mamidala, Polinedi, Rajesh, Vallamkonda, *et al.*, 2013., Raina, Chander, Bhardwaj, Kumar, Sharma, *et al.*, 2017). Juneja and Sairam (2018) have reported that the prevalence in rural areas was 0.90 per cent, 0.6 per cent in hilly regions, 1.01 per cent in urban areas, 0.1 per cent in tribal areas and 0.61 per cent in the coastal regions.

Etiology of Autism

Yet no known single cause for ASD has been reported. Numerous studies have demonstrated the role of both genetic and environmental factors. The risk factors are common in India and significantly influence the development outcome of the child. Pre- and perinatal events like disorders of pregnancy, labour complications, fetal distress, low birth weight and premature birth, advanced maternal age, fetal distress and gestational respiratory infections are associated with ASD (Mamidala *et al.*, 2013). Another attempt made by Verma, Chakraborti, Karmakar, Bandyopadhyay, Singh, *et al.* (2014) concluded that both male and female have a different genetic effect that might contribute to the sex-ratio differences and molecular pathology of the disorder. However, genetic association and gene-gene interaction analyses advocated probable involvement of ITGB3 and TPH2 in the pathophysiology of ASD (Singh, Chandra, Guhathakurta, Sinha, Chatterjee, *et al.*, 2013).

The American Psychiatric Association (APA) and DSM-V suggest that early diagnosis may exist before age six (Almulla, 2013). Though, most of the children don't receive a diagnosis until much later (Lord, Risi, DiLavore, Shulman, Thurm, & Pickles, 2006). The first ruling out is the diagnosis of intellectual development disorder or global developmental delay. Depending upon a broad range of symptoms, various models have been developed to understand the underlying reason for the development of ASD, as well as to treat it both at symptomatic level, along with at familial as well as societal level.

Intervention Programme for Autism Spectrum Disorder

Intervention is considered as a professional help given to the people who experience traumatic event or crisis. It is an external process that has an effect on modifying individuals affect, behaviour, and cognition. Latest scientific researches revealed that early identification and early detection have a pivotal role in management and treatment of ASD children (AAP: National Research Council, 2001; Dwason, 2008; Filipek *et al.*, 2000). Intervention should be planned, appropriate and must be sensitive to the needs and perception of a child with autism. Lam and Aman (2007) suggested that ASD consist of a wide array of symptoms and challenging behaviour. The behaviour is controlled by pharmacological treatments (Advokat, Mayville, & Matson, 2000; Singh, Matson, Cooper, Dixon, Sturmey, 2005), psycho-educational interventions (Dawson & Osterling, 1997; Smith, 1999). These psycho-educational interventions are the foremost treatment approach and are based on time and settings. The intervention should be organized, targeted, specific and operationally and maintaining consistency in programme. The primary task in intervention is to control challenging behaviour. The neuro-developmental theory has pointed out the increased brain plasticity of very young children and the potential opportunities for overcoming neuro-developmental deficits within early years (Huttenlocher, 1979; Nelson, Grether, Croen, Dambrosia, Dickens, Jelliffe, Hansen, & Phillips, 2001). Intensive intervention given in the first 3 to 4 years of age seemed to yield significant benefits despite its nature of severity in impairment (Landa & Garret-Mayer, 2006; Wetherby, Woods, Allen, Cleary, Dickinson, & Lord, 2004). A number of studies have reported significant gains by early intervention in various developmental domains for children with ASD (Ben, Itzchak & Zachor, 2007; Lord *et al.*, 2005; Magiati, Charman, & Howlin, 2007) that led to progress in cognitive skills, adaptive skills and reduced severity (Eikeseth, Smith, Jahr, & Eldevik, 2007; Zachor, Ben, Itzchak, Rabinovitch, & Lahat, 2007). Usually, goals of the intervention are related to social skills, communication, compliance, ritualistic and stereotypical behaviour (Matson, Dixon, & Matson, 2005; Matson, & Wilikins, 2007).

Apart from aforesaid therapeutic interventions, the child's focus and motivation are essential. To get the child to train or focus on the skills, different behavioural techniques are used. Further didactic training situation where the adult trainer or therapist follows and uses predefined activities and resources during the training session is encouraged. The specific behavioural techniques, such as prompts and reinforcement used in the session, are also planned strategically.

It becomes a challenge for families of children with ASD to teach social skills to children who are not able to assimilate these skills through naturally occurring reciprocal social interactions (Attwood, 1998; Bashe & Kirby, 2001; Holiday-Willey, 1999; Powers & Poland, 2003; Szatmari, Bremner, & Nagy, 1989; Shaked & Yirmiya, 2003). The literature has mentioned the extensive use of Applied Behaviour Analysis (ABA) on preschool children. This intensive behavioural programme is based on the concepts of operant conditioning through the use of a reward system in behavioural modification. While TEACHC (Treatment of Education of Autistic and related Communication Handicapped Children) and Picture Exchange Communication System (PECS) where visual cues are utilised in educational settings (Almulla, 2013). PECS is a systematic approach for training communication to autistic children. In this, visual graphic techniques are used for hand to hand exchange of pictures and also highly perspective user manual with its six levels to follow in the sequence.

However, many ASD children may benefit from occupational therapy, physiotherapy, and sensory integration therapy. Various other complementary and alternative treatments are biological therapies, diets, or chelation for the children, though; this has received less consideration for benefits (CDC, 2012).

Parents as an Essential Tool for Intervention

Parent-child interactions usually occur in different settings and parents impressions about their level of impairment may influence how they interact with their children (Konstantareas, Zazdeman, Homatidis, & McCabe, 1998). It appears that the parenting process has its subsequent role in the development of behaviour of children with ASDs (Carter *et al.*, 2007; Siller & Sigman, 2002). Parental involvement has a major role in the early intervention programme and the treatment of their child (Mahony & Wiggers, 2007). Ingersoll and Hambric (2010) reported the influence of the mental health of parents' too.

Parent-mediated training occurs throughout the day, hence facilitates generalization of acquired skills. In a comprehensive review Parsons, Cordier, Vaz, and Lee, (2017) reported that parents who get proper training, gain skills in the delivery of interventions, thereby improving joint attention, social communication and behaviours of their children with ASD.

In a very significant study of Jocelyn *et al.* (1998), parents of ASD children have received 12 weeks of intervention training through lectures and on-site consultation by the therapist. After the intervention period, the parents felt that they had acquired more knowledge on autism. The trained parents were satisfied and learned positive control in the parent-child relationship and their children progressed in the dimension of language acquisition. Ergnuer-Tekinolp and Akkok (2004) conducted a parents training programme (as a cognitive-behavioural training programme) including understanding their stress and coping strategies, problem-solving skills, relaxation training, positive thinking, and developing social support. It was found that after the training programme, the mother was more relaxed and revealed a more positive outlook.

The most common intervention for ASD is parental education. The most widely used education programmes are courses developed by the Canadian Hanen Centre (Hanen, 2012). This takes eight sessions for parents and three home visits by the speech-language pathologist. During this visit, the interaction between child and parent is videotaped, and feed-back are provided to parents to improve communication. The Hanen course is based on a developmental approach. It teaches responsive strategies to parents adding some behavioural techniques to stimulate communication learning within the frames of child-focused natural interaction at home (Hanan, 2012).

ComAlong named parental course include eight sessions focusing on responsive strategies and environmental teaching but also puts a significant focus on the use of augmentative communication strategies in-home setting (AKKtiv, 2012). The parents use aided language modelling with the help of picture boards (AKKtiv, 2012; Jonsson, Kristoffersson, Ferm, & Thunberg, 2011).

Effect of Parental Training on Children with ASD

Several models for intervening in parent-child interactions have been developed over the years (Marfo, Cynthia, Dedrick, & Barbour, 1998). Most of them were developed to aid in the stimulation of developmental competence in both the parents and the children. For the parents, the idea was to enhance interactive skills to develop higher levels of responsiveness in them, and for children, the hope was to facilitate their optimal psychological and social development.

Lovaas, Koegel, Simmons, and Long (1973) suggested that parental involvement in the treatment of their children is very urgent. Anan, Warner, McGillivary, Chong, and Hines (2008) reported that parents act as a therapist. Training of ABA to parents help children approves their cognitive and adaptive functioning. Gillet and LeBlanc (2007) trained parents for their non-verbal children with autism to elicit vocalization. Parents were trained to use videotapes for instructing their child with autism and the implementation of the procedure. Significant improvement was noted in terms of language acquisition.

Matson and Smith (2008) reported that intensive behavioural intervention for young children with autism is the inclusion of comprehensive package treatment of 20 to 40 hours per week over a year. Hence, teaching parents to use various strategies and involving them in intervention is very beneficial. Though the use of ABA is most effective and conventional approach (Matson, Mahan, & Matson, 2009), use of psychotropic drugs with a combination of other methods yields good results (Johnson *et al.*, 2007). Osborne *et al.* (2008) suggested that training to parents through behaviour management skill is an effective strategy. Butter (2007) reported that significant improvement in daily living skills and a decrement in non-compliance and irritation in ASD children was observed when training was given to parents for irritability, aggression, self-injury and tantrums. Similar findings that training to parents improved their children by being a good host at get together, handling of bullying, developing friendship, peer entry and exit skills was also reported by Laugesen, Frankel, Mogil, and, Dillon (2008).

This study utilizes multi-method therapeutic approaches and attempts to develop a sustainable intervention programme for children with ASD. Below this, a real case study has been presented with a wide array of a therapeutic programme that caused improvement in the child.

Case Report

The case study details a comprehensive sustainable treatment regime of an 11-year-old boy named Tejas (Pseudo name), diagnosed with ASD. The psychiatrist made the diagnosis and referred for psychotherapeutic interventions.

Presenting Complaints

When coming for the treatment, Tejas didn't respond when called by name. He didn't make any eye contact, was restless, moving all the time and didn't sit at any place for a while. He jumped constantly showing repetitive behaviour such as hand biting, tapping, rotating and shaking objects like pen and Echolalia. He was very nervous and showed less interest in talking to the therapist as the parents briefed the problem of the child. Parents reported that with a slight change in daily routine, he gets upset, frustrated, irritated and aggressive. He shows tantrums and crying.

Assessment

The follow-up assessments were conducted after every thirty days to monitor change in behaviour. Further, after meeting with the parents, it was confirmed by the psychologist that the child has the impairments of social interaction, social communication, social imagination, and tendency towards repetitive behaviour patterns which indicates ASD. The assessment was done using the following tools:

1. Childhood autism rating scale (15 items) was administered with the help of parents and severe level of autistic symptoms was observed.
2. The functional analysis of behaviour was done, and analysis revealed repetitive stereotypic behaviour was self-stimulatory and maintained by automatic reinforcement (occurs independently of the social mediation by others—bite relieves the itch). Temper tantrums and adamantine behaviour were maintained by positive reinforcement.

Case Conceptualization

The treatment was planned by integrating several approaches such as behavioural, sensory integration, occupational therapy, and psycho-educating parents. It was assumed that autistic behaviour was reinforced as the parents and family members are unaware of the problems. Further, it also satisfies some sensory need of the child that can be treated using negative reinforcement or by providing alternative behavioural interventions to meet those needs.

The Course of Treatment and Assessment of Progress

The initial pre-requisite goal was to improve seating behaviour, to establish and maintain eye-contact, to compliance to demands without getting distracted in therapeutic settings, and also to lessen the frequency of hand biting behaviour in a therapy setting. The problems that were taken into account during the intervention included aggressiveness or have tantrums (whenever he comes along with his father) continually running around, and self-injurious behaviour (hand biting).

Total ninety-six sessions of child and twenty-four sessions of parents were conducted over a period of six months. Play therapies, Sensory

Integration, Differential reinforcement, Occupational therapy, Social skills, Speech therapy, were included as an intervention programme. The intervention planned for parents were Cognitive Behaviour Therapy, Parent education related to disorder (Autism) and Family early intervention programme, Applied Behaviour Analysis (in collaboration with child), Eye movement desensitization and reprocessing (EMDR, in collaboration with the therapist).

First of all, in session one, the child demonstrated no preference to play with a particular toy. He did many activities, such as biting his hands, walking around the room. In the next fifteen sessions, sensory integration was given and was found child enjoying the same gradually. Sensory integration therapies utilizes play activities, and are designed to change how the brain reacts to touch, sound, sight and movement. It helps to calm down children when they are agitated.

Mother was instructed to use the Wilbarger brushing protocol, several times a day. Tejas's mother reported a decrease in sensory defensiveness and anxiety, decreased fear or discomfort of being touched after using this protocol. She also reported improved ability to transition between daily activity, improved attention and focus, enhanced coordination and better self-regulation. Differential reinforcement was given for appropriate response and extinction of undesired response. Hand biting activity was improved, and the mother was asked to provide chew gums to manage his self-stimulatory behaviour.

Jacobsen muscle relaxation and mindfulness were given to parents in session 36 as the parents were stressed out. Their thought pattern was also challenged. In further sessions, CBT and EMDR were administered on parents with the help of an expert. Almost all sessions, the parents were also participating in active and collaborated manner. Parents were asked to use cards and schedule to help the child overcoming his tantrums related to routine issues.

In session 65, ABA, social skills and occupational therapy [activities of daily living (ADLs) and instrumental activities of daily activities (IADLs)] was planned. In this session, the child was asked to tell stories with the help of therapist and parents, so that understanding of his interaction with his surrounding, including person and things will improve. ADLs and ISDLs activities and activities in Education, work, leisure, play and social participation were included. During a therapeutic session, the child used many occupational activities that helped him in resolving his sensory issues related to the tactile, proprioceptive, auditory, and visual, olfactory and vestibular system. His practices included jumping on the trampoline, jumping games, bicycle riding, throwing and catching a heavy ball, pulling and pushing activities, carrying or moving heavy objects, imitating animal walks that require substantial work (crab, bear), stimulated his proprioceptive system. For improving his tactile awareness, game based on clay type materials, drawing on mirror, finger painting, drawing shapes with fingers in sand, foam, massage, vibrating toys, using different textures for playing, playing hide and seek games, asking the child to explain shapes drawn on his/her back with fingers, finding objects from a bag were used. The child was asked to listen to his/her favourite soft music on headphones to reduce auditory sensitivity like OM chanting, Gaytri Mantra for reducing sensitivity against vestibular senses, games, for example, linear swinging on a swing or ball on facedown position, throwing and catching objects while swinging, jumping games and rolling activities were used. For improving his eye-hand co-ordination, i.e. ocular-motor control toys and pens with lights were used. The activities included such as, throwing balls at a target while swinging, ball throwing and catching, bubble-blowing which improved his ocular-motor control. Ball catching was played on the floor or a ball or while sitting in different positions to strengthen his postural control and motor skills. Activities, for instance, creating shapes by tearing papers with both hands, making shapes with play dough, cutting papers with scissors, making a necklace by placing beads through a string, improved his bilateral motor co-ordination.

In the session, 70 the child himself greeted everyone in the child, was oriented towards sessions and encouraged to learn "sorry" and "thank you".

In the session, 75 the child was made to interact with parents and peers of the same age group to learn and respond to the situation, despite his lack of interest.

In between session 90 to 96, the child made many friends, and talked voluntarily and played cooperatively with them. The eye contact was improved.

After 95 comprehensive sessions, significant improvement was observed in the boy. He finally got admission to a public school. The parents reported that he was ready to face challenges, but few sessions were continued with his parents.

With successful intervention in 120 sessions, the boy was able to sit in a place and learned to perform the assigned activities for 30 minutes. His other behaviour such as maintaining eye contact, responding to his name was improved while jumping and running around. Nail-biting was reduced significantly. The mother learnt the techniques of distracting and guiding him to other activity.

These all improved activities suggest that an ample therapeutic plan brings changes in the person with ASD. However, the available evidence from a variety of programme indicates that early intervention leads to better therapeutic outcomes (NIMH, 2004). The studies mentioned in the literature have emphasized on training and use of social skills of parents for sustainable rehabilitation. Researches have suggested a various multi-skills approach where a range of teaching methods are available, e.g., Speech and Language Therapy, Occupational Therapy, Applied Behaviour Analysis (ABA) etc. The present study has utilized various interventions such as ABA, CBT, Occupational therapy, Family therapy, and Social skills which have also received considerable attention by the researchers too (Attwood, 2004; Moree & Davis, 2010; Sze & Wood, 2008). In the present case study, the child was of eleven years old, and numerous studies have demonstrated that the therapeutic interventions have promising effect if the child enters in the programme at a very early age (Panerai *et al.*, 2009).

Discussion

Autism spectrum disorder (ASD) is considered as a heterogeneous group of disorders that need accurate and detailed assessment. It requires a complete history from family and an adequate observation period for improvement. The success of the therapy depends not only on a single treatment but various therapies or treatment is used to resolve different problems. Therefore, early diagnosis and subsequent intervention are suggested. Early diagnosis of autism allows the design of early and effective intervention programmes for better long-term outcome of the individual (Fernell, Eriksson, & Gillberg, 2013). Planning of the therapy or treatment needed the involvement of social connections. Raising an ASD child puts a lot of strain on the parents and caregivers due to increased responsibility and social stigma. The stress of caring for an ASD child can influence the psychological and emotional wellbeing of parents (Divan, Vajaratkar, Desai, Strik-Lievers, & Patel, 2012).

Various studies report successful outcome using comprehensive eclectic interventions (Magiati, Tay & Howlin, 2012). However, these programmes are based on the cognitive, communicative and neurophysiological development, but the approaches based on the behavioural tradition or Applied Behaviour Analysis helps in improving that learned behaviour. The viability of the programmes should be more child-focused. It may focus on a child's motivation and interest and emphasises the communication between the parent and the child and are implemented in-home setting, and clinic sessions.

The finding of this study is in line that early diagnosis (Chambers, Wetherby, Stronach, Njongwe, Kauchali, & Grrinker, 2017; Chinawa, Manyike, Aniwada, *et al.*, 2016; Wetherby, Guthrie, Woods, *et al.*, 2014) and intervention (Bal, Kim, Cheong, & Lord, 2015; Smith, 1999) are imperative to facilitate development in persons with ASD. The present study has used a multi-skill training approach for the effective intervention of the child. Literature mentions that ASD children are often found inattentive, non-cooperative, aggressive and feels difficulty in engaging themselves.

Therefore, parents and school staffs are required to engage these children in significant and positive skill development to decrease disruptive behaviour. Another case by Agazzi, Tan, and Tan, (2013) on ASD children has reported the effectiveness of parent-child interaction and evidenced-based intervention. The results of the study described above suggested progress in child compliance and a decrease in disruptive behaviours. Additionally, parents improved their use of positive parenting strategies that helped to improve the parent-child relationship.

In conclusion, ASD is an extensive condition and can influence many factors of a child's life. There is a wide variety of treatment approach for ASD. The multi-method method with sensory-based interventions is used (Wilberger approach) to treat ASD children with the best care. The child and the family not only gets affected by ASD but also has straight and indirect cost implications on the nation as resources have to be utilized in providing health care, support for education, and rehabilitative services for these children (Barnett, & Masse, 2007). Therefore, it is recommended further, that psycho-education and proper training to families about autism such as how to manage and cope with it is essential. Support groups for the families might be of great benefit. Through education to families and giving them training, the stigma surrounding the disorder may be tackled. Increased awareness in communities about ASD may decrease stigma and encourage caregivers to seek help for children displaying symptoms of ASD.

References

Advokat, C.D., Mayville, E.A., and Matson, J.L. (2000). "Side effect profiles of atypical antipsychotics, typical antipsychotics or no psychotic medications in persons with mental retardation", *Research in Developmental Disabilities, 21*, 75–84.

Agazzi, H., Tan, R., and Tan, S.Y. (2013). "A Case Study of Parent-Child Interaction Therapy for the Treatment of Autism Spectrum Disorder", *Clinical Case Studies, 12*(6).

AKKtiv. http://www.akktiv.se (accessed 23 October 2012).

Almulla, N. (2013). "Diagnosis and Management of a 7-year Old Child with an Autism Spectrum Disorder (ASD) in Bahrain: A Case Study", *International Journal of Scientific Study, 1*(1), 33-37.

Anan, R.M., Warner, L.J., McGillivary, J.E., Chong, I.M., and Hines, S.J. (2008). "Group intensive family training (GIFT) for pre-schoolers with autism spectrum disorders", *Behavioural Interventions, 23*, 165–180.

Attwood, T. (1998). *Asperger's Syndrome: A guide for parents and professionals*, London: Jessica Kingsley Publishers.

Bal, V.H., Kim, S.H., Cheong, D., and Lord, C. (2015). "Daily living skills in individuals with autism spectrum disorder from 2 to 21 years of age", *Autism, 19*(7), 774-784.

Barnett, W.S., and Masse, L.N. (2007). "Comparative benefit-cost analysis of the Abecedarian programme and its policy implications", *Econ Educ Rev, 26*,113-25.

Baron-Cohen, S. (1998). "Does Autism Occur More Often in Families of Physicists, Engineers, and Mathematicians?", *Autism, 2*(3), 296-301.

Bashe, P.R. and Kirby, B.L. (2001). "The oasis guide to Asperger Syndrome: Advice, support, insight, and inspiration", New York: Crown Publishers.

Ben-Itzchak, E., Zachor, D.A. (2007). "The effects of intellectual functioning and autism severity on outcome of early behavioural intervention for children with autism", *Research in Developmental Disabilities, 28,* 287–303.

CDC, USA. (2012). "Facts, Autism Spectrum Disorders (ASD)", Centre for Disease Control and Prevention: Retrieved from https://www.cdc.gov/ncbddd/autism/index.html

Chambers, N.J., Wetherby, A.M., Stronach, S.T., Njongwe, N., Kauchali, S., and Grrinker, R.R. (2017). "Early detection of autism spectrum disorder in young Zulu-speaking children in South Africa", *Autism, 21*(5), 518-526.

Chinawa, J.M., Manyike, P.C., Aniwada, E.C., *et al.* (2016). "Prevalence and socioeconomic correlates of autism among children attending primary and secondary schools in South East Nigeria", *Afri Health Sci. 16*(4), 936-942.

Daley, T.C. (2004). "From symptom recognition to diagnosis: Children with autism in urban India", *Social Science Medicine, 58*, 1323-1335.

Dawson, G. (2008). "Early behavioural intervention, brain plasticity, and the prevention of autism spectrum disorder", *Development and Psychopathology, 20*, 775.

Dawson, G., and Osterling, J. (1997). "Early intervention in autism", In M. Guralnick (Ed.). *The Effectiveness of Early Intervention*. Baltimore: Brookes.

Divan, G., Vajaratkar, V., Desai, M.U., Strik-Lievers, L., Patel, V. (2012). "Challenges, coping strategies, and unmet needs of families with a child with autism spectrum disorder in Goa, India", *Autism Research, 5,* 190-200.

Eikeseth, S., Smith, T., Jahr, E., and Eledevik, S. (2007). "Outcome for children with autism who began intensive behavioural treatment between age four and seven: A comparison controlled study", *Behaviour Modification, 31*, 264–278.

Fernell, E., Eriksson, M.A., and Gillberg, C. (2013). "Early diagnosis of autism and impact on prognosis: A narrative review", *Clinical Epidemiology, 5,* 33-43.

Filipek, P.A., Accardo, P.J., Ashwal, S., Baranek, G.T., Cook, J.E. H., Dawson, G., *et al.* (2005). "Practice parameter: Screening and diagnosis of autism", *Neurology, 55*(4), 468–479.

Gillett, J., and Leblanc, L. (2007). "Parent-implemented Natural Language Paradigm to increase language and play in children with autism", *Research in Autism Spectrum Disorders, 1*, 247-255. 10.1016/j.rasd.2006.09.003.

Hanen centre. http://www.hanen.org (accessed 23 October 2012).

Holiday-Willey, L. (1999). *Pretending to be normal: Living with Asperger's Syndrome*. London and Philadelphia: Jessica Kingsley Publishers.

Huttenlocher, P.R. (1979). "Synaptic density in human frontal cortex-developmental changes and effects of aging", *Brain Res, 163*, 195–205.

Johnson, C.R., Handen, B.L., Butter, E., Wagner, A., Mulick, J., Sukhodolsky, D.G., Williams, S., Swiezy, N.A., Arnold, L.E., Aman, M.G., Scahill, L., Stigler, K.A., McDougle, C.J., Vitiello, B., and Smith, T. (2007). "Development of a parent training programme for children with pervasive developmental disorders", *Behavioural Interventions, 22*, 201-221.

Jonsson, A., Kristoffersson, L., Ferm, U., Thunberg, G. (2011). *The ComAlong communication boards: Parents' use and experiences of aided language stimulation. Augment Altern Commun., 27*(2), 103-16. doi: 10.3109/07434618.2011.580780.

Juneja, M., and Sairam, S. (2018). "Autism Spectrum Disorder: An Indian Perspective", *Creative Commons Attribution* 4.0.

Kumar, A., Juneja, M., and Mishra, D. (2016). "Prevalence of Autism Spectrum Disorders in Siblings of Indian Children with Autism Spectrum Disorders", *Journal of Child Neurology, 31*, 873-878.

Lam, K.S. L., Aman, M.G. (2007). "The Repetitive Behaviour Scale—Revised: Independent validation in individuals with autism spectrum disorders", *Journal of Autism and Developmental Disorders, 27*, 855–866.

Landa, R., and Garrett-Mayer, E. (2006). "Development in infants with autism spectrum disorders: A prospective study", *Journal of Child Psychology and Psychiatry, and Allied Disciplines, 47*, 629–638.

Laugesen, E.A., Frankel, F., Mogil, C., and Dillon, A.R. (2008). "Parent-assisted social skills training to improve friendships in teens with autism spectrum disorders", *Journal of Autism and Developmental Disorders 10.*1007/s10803-008-0664-5.

Lord, C., Risi, S., DiLavore, P. S, Shulman, C., Thurm, A., and Pickles, A. (2006). "Autism from 2 to 9 Years of Age", *Arch Gen Psychiatry, 63*(6), 694-701.

Lord, C., Wagner, A., Rogers, S., Szatmari, P., Aman, M., Charman, T., *et al.* (2005). "Challenges in evaluating psychosocial interventions for autistic spectrum disorders", *Journal of Autism and Developmental Disorders, 35*, 695–708.

Lovaas, O.I., Koegel, R. L, Simmons, J.Q., and Long, J.S. (1973). "Some generalization and follow-up measures on autistic children in behaviour therapy", *Journal of Applied Behaviour Analysis, 6*(1), 131-166.

Magiati, I., Charman, T., and Howlin, P. (2007). "A two-year prospective follow-up study of community-based early intensive behavioural intervention and specialist nursery provision for children with autism spectrum disorders", *Journal of Child Psychology and Psychiatry, 48*, 803–812.

Magiati, I., Tay, W.X., and Howlin, P. (2012). "Early comprehensive behaviourally based interventions for children with autism spectrum disorders: A summary of findings from recent reviews and meta-analyses", *Neuropsychiatry, 2*(6), 543-570.

Mamidala, M.P., Polinedi, A, P.T. V.P. K., Rajesh, N., Vallamkonda, O.R., *et al.* (2013). "Prenatal, perinatal and neonatal risk factors of Autism Spectrum Disorder: A comprehensive epidemiological assessment from India", *Res Dev Disabil. 34,* 3004-3013.

Marfo, K., Cynthia, F.D., Dedrick F, Barbour N. (1998).) "Mother-child interactions and the development of children with mental retardation", In: A.B. Burack., R.M. Hodapp E. and F., Zigler (Eds.). *Handbook of Mental Retardation and Development*. Cambridge: Cambridge University Press, pp. 637–668

Matson, J.L., and Smith, K.R. M. (2008). "Current status of intensive behavioural interventions for young children with autism and PDD-NOS", *Research in Autism Spectrum Disorders, 2*, 60–74.

Matson, J.L., and Wilkins, J. (2007). "A critical review of assessment targets and methods for social skills excesses and deficits for children with autism spectrum disorders", *Research in Autism Spectrum Disorders, 1,* 28–37.

Matson, J.L., Dixon, D.R., and Matson, M.L. (2005). "Assessment and treatment of aggressive behaviour in children and adolescents with developmental disabilities", *Journal of Educational Psychology, 25*, 151–181.

Matson, M.L., Mahan, S., and Matson, J.L. (2009). "Parent training: A review of methods for children with autism spectrum disorders", *Research in Autism Spectrum Disorders, 3*, 868-875.

National Research Council. Committee on Educational Interventions for Children with Autism, Division of Behavioural and Social Sciences and Education. In C, Lord and J.P. McGee (Eds). *Educating Children With Autism. (2001).* Washington, DC: National Academy Press.

Nelson, K.B., Grether, J.K., Croen, L.A., Dambrosia, J.M., Dickens, B.F., Jelliffe, L.L., Hansen, R.L., Phillips, T.M. (2001). "Neuropeptides and neurotrophins in neonatal blood of children with autism or mental retardation", *Annals of Neurology, 49,* 597–606.

Osborne, L.A., McHugh, L., Saunders, J., and Reed, P. (2008). "Parenting stress reduces the effectiveness of early teaching interventions for autistic spectrum disorders", *Journal of Autism and Developmental Disorders, 38,* 1092-1103.

Parsons, D., Cordier, R., Vaz, S., and Lee, H.C. (2017). "Parent-Mediated Intervention Training Delivered Remotely for Children With Autism Spectrum Disorder Living Outside of Urban Areas: Systematic Review", *J Med Internet Res. 19*, e198.

Powers, M.D. and Poland, J. (2002). "Asperger Syndrome and your child, a parent's guide: Unlocking your child's potential", New York: Harper Collins.

Raina, S.K., Chander, V., Bhardwaj, A.K., Kumar, D., Sharma, S. *et al.* (2017). "Prevalence of Autism Spectrum Disorder among Rural, Urban, and Tribal Children (1-10 Years of Age). *J Neurosci Rural Pract. 8,* 368-374.

Ronald, A. (1994). "Problem children problem parents", *Indian Journal of Pediatrics, 11,* 20-29.

Rudra, A., Belmonte, M.K., Soni, P.K., Banerjee, S., Mukerji, S., *et al.* (2017). "Prevalence of autism spectrum disorder and autistic symptoms in a school-base cohort of children in Kolkata, India", *Autism Res. 10,* 1597-1605.

Shah, A., and Frith, U. (1993). "Why do autistic individuals show superior performance on the block design task?" *Journal of Child Psychology and Psychiatry, 34*(8), 1351-1364.

Shaked, M. and Yirmiya, N. (2003). "Understanding Social Difficulties", In M. Prior, (Ed.), *Learning and Behaviour Problems in Asperger Syndrome.* New York and London: The Guilford Press. pp. 104-125.

Singh, A.N., Matson, J.L., Cooper, C.L., Dixon, D., and Sturmey, P. (2005). "The use of risperidone among individuals with mental retardation: Clinically supported or not?", *Research in Developmental Disabilities, 26,* 203–218.

Singh, A.S., Chandra, R., Guhathakurta, S, Sinha, S., Chatterjee, A., *et al.* (2013). "Genetic association and gene-gene interaction analyses suggest likely involvement of ITGB3 and TPH2 with autism spectrum disorder (ASD) in the Indian population", *Prog Neuropsychopharmacol Biol Psychiatry, 45,* 131-143.

Smith, T. (1999). "Outcome of early intervention for children with autism", *Clinical Psychology: Science and Practice, 6,* 33–49.

Szatmari, P., Bremner, R., and Nagy, J. (1989). "Asperger's Syndrome: A review of clinical features", *Canadian Journal of Psychiatry, 34,* 554-560.

Taylor, B., Jick, H., and MacLaughlin, D. (2013). "Prevalence and incidence rates of autism in the UK: Time trend from 2004–2010 in children aged 8 years", *BMJ Open, 3*(10), e003219.

Verma, D., Chakraborti, B., Karmakar, A., Bandyopadhyay, T., Singh, A.S., *et al.* (2014). "Sexual dimorphic effect in the genetic association of monoamine oxidase A (MAOA) marker with autism spectrum disorder", *Prog Neuropsychopharmacol Biol Psychiatry, 50,* 11-20.

Wetherby, A.M., Guthrie, W., Woods, J., *et al.* (2014). "Parent-implemented social intervention for toddlers with autism: An RCT", *Paediatrics, 134*(6), 1084-1093.

Zachor, D.A., Ben-Itzchak, E., and Rabinovich, A.L. (2007). "Change in autism core symptoms with intervention", *Research in Autism Spectrum Disorders, 1,* 304–317.

Zwaigenbaum, L. (2001). "Autistic spectrum disorders in preschool children", *Canadian Family Physician, 47,* 2037-42.

19

Contemplating the Lives of Visually Impaired

A Review of Studies

Vatsala Pathak and *Anubhuti Dubey*

Introduction

Disability affects an individual's life and changes one's perception towards everything. The problems of individuals with any disability are totally different. It is a condition that makes it difficult for a person to excel in certain activities. The impairments that lead to disability may be cognitive, physical, sensory or combination of multiple factors. The World Health Organization proposes the following definition of disability:

Disability is an umbrella term, covering impairments, activity limitations, and participation restrictions. Impairment is a problem in body function or structure; an activity limitation is a difficulty encountered by an individual in executing a task or action; while a participation restriction is a problem experienced by an individual in involvement in life situations. Disability is thus not just a health problem. It is a complex phenomenon, reflecting the interaction between features of a person's body and features of the society in which he or she lives.

One of the most important areas of disability seems to be rising worldwide—the area of Visual Impairment (VI). It has been reported that Blindness and vision impairment affect at least 2.2 billion people around the world. Of those, one billion have preventable vision impairment or one that has yet to be addressed. Reduced or absent eyesight can have major and long-lasting effects on all aspects of life, including daily personal activities, interacting with the community, school and work opportunities and the ability to access public services. In 1992, the World Health Organization (WHO) added a functional dimension to the definition of VI. This definition is stated as: a person with low vision is one who has impairment of visual functioning even after treatment and/or standard refractive correction, and has visual acuity (VA) of less than 6/18 to light perception, or a visual field of less than 10 degrees from the point of fixation.

Prevalence of Visual Impairment Worldwide

The prevalence of Visual Impairment differs depending on whether presenting vision or best-corrected vision is reported or not (Murthy & Johnson, 2012). In the year 2002, it was rated that with best-corrected vision there were 161 million individuals with Visual Impairment globally (Resnikoff *et al.* 2002). However, when the prevalence of uncorrected refractive error was included, this value increased substantially to 314 million individuals with Visual Impairment. This reflects that extra 153 million individuals were visually impaired from uncorrected refractive error alone. The categories of visual impairment in ICD are shown in Table 19.1. Globally the number of people of all ages visually impaired is estimated to be 285 million, of whom 39 million are blind. People aged 50 years and older are 82 per cent of all blind.

Table 19.1: Categories of severity of visual impairment according to the International Statistical Classification of Diseases

Category of visual impairment	*Visual acuity with best possible correction*		*Or central visual field*	*Classified as*
0	Maximum less than	Minimum equal to or better than	-	-
1	6/18 3/10(0.3) 20/70	6/60 1/10(0.1) 20/200	-	Low vision
2	6/60 1/10(0.1) 20/200	3/60 1/20(0.05) 20/400	-	Low vision
3	3/60 1/20(0.05) 20/400	1/60 (finger counting at 1 metre) 1/50 (0.02) 5/300 (20/1200)	10° or less but more than 5°	Blindness
4	1/60 (finger counting at 1 metre) 1/50 (0.02) 5/300	Light perception	5° or less	Blindness
5	No light perception	-	-	Blindness
6	Undetermined or unspecified	-	-	Unspecified

Source: Pascolini, Mariotti (2010).

Causes of Visual Impairment

The specific cause of visual impairment varies for every individual. As a result of prevalence of cataract being lowest and macular degeneration being greatest in high-income regions, the causes of visual impairment differs. (Bourne *et al.*) Worldwide, the leading causes of blindness and moderate and severe Visual Impairment include uncorrected refractive error, cataract and macular degeneration. Bourne *et al.* further reported that the magnitude of individuals affected by blindness and moderate and severe Visual Impairment caused by uncorrected refractive error increased from 6.3 million and 88.0 million in 1990 to 6.8 million and 101.2 million in 2010, respectively. The data in Table 19.2 reflects studies that have reported on the distribution of the major causes of VI. There may be

Table 19.2: Summary of Studies Reporting on the Major Causes of Visual Impairment

Author	Area	Course of Moderate and severe visual impairment	Course of Blindness
Resnikoff et al.	Global	Cataract	Cataract, glaucoma, ARMD, trachoma, corneal opacity, childhood blindness, diabetic retinopathy
Pascolini and Mariotti	Global	Uncorrected refractive error, cataract, glaucoma	Cataract, glaucoma, ARMD, childhood blindness, corneal opacity
Pizzarello et al.	Africa	NR	Cataract, trachoma, onchocerciasis, childhood blindness, refractive error.
Oduntan	Africa	Cataract, Corneal and Retinal Diseases	NR
Bourne et al.	Sub-Sahara Africa (Southern)	Uncorrected Refractive Error, cataract, macular degeneration	Cataract, uncorrected refractive error, macular degeneration
Oduntan	South Africa	Cataract, corneal, opacity and Glaucoma	NR
Sacharowitz	South Africa	Cataract, glaucoma, refractive error, retinal diseases	Corneal scarreing
Naidoo et al.	South Africa	NR	Cataract, refractive error, glaucoma
Cockburn et al.	Cape Town	Cataract, Posterior segment diseases, refractive error	Posterior segment diseases, cataract, glaucoma, ARMD
Maake and Oduntan	Limpopo	Uncorrected refractive error, cataract, glaucoma	Cataract, glaucoma, corneal anomalies

number of factors related to reduced eyesight which may include diseases like diabetes and trachoma, trauma to the eyes, age-related macular degeneration and cataracts. The majority of people with vision impairment are over the age of 50 years; however, vision loss can affect people of all ages. Vision loss is one of the leading causes of disability in older adults, which is also related with reduced quality of life and increased depressive and anxiety symptoms. The depression and anxiety may further become a cause for decline in quality of life, may aggravate disability caused by the visual impairment, and may increase vulnerability for health decline.

A Glance at Mental Health of Visually Impaired Population

Marginalized group seems to be restricted from enjoying all facilities of life which makes it difficult for them to accept the fact easily sometimes and thus, it becomes important for a researcher to explore the type of mental health one undergoes because of it. Mental health, which refers to cognitive, behavioural, and emotional well-being, is all about how people think, feel, and behave. People sometimes use the term "mental health" to mean the absence of a mental disorder. However, this link also works in the other direction. Various factors in people's lives, like interpersonal connections, and physical factors may all contribute to mental health disruptions. Depression, anxiety, stress, poor wellbeing, poor quality of life, emotional imbalance, poor psychosocial development, are indicators of one's poor mental health. This grounds the presence of negative like attitude and difficulty in coping with the stress perceived by a visually impaired person. This perceived stress in turn enhances the severity of negative mental health. The researches in areas of visual impairment seem to be mainly focused on symptoms of depression and anxiety in adults using screening questionnaires; showing that approximately one-third of visually impaired older adults experience clinically significant symptoms of depression and/or anxiety (also called sub-threshold depression and/or anxiety). This is twice as high as the prevalence found in general elderly populations (approximately 16%). Only a few studies have focused on assessing major depressive and/or anxiety disorders according to the criteria of the diagnostic statistical manual (DSM) in visually impaired older adults. However, none of those studies gave a complete picture of threshold and sub-threshold symptoms of depression and anxiety, and none distinguished between different anxiety disorders. Co-occurring mental disorders are common for those living with visual impairment. The sudden loss of eyesight associated with acquired blindness has statistically been known to accompany other issues such as anxiety, depression, phobias, Post-Traumatic Stress Disorder (PTSD), and even suicidal thoughts. Visual impairment in 2010 was a major global health issue: the preventable causes were as high as 80 per cent of the total global burden. Different areas that contribute towards determining an individual's mental health are quality of life, wellbeing, emotional health, psychosocial development, perceived social support, etc. Some of these have been discussed in this review paper.

Quality of Life

Quality today has come in the centre for study and research as a result for the ultimate goal of a better future for an individual's life. For researchers, the direct interest in the quality of life lies in the fact that it is one of the most important indicators of the progress of societies. This is usually reflected in the satisfaction of the individual and the sense of happiness and the desire for living. In this era, it is but obvious for human beings that they will not be confined only to their primary and essential element to address their survival needs; they perceive much beyond that and which includes everything that improves the quality of life. The ingredients of mental, psychological, emotional, social, religious beliefs, cultural and values, economic conditions enable one to determine what things bring him happiness and contentment in life and all these put together form one's quality of life. Disease and disability are of concern because they affect either life expectancy or life quality. Thus, it becomes important for a researcher to know about the quality of life of individuals concerned with different challenges in life.

Many studies have been done covering different aspects of visually impaired people. The life of such people is full of struggles as they are dependent on others for things in their lives, which in turn severely affects their quality of life. Regarding this, many studies have been done. One of the studies was done by Broman, Munoz, Rodriguez, Sanchez, Quigley, Klien, Snyder and West (2002) to understand the impact of visual impairment and eye disease on Vision-Related Quality of Life in a Mexican-American Population concludes that Mexican-American persons aged 40 or more, monocular impairment and better-eye acuity was associated with a decrease in most domains representing quality of life. Subjects with uncorrected refractive error, cataract, diabetic retinopathy, and glaucoma associated with poor quality of life, many not explained by loss of acuity. Further work on the specific measures of vision associated with reported decreases in quality of life, such as visual field or contrast sensitivity is warranted. Langelaan, Boer, Nispen, Wouters, Moll and Rens

(2007) conducted a research to understand the difference between quality of life between Visual Impaired population and general population with other chronic conditions. The results revealed that Visual impairment had a substantial impact on the quality of life compared with other chronic conditions, it seemed to affect the health related quality of life, spoiling the quality of life more than diabetes type II, coronary syndrome, and hearing impairments, but less than stroke, multiple sclerosis, chronic fatigue syndrome, major depressive disorder, and severe mental illness. A great contribution is found in this area by Varma *et al.* (2006) to assess the impact of unilateral and bilateral visual impairment and its severity on health-related quality of life in Latinos. The results revealed that relative to persons with no visual impairment, persons with bilateral mild and unilateral or bilateral moderate/severe visual impairment report greater difficulties in performing most vision-dependent routine activities and experience vision-related dependency and poorer vision-related mental health. Because most visual function subscale scores were significantly lower in persons with bilateral mild and/or unilateral/bilateral moderate/severe visual impairment, health care providers should consider intervention in these persons.

Emotional Consequences

Emotional health is a prime aspect of overall health of a person. Those who are emotionally healthy are in control of their thoughts, feelings, and behaviours. They're able to cope with life's struggles and challenges. They can keep problems in perspective and bounce back from setbacks i.e. they have a good resilience. Emotional health makes it easy for one to work productively. It also affects the physical health of a person. Therefore, emotional adjustment also plays a major role for an individual. Emotional adjustment refers to the maintenance of emotional equilibrium in the face of internal and external stressors and this is facilitated by different cognitive processes of acceptance and adaptation. Evidences found in researches show a link between an upbeat mental state and physical signs of good health. These include lower blood pressure, reduced risk of heart disease, and a healthier weight. People with visual impairment are also found to have emotional and social consequences. The definition of emotional adjustment also includes a decline in mental health, especially the occurrence of depression, as well as less severe manifestations of emotional disturbance. Empirical research on these topics strongly and consistently confirms difficulties in emotional functioning among visually impaired elders. In particular, a considerable body of research using different methodologies has reflected the prevalence of depression in visually impaired groups to be at least twice as high as that found in normal populations. Social adjustment to vision loss is construed to involve difficulties in social functioning, changes in social support, and loneliness. Although research findings indicate loss of social activity and, to a lesser extent, loss of social support among the visually impaired, the relationship between vision loss and loneliness remains unclear (Burmedi, Becker, Heyl, Wahl & Himmesbach, 2002). There are, however, firm indications that social support can provide an effective buffer against age-related vision loss.

Psychosocial Development

Psychosocial development is one of the necessary developments that need to be taken care of. "Psychosocial" refers to the relation between one's psychological development and interaction with social environment involving both psychological and social aspects in human development. In case of visually impaired individuals this is another majorly affected area and different studies have been conducted to see the level of psychosocial development in such individuals. In this series Huurre and Aro (1998) presented some key results in which it was found that the psychosocial developmental outcomes of adolescents with visual impairment were similar to their peers without visual impairment. The study also revealed that adolescents with visual impairment often undergo feeling of loneliness and find difficulty in making friends. Another interesting result was in the same study which revealed that Self-esteem, school achievement and social skills were lower in girls with visual impairment in comparison to boys and different studies done in this area also comes with a fact that girls need more psychosocial support than boys. Many review articles have focused on the impact of age-related low vision on behavioural competence, including activities of daily living, mobility, and leisure pursuits. In particular, age-related low vision is shown to be a significant and unique predictor of performance on activities of daily living, stronger than hearing impairment, yet less influential than many other age-related health problems. Age-related low vision also seems to be highly detrimental to mobility and the pursuit of vision-dependent leisure activities, however, evidence also suggests that the visually impaired elderly can effectively compensate for or otherwise adapt to decline in competence domains (Burmedi, Becker & Himmesbach, 2002).

Social Support

Another stream of studies has proved the relationship between social support, good health, lower mortality rates and faster recoveries. (Cohen, Syme, 1985; Hale, Hannum, & Espelage, 2005; Hurdle, 2001). Some other researches have emphasized on the relationship between social support and mental health. Cohen and McKay (1984) theorized that social support acts as a buffer to protect individuals from the harmful physical and mental effects of stressful life events. For disabled people, social support is another significant area that plays a major role. Thus, it becomes important for researchers to explore the role of social support in such individual's life. Also the fact that chronic conditions have the potential to give rise to both physical as well as mental components makes it more important (Levine & Blackburn, 1946; Seybold, 2005). Li and Moore (1998) investigated the social variables that help an individual to accept his or her disability. They perceived social discrimination was one of the important factors towards contributing negative outcomes and that subsequent social integration improved an individual's psychological well-being. Kef (2002) studied the effect of the size and composition of social support networks among visually impaired adolescents. Reviewing these studies brings us the knowledge that social support plays a major role in visually impaired people's life.

Dr. Mhairi Thurston, a senior lecturer in counseling and who also served as a Chair of the Research Governance Committee for BACP, has contributed in the area of visual impairment where he investigated the impact of acquired sight loss in four core areas—mood, self concept, social connectedness and loss. His work indicated that participants experienced reduced mental health and decreased social functioning as a result of sight loss. It was also reflected that participants shared common socio-emotional issues during transition from sight to blindness, relating to diagnosis, coping with deterioration of sight, experiencing loss, experiencing changed perceptions of self in relation to society. Thurston further examined this issue and considered the need for psychological support amongst individuals with visual impairment (Thurston, 2010). He reported negative perception of counseling among visually impaired participants and lack of counseling opportunities in relation to their sight loss.

Some psychologists tried to explore the relationship between the positive variables of mental health like hope, resilience, optimism etc. and its functioning in visually impaired population but, very few studies have been reported under this mainly it includes studies related to mindfulness and hope. Mindfulness is one of the forms of meditative practice which includes paying attention to the present moment experiences in a non-judgmental way. In this, an individual is in a stable and non-reactive awareness. Mindfulness has been studied in relation to various health conditions, but no specific study is published that considers mindfulness in context of visual impairment. Lorna (2014) conducted a semi-structured interview for blind and partially sighted individuals who participated in regular mindfulness practice. Their narratives were then analyzed. It was found that mindfulness enhanced spiritual well-being by increasing their sense of intrapersonal, interpersonal, and transpersonal 'connectedness', which was seen to be related to a self-perceived increase in emotional, social, and physical health. The findings of this study call for further research into the utility of mindfulness as a well-being resource for individuals with a visual impairment. Another interesting result is found in one of the studies conducted by Warren *et al.* The study aimed towards examining the relationship between hope and self-reported functional ability level. A mediating role for hope in relation between a proactive sociable style and perceived level of functional ability was found in results. This study focuses on the importance of one of the area from positive psychology but less studies with such context reflects a need to enhance the quality of study with the concepts of positive psychology in context to visual impairment. In this context, a study done by Glenda *et al.* (2010) captures our attention as the study tried to explore the importance of leisure activities fostering resilience in blind people. This study explored the benefits of leisure activities blind people and these activities provided them with supportive relationships, a desirable identity, experiences of power and control, and experiences of social justice which in turn enabled the young people under the study to thrive despite adversity. A research in South Africa was conducted by Heidi and Abraham (Heidi & Abraham, 2011) to see the resilience of parents with visually impaired children. The results showed that familial values such as attitude toward the disability, religious faith, and familial closeness permitted a process of inclusion through the use of resources and acceptance of help and the development of a sense of accomplishment.

Conclusion

People belonging to marginalized group suffer in many areas and face multiple deprivations in life. Such people do not enjoy the same privileges as that of rest of the society and this makes them susceptible for many challenging situations that affect their mental peace. Persons with visual impairment express a variety of emotional, cognitive, behavioural and social responses to this significant loss. This review paper focused on the social, emotional, behavioural and the psychological facets such people go through. It is crystal clear that the intensity of this disability possesses a direct relation with one's mental health. When such people fail in excelling in daily activities, they feel frustrated and depressive. Not being able to work in every field gives rise to anxiety, depression, stress and many other symptoms of negative mental health. Different studies have shown that there is an importance of social and psychological support in such individual's life. Other side of the researches has reflected that positive variables like support and counseling with such individuals gives rise to positive variables of mental health like hope, resilience, optimism etc. Further in-depth research in the area of visual impairment in context to positive variables of mental health across different age groups is required.

References

Broman, A.T., Munoz, B., Rodriguez, J., Sanchez, R., Quigley, H.A., Klein, R., and West, S.K. (2002). "The impact of visual impairment and eye disease on vision-related quality of life in a Mexican-American population: Proyecto VER", *Investigative Ophthalmology and Visual Science*, *43*(11), 3393-3398.

Burmedi, D., Becker, S., Heyl, V., Wahl, H.W., and Himmelsbach, I. (2002). "Emotional and social consequences of age-related low vision", *Visual Impairment Research*, *4*(1), 47-71.

Bourne, R.R., Stevens, G.A., White, R.A., Smith, J.L., Flaxman, S.R., Price, H., … and Pesudovs, K. (2010). "Causes of vision loss worldwide, 1990–2010: A systematic analysis", *Lancet Glob Health*, 2013; 1 (6): e339–49.

Cockburn, N., Steven, D., Lecuona, K., Joubert, F., Rogers, G., Cook, C., and Polack, S. (2012). "Prevalence, causes and socio-economic determinants of vision loss in Cape Town, South Africa", *PloS one*, *7*(2), e30718.

Cohen, S., and Syme, S.L. (1985). "Issues in the study and application of social support", In Cohen, S., and Syme, S.L. (Eds.), *Social Support and Health* (pp. 3–22). Orlando, FL: Academic.

Cohen, S., and McKay, G. (1984). "Social support, stress and the buffering hypothesis: A theoretical analysis", In Baum, A., Stinger, J.E., and Taylor, S.E. (Eds.), Handbook of Psychology and Health (Vol. 4, pp. 253–267). Hillsdale, NJ: Lawrence Erlbaum.

De Klerk, H., and Greeff, A.P. (2011). "Resilience in parents of young adults with visual impairments", *Journal of Visual Impairment and Blindness*, *105*(7), 414-424.

"Disabilities". World Health Organization. Retrieved October 28, *2016.*

Huurre, T.M., and Aro, H.M. (1998). "Psychosocial development among adolescents with visual impairment", *European Child and Adolescent Psychiatry, 7*(2), 73-78.

Hale, C.J., Hannum, J.W., and Espelage, D.L. (2005). "Social support and physical health: The importance of belonging", *Journal of American College Health,* 53, 276–284.

Hurdle, D.E. (2001). "Social support: A critical factor in women's health and health promotion", *Health and Social Support,* 26, 72–79.

Jackson, W.T., Taylor, R.E., Palmatier, A.D., Elliott, T.R., and Elliott, J.L. (1998). "Negotiating the reality of visual impairment: Hope, coping, and functional ability", *Journal of Clinical Psychology in Medical Settings, 5*(2), 173-185.

Jessup, G.M., Cornell, E., and Bundy, A.C. (2010). "The treasure in leisure activities: Fostering resilience in young people who are blind", *Journal of Visual Impairment and Blindness, 104*(7), 419-430.

Kef, S. (2002). "Psychosocial adjustment and the meaning of social support for visually impaired adolescents", *Journal of Visual Impairment and Blindness,* 96, 22–37.

Langelaan, M., De Boer, M.R., Van Nispen, R.M., Wouters, B., Moll, A.C., and Van Rens, G.H. (2007). "Impact of visual impairment on quality of life: A comparison with quality of life in the general population and with other chronic conditions", *Ophthalmic Epidemiology, 14*(3), 119-126.

Li, L., and Moore, D. (1998). "Acceptance of disability and its correlates", *Journal of Social Psychology,* 138, 13–25.

Levine, J., and Blackburn, A.R. (1946). "Rehabilitation of the newly blinded", *Journal of Clinical Psychology,* 2, 140–145.

Marquès-Brocksopp, L. (2014). "Mindfulness, spiritual well-being, and visual impairment: An exploratory study", *British Journal of Visual Impairment, 32*(2), 108-123.

Murthy, G.V. S., and Johnson, G.O. R.D. O.N. (2012). "Prevalence, incidence and distribution of visual impairment", *The Epidemiology of Eye Disease,* 3-61.

Naidoo, K.S., Sweeney, D., Jaggernath, J., and Holden, B. (2013). "A population-based study of visual impairment in the Lower Tugela health district in KZN, SA", *African Vision and Eye Health, 72*(3), 110-118.

Ndlovu, M.Z., Mothapo, K.T., Kgatla, M.H., Tshihomu, M.S., and Mathebula, S.D. (2019). "Agreement between distance and near minus-lens-to-blur amplitude of accommodation in pre-presbyopic subjects", *African Vision and Eye Health, 78*(1), 1-7.

Oduntan, A.O. (2005). "Prevalence and causes of low vision and blindness worldwide", *African Vision and Eye Health, 64*(2), 44-57.

Pascolini, D., and Mariotti, S.P. (2012). "Global estimates of visual impairment: 2010. *British Journal of Ophthalmology, 96*(5), 614-618.

Pizzarello, L., Abiose, A., Ffytche, T., Duerksen, R., Thulasiraj, R., Taylor, H., … and Resnikoff, S. (2004). "VISION 2020: The Right to Sight: a global initiative to eliminate avoidable blindness", *Archives of Ophthalmology*, *122*(4), 615-620.

Resnikoff, S., Pascolini, D., Etya'ale D, *et al.* (2004). "Global data on visual impairment in the year 2002." *Bulletin of the World Health Organization*, 82(11), 844–551.

Resnikoff, S., Pascolini, D., Mariotti, S.P., and Pokharel, G.P. (2008). "Global magnitude of visual impairment caused by uncorrected refractive errors in 2004. *Bulletin of the World Health Organization*, *86*, 63-70.

Sacharowitz, H.S. (2005). "Visual impairment in South Africa: Achievements and challenges", *African Vision and Eye Health*, *64*(4), 139-149.

Seybold, D. (2005). "The psychosocial impact of acquired vision loss—Particularly related to rehabilitation involving orientation and mobility", *International Congress Series*, 1282, 298–301.

Thurston, M. (2010). "An inquiry into the emotional impact of sight loss and the counselling experiences and needs of blind and partially sighted people", *Counselling and Psychotherapy Research*, *10*(1), 3-12.

Varma, R., Wu, J., Chong, K., Azen, S.P., Hays, R.D., and Los Angeles Latino Eye Study Group. (2006). "Impact of severity and bilaterality of visual impairment on health-related quality of life", *Ophthalmology*, *113*(10), 1846-1853.

World Health Organization (1992). *International Statistical Classification of Diseases and Related Health Problems:* 10th revision (ICD-10).

World Health Organization, (2007). Global Initiative for the Elimination of Avoidable Blindness: Action Plan 2006-2011.

20

Relationship between Attachment and Wellbeing in Children and Adolescents

A Critical Review

Gunjan Joshi

Introduction

Formation of Attachment

The bond established between the caregiver and the child early during infancy is crucial because it influences several aspects. This bond formed early during childhood is what is called attachment and this forms the pillar of the relationship.

According to Bowlby (1977), the construct of attachment is defined as an enduring emotional bond that an individual forms over time and space with another person. The quality and timing of this bond determines an individual's development later in life.

Considering the process of socialization and formation of attachment; caregivers act as the first source which is then followed by significant others like relatives and peers (Bowbly, 1977). Consistent availability of the attachment figure during the time of need and distress serve as a source of healthy attachment because the child is comfortable knowing that there is someone to count on. Apart from the consistent availability of the attachment figure, it's the essence of the kind of bond shared between parent-child sets the foundation for development later in life. This type of attachment is secure and is related to better adaptation. When the attachment is secure with the caregiver, it is easier for the child to become independent and build good relations with other people specially the peer in school which act as a second source for the child to socialize (Malekpour, 2007). On the contrary, insecure attachment is related to maladaptive adjustment thereby increasing the risk for experiencing clinical distressful symptoms (Brumariu, 2015).

The kind of attachment security established during childhood years exerts tremendous influence on the subsequent attachment formed during adolescence as a secure attachment will foster better health and well-being. Adolescence is a time when individuals undergo major transition and during this time attachment is crucial for dealing with stress and coping, facing negative encounters (Malekpour, 2007). Due to this reason; the kind of attachment formed influences various aspects such as psychological, emotional, psychosocial and subjective sense of wellbeing and its development later in life. Disturbances in attachment patterns have been often reported in association to distress and maladaptive behaviour. These disturbances can become evident at any point and irrespective of any specific time period. Moreover dysfunctional attachment provides explanations related to developmental pathology. There are certain behaviours that are a result of poor attachment styles which may increase the experience of distress and vulnerability in an individual.

Based on this fact, the aim of this conceptual paper is to review attachment and wellbeing during lifespan of an individual.

Understand Self and the World: Individual's Internal Working Model

According to John Bowlby (1977), an individual makes sense of their world through an internal working model. The way this working model develops depends on the kind of attachment pattern formed with the primary caregivers. At this point the concept of attuned parenting (Bowlby, 1969) becomes very important. It helps the child learn that caregivers are responsive to the needs and helps build the trust, empathy and an effective communication between the child and the caregiver. Thus, anything that disrupts the cycle of attunement early in childhood bears subsequent consequences on the attachment that's formed (Rees, 2001). If the caregiver is there to respond to the child's need and is available consistently in times of distress; the child develops a sense of security which leads to building of a secure attachment style with the caregiver. According to Elicker *et al.* (1992), securely attached infants are social with friends and unknown people compared to their counterparts who are anxiously attached.

However, if the caregiver is negligent and insensitive, it leads to an insecure working model of attachment thus causing to a worthless image of self and insecure and unreliable image of the others; therefore leading to the perception of the world as insecure place. Once formed, the internal model of working becomes stable throughout life. Thus, it is justified to say that the attachment pattern impacts the wellbeing of an individual (Chauhan & Verma, 2014).

The Present Study

Attachment is a well-researched concept which has its roots of origin in Bowbly's attachment theory. Since then a plethora of work has been done to assess the impact of attachment on various aspects of individual wellbeing. Therefore, the rationale of the study is to review the extensive literature which has immensely contributed to the body of knowledge about how attachment impacts the wellbeing. This review will cover results of the reported studies done from 1995-2017 on attachment and wellbeing. It will highlight how problems in attachment act as a precursor to psychological and behavioural issues in children and adolescents. Family and home being the first source for socialization becomes very important as children learn wide variety of behaviour and values from there. School is the next stepping stone which exposes the child to people of similar age group. Many of the behavioural issues which include both internalizing and externalizing behaviours can therefore be seen from as developing due to attachment issues with both parents and peers. Thus, attachment can then interfere with child's ability to perform in school which leads to significant concerns about the child. Thus, the goal of this review is to report studies related to attachment with both parents and peers and its subsequent influence on child's wellbeing.

Method

Using Ebsco, Proquest, jSTOR and Google scholar as search engines literature on attachment and wellbeing from 1990 to 2017 was retrieved using keywords 'attachment', 'psychosocial functioning', 'wellbeing', 'attachment related disorder' and 'transition in attachment'. A total of 35 articles on attachment and wellbeing were reviewed. From a methodological viewpoint, the retrieved articles can be divided into the following: Empirical studies carried out on attachment and wellbeing done both clinical and non-clinical samples, Case reports, review papers, journal articles and theoretical papers on attachment and its relationship to wellbeing.

Findings

Attachment and Psychosocial Functioning

Mothers being the primary caregiver have an important role in the kind of attachment formed during early infancy and childhood years. Secure attachment is considered as a healthy model of upbringing wherein the caregiver is concerned and receptive to the needs and demands of the child. In contrast insecure attachment signifies that certain issues of trust, responsiveness and sensitivity are missing between the child-caregiver relationships (Grossman & Grossman, 1991).

Studies done in the past have shown that the quality life of mentally healthy children is positive and they do well in terms of their performance in home, schools and in their communities. Moreover such children tend to stay symptom free and are not vulnerable to developing pathology in further life (Hoagwood, Jensen, Petti & Burns, 1996).

Moreover, various studies have shown attachment as a correlate of psychosocial functioning. A study conducted by Brown and Whiteside (2007) found that those children who reported insecure attachment also rated high on degree of their anxiety and distress. Findings also reported that insecure attachment was shown to bear impact on child's level of worry. Children who are securely attached strike a balance in autonomy and the way they relate to their parents. Moreover such children are more confident about their actions and at the same time can trust others.

In contrast, children who develop insecure attachment are anxious and show submissive behaviour. Because securely attached children report better quality of life; such an attachment pattern is related to healthy social and psychological functioning and reduced psychological problems. Adolescents with insecure attachment report higher degree of distress and internalizing behaviours (Chauhan & Verma, 2014). Another Study, conducted by Elgar, Knight, Worrall and Sherman (2003) assessed the self-reported attachment, substance abuse and behavioural problems of 68 male juvenile delinquents and the findings reported that insecure attachment was linked to behavioural issues, increased substance abuse and dysfunctional families.

Moreover as internal working model of attachment determines important aspects of later life by acting as a pillar to future experiences encountered like how the children views their surrounding and the kind of attachment that is formed with other people; Rutter (1995) conducted a study on the similar lines wherein he investigated whether the attachment once formed can be changed over time or whether it lays the foundation for further development. He found that the pattern of attachment formed during early years remains stable for the rest of the life. This pattern of attachment then forms the basis for how an individual views their social world and form expectations from the other people. Thus, attachment is not only important during childhood years but bears significant effect throughout entire lifespan. The pattern of attachment formed during children effects how they perceive their mental health and psychosocial wellbeing later in life.

Konstantinos and Georgios (2006) investigated the relationship between attachment and wellbeing. Findings reported that anxious attachment and wellbeing were negatively correlated. Moreover negative correlation was found between avoidant attachment and perceived support satisfaction.

Carr, Colthurst, Coyle and Elliott (2013) conducted a study to investigate how attachment predicts various aspects of psychosocial wellbeing and mental health. Results indicated that those students who scored higher in the insecurity aspect of the vulnerable attachment style questionnaire reported negative mental and psychosocial health. Findings of this study were significant as it revealed insecure attachment as a predictor of negative psychosocial wellbeing.

Attachments starts with parents however attachment with peers during the time of adolescents plays a very important role. Adolescents who reported secure attachment with both parents and peers separately reported good overall adjustment (Sasikala & Cecil, 2016). Thus, adolescents can be made to handle stress and adjust well by increasing their bond not only with the parents as their caregiver but also their peers as they become a major source of socialization during this age. A balance of good relations with both can make things better for adolescents as they will feel confident to deal with issues by themselves.

Another study conducted by Muris, Meesters, Melick, and Zwambag (2001) investigated perceived attachment style and quality amongst adolescents and assessed and how this is related to symptoms of anxiety and depression. Finding revealed that those adolescents who perceived their attachment as secure reported higher trust levels and alienation in comparison to their counterparts who reported insecure attachment. Moreover; low levels of communication, trusts and high alienation were associated with increased anxiety and depression in this population. With this the overall health and the quality of life of the adolescent would be drastically be affected. This makes me bring up the point that addressing attachment related issue will act as a rescue for treating depression and anxiety.

Apart from mental health, attachment is also linked to academics performance in school. Chen (2017) conducted a study which revealed that attachment to mother and father was related with higher academic achievement amongst adolescents. Moreover he also investigated the role of self worth as a mediating variable and the findings revealed that those adolescents who rated higher degree of attachment with parents were more likely to have high self-esteem. Thus, poor academic performance can be traced back to the attachment with parents. There is a possibility of improving academic performance by fixing attachment issues.

Schneider and Younger (1996) in their study investigated whether secure parental attachment led to higher inter-personal relational competence skills amongst school children. Results revealed that parent-child attachment was positively related to social competence in adolescents. Trust and communication subscales were highly correlated with the same parent. With respect to alienation from parents, it was found that alienation from father was negatively correlated to adolescents self-reported interpersonal competence.

Attachment and Psychological Wellbeing

Researches in the past have shown that individuals who score high on insecure attachment or either of the two dimensions i.e. attachment anxiety or avoidance; experience low self-esteem and self-worth. Thus, the attachment pattern formed with the caregiver becomes very crucial in terms of the wellbeing of the child. Communication with a caregiver who is generally unavailable or inconsistent leads to insecure attachment. Moreover caregivers who are too critical of their children, and show disapproval and rejection increase the likelihood for psychopathology later in life (Mikulincer & Shaver, 2007).

Studies have also shown that a secure child is more likely to be confident and can deal with stress and peer pressure in a resilient manner. Secure attachment leads to psychological wellbeing and helps deal with stress throughout life (Malekpour, 2007).

Lucktong, Salisbury and Chamratrithirong (2017) conducted a cross-sectional study to assess the effects of attachment (parents, peers and school) on psychological well-being of adolescents aged 12 to 15 years with self-esteem as the mediating variable. Results revealed that parental attachment and school attachment were positively related to life satisfaction and greater parental and peer attachment was negatively related to psychological difficulties and externalizing and internalizing problems.

Flouri and Buchanan (2003) based on their study on 2722 adolescents between the age group 14-18 years reported that parents' degree of involvement significantly affected adolescents psychological wellbeing. Love and Murdock (2004) in their study reported attachment to parents as a significant predictor of wellbeing. Thus, forming secure attachment during childhood years has a predictive value for later adjustments.

Parents being the primary caregivers do play crucial role however apart from parents, attachment with peers also has great importance. Berndt (1979) proposed a viewpoint on the attachment wherein he describes how family and peers act as two entirely different social worlds. These two social worlds may be independent that is attachment to family and peers may be independent of each other and the relative importance adolescent's place of each of these depends on which context they view as important for their self-evaluation. Thus, in stressful situations if the adolescent has poor attachment with family members it will be compensated by attachment with friends and vice-versa. Another viewpoint states that in adolescents the attachment undergoes a major shift from parents to peers. With time this view has been revised and studies show that when taking decisions pertaining to future, parents are more likely to ask rather than their peers.

Raja, McGee and Stanton (1992) conducted a study on 935 adolescents wherein they assessed how perceived attachment with parents and peers separately contributes to their psychological wellbeing. Findings reported that lower perceived attachment with parents was related to lower scores on adolescents' wellbeing. Those adolescents who reported high on both parent and peer attachment, scored highest on their perceived strength. The results also found that attachment to both parents and peers plays a crucial role and that attachment with parents cannot be compensated by peers altogether with regard to their mental health.

Therefore, high perceived attachment with parents is very important in predicting the psychological wellbeing of adolescents. From the findings of this study, rather than the shift the adolescents maintain their relationship with both parents and peers however there are some situations where relationship with parents are better (Raja, 1992).

Attachment and Emotional Regulation

Emotional regulation is defined as 'the ability to inhibit, enhance, maintain, and modulate emotional arousal to accomplish one's goals' (Eisenberg *et al.*, 1997, p. 642). Emotional regulation is not only awareness and modulation of one's own emotions but also regulating these emotions in a productive manner (Denham, Bassett, Way, Mincic, Zinsser, & Graling, 2012).

Bowlby's theory of attachment has highlighted how attachment is related to emotions. According to his theory; caregivers who are sensitive to the needs of the child and are responsive when the child needs them; help the child in regulating their feelings which is directly related to child's sense of emotional wellbeing and enabling the aspect of felt security in the child (Sroufe & Waters, 1977).

Studies in the area of attachment and emotional regulation have shown that insecure parental attachment is closely linked to emotional difficulties and also predicts conduct problems in later life. Thus, the role of parental attachment becomes very crucial in reducing such negative behaviours (Oldfield, Humphrey and Hebron; 2016).

Pauli-Pott, Haverkock, Pott and Beckmann (2007) conducted a study to assess relation between the quality of attachment and infant negative emotionality and how this affects the subsequent behaviour problem. Results revealed that secure attachment and disorganized attachment early in infancy were significantly related to the behavioural problems. Disorganized attachment is directly related to poor adjustment and is higher in infants who displayed negative emotionality.

Being able to regulate one's emotions to able to understand the concerns of other requires formation of secure attachment bond. In his study Laible (2007) found that adolescents who develop secure attachment with their parents engage in more pro-social behaviour which involves being more emotionally aware and sympathetic.

Various other studies have clearly shown that the way parents bring up their children is related to the emotional capacity of children. Akhtar (2012) conducted a study to examine how parenting styles affect the subsequent attachment in a sample of 179 undergraduate students ranging between the ages 15-18 years. To assess parenting styles of mother and father the parental authority questionnaire was used and to tap onto attachment styles of students, the adult attachment scale was used. Using Pearson's correlation results revealed that parenting style is related to the subsequent attachment between parent-child.

Authoritarian parenting style by both parents was related to anxious attachment. Permissive parenting by father and mother was significantly correlated with avoidant and anxious attachment respectively. Hence both parenting and attachment go hand in hand. The attachment formed between parent-child then impacts process of emotional regulation in children.

As parenting and attachment are intertwined concepts; the type of parenting is directly related to the attachment formed between parents and the child. Bad parenting affect children's capacity to regulate their emotions leading to maladaptive and dysfunctional ways of regulation emotions (Eisenberg *et al.*, 1999).

Brenning *et al.* (2015) in their longitudinal study reported that adolescents' perception of their mother as autonomy supportive is related to their use of adaptive emotional regulation strategy which then leads to better adjustment. On the contrary; those adolescents who reported the use of dysregulation as a strategy perceived decreased autonomy—supportive parenting.

Another study conducted by Jabeen, Anis-Ul-Haque and Riaz (2013) examined how maternal and paternal parenting styles predict emotional regulation in adolescents. Results revealed that authoritative parenting by mother and father had significant positive effects on emotional regulation of adolescents and that permissive parenting style by father had negative effect on emotional regulation.

Behaviours/Problems/Symptoms/Conditions Linked to Poor Attachment Pattern

Studies in the area of attachment and its long term effects; have shown poor attachment as a predictor of certain behavioural problems. These behavioural difficulties arise due to reason of distrust, desire for or wanting attention, fear of rejection, parents being unresponsive or unavailable or because of some associated trauma (Rees, 2005).

According to Rees (2007) poor attachment or problems with forming healthy attachment can lead to development of consequences like difficulty understanding what to expect from the world around them, understanding their own emotions, relationships, poor regulation and monitoring of stress and exhibit lack of concern and empathy for others.

Dysfunctional attachment is directly related to such prominent consequences. Some of the disorders that have been speculated for evidence include conduct disorder, ADHD, Asperger's syndrome and OCD. ADHD is one condition that is closely related to problems with attachment. There is also evidence to support the fact that disturbances in attachment early in the childhood impacts the immunity and predisposes a person to developing psychosomatic illness.

Cooper, Shaver and Collins (1998) in their study investigated attachment style and how it is related to symptomatology in a sample of 1,989 adolescents ranging between ages 13 to 19 years. The findings of the study reported that adolescents who reported secure attachment were best adjusted and those who reported anxious attachment were worst adjusted and had very poor self-concept as well as reported highest levels of symptomatology and indulging in risky behaviours.

Another study conducted by Howard and Medway (2004) examined how attachment was related to coping strategy in a sample of 75 high school students. Findings revealed that high attachment security was positively related to communication with parents. Moreover they attachment security was negatively related to maladaptive avoidance behaviours. Thus, securely attached adolescents were less likely to indulge in risky behaviours including excessive drinking and drug use. Insecure attachment even predicted symptoms of depression amongst younger adolescents (Sund & Wichstrøm, 2002).

Discussion

Implications for Practice

Based on the review, where a number of studies have been conducted on attachment and its relationship with wellbeing, one thing that becomes very clear is the predictive nature of unhealthy attachment style in leading to various mental health issues amongst school aged children and adolescents. Utilizing the predictive nature this relationship, behavioural issues and mental health problems can be more effectively dealt with by addressing attachment issues in school by the counselors or other health care providers. Interventions targeted at addressing or resolving issues pertaining to attachment with the caregiver can lead to profound improvement in the socialization of the child in school and later during adolescence. Another perspective to this is that the behaviour of the child in school can determine what's going wrong in the family. Many externalizing behaviours like aggression and bullying amongst children have its roots in attachment issues either within family or with peers especially during adolescents. Therefore, working on resolving the source of these behavioural problems will eventually lead to handling these problems effectively. The role of counselors and mental health professionals becomes important here as they may intervene to dwell more into each case and come up with the possible solution. If the child has attachment issues with parents then the case can be dealt by referring it to mental health professional. The child can undergo sessions of therapy, counseling and in some cases parenting education could also be considered. Depending on the nature of problem which requires involvement of the family members during sessions, family therapy could also be considered as an option. However, when attachment with peers is the source to behavioural issues exhibited by the child, intervention by the counselors in school can make the situation better. Establishing a safe environment for the child so that there is enough room for sharing confidential information becomes important. Counselors in school can act as a support system for the child if he has problems with attachment at home or with peers.

Conclusion

Attachment plays a very crucial role from the beginning of infancy as it exerts substantial influence over later development. As parent-child attachment forms the base through which the child views the world, disruption in attachment leads to issues pertaining to trust about self as well as the world around. Securely attached individuals have high self-concept, are self-competent, resilient, monitor and regulate their emotions appropriately and are able to share close bonds with others. This helps foster their wellbeing and lead a healthy life. Even during times of stress and unfamiliar environment such individuals are able to deal effectively in contrast to anxious people who generally have problems with attachment.

Moreover as people with insecure attachment tend to report high on the dimensions of anxiety, depressive thoughts and display risky behaviours, working on establishing secure attachment and modifying the existing maladaptive attachment becomes very important. The negative consequences of dysfunctional attachment can be dealt by dealing with the underlying cause i.e. working on attachment related issues.

References

Akhtar, Z. (2012). *Strength for Today and Bright Hope for Tomorrow*, 12(January), 555–566.

Bowlby, J. (1969). *Attachment and Loss*. London: Hogarth Press.

Bowlby, J. (1977). "The making and breaking of affectionate bonds", *British Journal of Psychiatry*, 130, 201-210.

Brenning, K., Soenens, Van Petegem S., and Vansteenkiste, M. (2015). "Perceived Maternal Autonomy Support and Early Adolescent Emotional Regulation: A longitudinal Study", Social Development [serial online], *24*(3):561-578.

Available from: Psychology and Behavioural Sciences Collection, Ipswich, M.A. Accessed August 23, 2017

Brown, A.M., and Whiteside, S.P. (2007). "Relations among perceived parental rearing behaviours, attachment style, and worry in anxious children", *Journal of Anxiety Disorders*, 22, 263-272.

Brumariu, L.E. (2015). "Parent-Child Attachment and Emotion Regulation", *New Directions for Child and Adolescent Development*. https://doi.org/10.1002/cad.20098.

Carr, S., Colthurst, K., Coyle, M., and Elliott, D. (2013). "Attachment dimensions as predictors of mental health and psychosocial well-being in the transition to university", *European Journal of Psychology of Education*, Springer. https://doi.org/10.2307/23421888.

Chauhan, R., and Verma, S. (2014). "Attachment and Psychosocial Functioning: an Overview", *Social Science International*, *30*(2), 331–344. Retrieved from http://ovidsp.ovid.com/ovidweb.cgi?T = JS & PAGE = reference & D = psyc11 & NEWS = N & AN = 2 014-39906-008

Chen, B. (2017). "Parent-Adolescent Attachment and Academic Adjustment: The Mediating Role of Self-Worth", *Journal of Child and Family Studies*, *26*(8), 2070-2076.

Chisolm, K.S. (2012). "The relationship between attachment, coping, and psychological distress in a sample of adolescent females in foster care (Order No. 3569213). Available from ProQuest Dissertations and Theses Full Text. (1348169442). Retrieved from https://search.proquest.com/docview/1348169442?accountid = 38885

Cooper, M.L., Shaver, P.R., and Collins, N.L. (1998). "Attachment styles, emotion regulation and adjustment in adolescence", *Journal of Personality and Social Psychology*, 74, 1380–97.

Denham, S., Bassett, H., Way, E., Mincic, M., Zinsser, K., and Graling, K. (2012). "Preschoolers' emotion knowledge: Self-regulatory foundations, and predictions of early school success", *Cognition and Emotion*, *26*(4), 667-679. doi: 10.1080/02699931.2011.602049

Eisenberg, N., Fabes, R.A., Shepard, S.A., Guthrie, I.K., Murphy, B.C., and Reiser, M. (1999). "Parental reactions to children's negative emotions: A longitudinal relation to quality of children's social functioning", *Child Development*, 70, 513-534. doi: 10.1111/1467-8624.00037.

Elgar, F.J., Knight, J., Worrall, G.J., and Sherman, G. (2003). "Attachment Characteristics and Behavioural Problems in Rural and Urban Juvenile Delinquents", Retrieved from https://search.proquest.com/docview/821826678/62AB38056A74C0CPQ/1?accountid = 3888 5.

Elicker, J., Englund, M. and Sroufe, L.A. (1992). "Predicting peer competence and peer relationships in childhood from early parent-child relationships", In R. Park and G. Ladd (Eds.), *Family-Peer Relationships: Modes of Linkage* (pp. 77-106). Hillsdale, New Jersey: Erlbaum.

Flouri, E., and Buchanan, A. (2003). "The role of father involvement and mother involvement in adolescents' psychological well-being", *British Journal of Social Work*, 33, 399–406.

Garber, J. and Flynn, C. (2001) Predictors of depressive cognitions in young adolescents", *Cognitive Theory and Research*, 25, 353–376.

Grossmann, K.E., and Grossmann, K. (1991). "Parent-infant attachment relationship in Bielefield," in K. Immelmann, G. Barlow, L. Petrovitch, and M. Men (Eds.), *Behavioural Development: The Biefield interdisciplinary project* (694-699). New York: Cambridge University Press.

Hoagwood, K., Jensen, P.S., Petti, T., and Burns, B.J. (1996). "Outcomes of mental health care for Social children and adolescents: I. A comprehensive conceptual model", *Journal of the American Academy of Child and Adolescent Psychiatry*, 35, 1055–1063.

Howard, M.S. and Medway, F.J. (2004), Adolescents' attachment and coping with stress", *Psychology Schools*, 41, 391–402.

Jabeen, F., Anis-Ul-Haque, M., and Riaz, M.N. (2013). "Parenting Styles as Predictors of Emotion Regulation Among Adolescents", *Pakistan Journal of Psychological Research*, *28*(1), 85–105.

Laible, D. (2007). "Attachment with parents and peers in late adolescence: Links with emotional competence and social behaviour", *Personality and Individual Differences*, 43, 1185—1197.

Love, K.M., and Murdock, T.B. (2004). "Attachment to parents and psychological well-being: An examination of young adult college students in intact families and stepfamilies", *Journal of Family Psychology*, *18*(4), 600-608. doi:10.1037/0893-3200.18.4.600

Lucktong, A., Salisbury, T.T., and Chamratrithirong, A. (2017). "The impact of parental, peer and school attachment on the psychological well-being of early adolescents in Thailand", *International Journal of Adolescence and Youth*, 1–15. https://doi.org/10.1080/02673843.2017.1330698.

Malekpour, M. (2007). "Effects of Attachment on Early and Later Development", *The British Journal of Development Disabilities*, *53*(105), 81–95. https://doi.org/10.1179/096979507799103360

Mikulincer, M. and Shaver, P.R. (2007). *Attachment in Adulthood: Structure, Dynamics, and Change",* New York, NY: The Guilford Press.

Muris, P., Meesters, C., van Melick, M. and Zwambag, L. (2001). "Self-reported attachment style, attachment quality and symptoms of anxiety and depression in young adolescents", *Personality and Individual Differences*, 30, 809-818.

Nada-Raja, S., McGee, R., and Stanton, W.R. (1992). "Perceived attachments to parents and peers and psychological well-being in adolescence", *Journal of Youth Adolescence,* 21, 471–85.

Oldfield, J., Humphrey, N., and Hebron, J. (2016). "The role of parental and peer attachment relationships and school connectedness in predicting adolescent mental health outcomes", *Child and Adolescent Mental Health*, *21*(1), 21-29.

Pauli-Pott, U., Haverkock, A., Pott, W., and Beckmann, D. (2007). "Negative emotionality, attachment quality, and behaviour problems in early childhood",

Infant Mental Health Journal, 28, 39–53. https://doi.org/Doi 10.1002/Imhj.20121

Rees, CA. (2005). "Thinking about children's attachments", *Arch Dis Child*, *90*(10):1058–1065.

Rees, C. (2007). "Childhood attachment", *The British Journal of General Practice*, *57*(544), 920–922.

Rutter, M. (1995). "Clinical Implications of Attachment Concepts: Retrospect and Prospect", *Journal of Child Psychology and Psychiatry*, *36*(4), 549–571.

Raja, N. (1992). "Perceived Attachments to Parents and Peers and Psychological Well-being in Adolescence", *Journal of Youth and Adolescence*, *21*(4).

Sasikala, S., and Cecil, N. (2016). "Parental Bonding, Peer Attachment and Psychological Well-being among Adolescents: A Mediation Analysis", *Journal of Psychological Research*, *11*(1), 21–31.

Sroufe, A., and Waters, E. (1977). "Attachment as an organizational construct", *Child Development*, 48, 1184-1199.

Sund, A.M. and Wichstrom, L. (2002). "Insecure attachment as a risk factor for future depressive symptoms in early adolescence", *Journal of American Academic Child Adolescents Psychiatry*, 4, 1478–85.

Thompson, R.A. (2000). "New directions for child development in the twenty-first century: The legacy of early attachments", *Child Development*, 71, 145-152.

21

Mental Health Promotion Among Students

A Holistic School-based Approach

Vandana Singh and *Anubhuti Dubey*

Background

Mental health is defined as a subjective state of well-being. It incorporates individuals' feelings about their potentials, strengths, and weakness, how to deal with the daily hassles of life, and can contribute to society (WHO, 2004). Mental health builds the ability to perceive self-efficacy, autonomy, competence, and self-actualization that deals with the individual's awareness, attitude, and belief about mental illnesses. The positive dimension of mental health is described in the definition of health of WHO: 'Health does not just mean by the absence of physical illness or disease, rather, it is an umbrella term which includes people's physical, mental as well as social health and wellbeing' (WHO, 2001, p. 1). Mental Health and positive living styles are the abilities for adaptive and positive behaviours and need to be mandated for helping children and adolescents to effectively deal with the demands and challenges of everyday life. A transition from childhood to adolescence leads to major physiological, mental, emotional, and behavioural changes. Though most children adjust themselves in these transitions but some of them become stressed and they have difficulty adjusting in these kinds of changes (Collins et al., 2018). If they fail to get proper support then several personalities and psychological problems i.e. anxiety, depression, eating disorders, ADHD, arise (Grover, *et al.,* 2019). Therefore, it is important to provide them a very healthy and nurturing atmosphere to boost their mental health.

Mental Health Issues Among Children and Adolescents

Mental Health is defined as the ability to achieve and sustain the supreme psychological strength and well-being. It is directly related to the students' capability in psychological and social functioning. It is not just the absence of mental illness, but also covers social, emotional, and behavioural health and the ability to cope with life's challenges (WHO, 2018). Mental health problems are linked to severe negative outcomes such as academic and behavioural problems, dropout, and delinquency, etc. (Pedrelli, 2015). Mental health problems among children and young people manifest in many ways, including emotional problems such as anxiety and depression, hyperactivity, conduct disorders, and peer problems. These problems have increased rapidly among children and adolescents, particularly behaviour-related problems and suicidal tendencies have dramatically increased in India (Radhakrishnan & Andrade, 2012). Most of the risk-taking behaviours and psychological problems among children and adolescents appear during the adolescent period. Crime, sexual permissiveness, drug abuse, rule violation, bullying, and school dropouts are on the rise among the youth. These problems have a strong impact on their participation in the classroom, academic achievement, interpersonal relationships, mental health, and psychological well-being. Promoting healthy competence has the potential to prevent high-risk behaviours, psychological problems and enhance good spirit among children and adolescents. It can be preventable through school mental health programmes which can boost mental health and well being among children and adolescents (Patel, *et al.*, 2012).

What Statistics Say?

It is estimated that approximately 20 per cent of adolescents in the world have mental health or some sort of behavioural issues. Up to 50 per cent of mental, behavioural, and psychological problems occur during adolescence (Kessler & Berglund *et al.*, 2005). A study conducted in Bangalore in 2005 indicated that the prevalence rate of psychiatric disorders in the neonate to 16-year-old children was 12.5 per cent with no significant difference in prevailing rates in the urban middle class, slum and rural areas. An assessment of felt treatment needs indicated that only 37.5 per cent of the families considered that their children had any psychiatric condition (Srinath, 2005). In the psychiatric morbidity profile of 2544 children from central India, the researcher found that 6.8 per cent of them had psychiatric morbidity. Most of them were aged between 11–16 years. Mental retardation was the most common disorder with 64 per cent, followed by epilepsy (7%), ADHD (5.7%), schizophrenia and other psychosis disorders (5.7%), depression (4%) and autism (1.1 per cent) (Solanki & Rastogi, 2017). Keyho and his colleague (2019) conducted a research in Nagaland and they found that the prevalence rate of severe mental illness was 17.2 per cent and approximately 28.8 per cent students were at the borderline level. The study also revealed that 17.1 per cent students were suffered from emotional problems, 16.1 per cent have hyperactivity and 15.2 per cent have some sort of conduct disorder. Now the situation has become worse. The stress faced by children and adolescents is massive. In a report of WHO (2011), it is claimed that 'near about 7.5 per cent of the Indian population suffers from some kind of mental disorder. India accounted for nearly 11.6 per cent of global mental, neurological, substance abuse disorder and it also predicts that by 2020 the percentage will be increased from 7.5 to 20 per cent'. If these data are to be relied upon, then the result would be terrific because there is no systematic understanding of prevalence and risk factors are readily available in every state of India (India State Level Distance Burden Initiative Mental Disorders Collaborators, 2017). A meta-analysis was performed on mental health issues and it was found that the estimated prevalence rate of mental disorders was 12.1 per cent, whereas disease-specific prevalence was 4.16 per cent for nocturnal enuresis, 2.38 per cent for pica disorder, 1.78 per cent for behaviour disorders, and 1.26 per cent for other developmental disorders among children and adolescents in India (Malhotra, 2014). Another study conducted on students from rural schools in Haryana and West Bengal found that the prevalence rates of mental disorders were 20.7 per cent and 33.33 per cent respectively (Hossain & Purohit, 2019). Suicide rates among Indian youths especially among the student population appear to be quite higher than anywhere else in the world, accounting for 12.2 per cent per 100,000 male population and 9.1 per cent per 100,000 female population ages ranged between 10-19 years (WHO, 2014). It shows some sort of gender differences in behaviour problems and suicidal tendency as well. Thresholds for mental health services have been rising, with the result that some young people in need do not receive any specialist support, while those who do are often forced to wait many months before getting treatment without being directed to alternative forms of support in the meantime. The tragedy of this growing mental health crisis is underlined by the fact that there is good evidence to suggest that early access to appropriate health services has the potential to improve outcomes of mild, moderate and more serious mental health problems, yet services are currently unable to cope with demand.

Mental Health Programmes in Schools

Mental health programmes for young people can only be successful if it is flexible, culturally appropriate and more specifically centred on their needs and concerns (Vranda, 2015). The ideal place for such programmes is the school where there is ample opportunity to promote the mental health of young people (Weist & Murray, 2008). Stress, anxiety, and depression are the most frequently identified mental health problems among students. Psychoses, substance abuse disorders and self-harm tendencies, which are less common and are poorly addressed, but often much more serious and enduring. Many of the mental, behavioural and psychological problems among children and adolescents can be prevented, if it is diagnosed and intervened at an early stage. There is considerable potential for school-based interventions to mitigate risk factors and enhance protective factors to promote mental health and wellbeing of children and adolescents. A well-inclusive programme has the potential to build efficiency among children and adolescents in schools if it incorporates teachers as facilitators and this yields long-term outcomes on investment (Parikh, *et al.* 2019). Good mental health is vital to children and adolescents' success in school and social life. Researches confirmed that students who receive social-emotional and mental support always achieve better academically. It also improves the perception of healthy a School climate, classroom behaviour, on-task learning, and students' sense of connectedness and well-being as well (Thapa, Cohen, Guffey, & Alessandra, 2013). So, schools must recognize and respond to the diverse mental health and well-being needs of students and thereby ensuring quality education to all through the appropriate curriculum, organizational arrangements, teaching strategies, and resource supports.

In this context, schools have a unique opportunity to improve the lives of students. Progressively, schools should expand their role in providing services for the overall child and adolescent development and well-being. As a powerful socialization agent, the school plays an important role in the transformation of cognitive, linguistic and psychosocial competencies. The school is not only a place for academics, but also an important environment where students form peer-group relationships, develop social skills and become familiar with many social and personal possibilities. A climate of the school, which is a place for learning and modelling, also has the potential to contribute positively to the mental health and well-being of students. It is important to build happy, healthy and harmonious schools for students' mental health welfare, which are significant demographic dividends and most important national assets. It is to be noted that India does not yet have a comprehensive approach and practices for school mental health promotion.

Existing Policies and Services for Mental Health Promotion in India

In India, there is no separate all-encompassing policy to deal with mental health issues in children. Children's mental health policy is limited, and the behavioural and emotional support needs and aspects of special students are completely ignored. In the five-year plans, the government has earmarked only a few million rupees to provide mental health facilities for the entire country, in which mental health promotion of the children has received very little priority (Bhat, 2012). Several mental health and other disabilities programmes and policies have lots of complications related to its nature, administration, or access to a targeted group of people. Mental health facilities are limited in India (Lahariya, 2018) and primary health care doctors and nurses have no official in-service training in the mental health sector. Mental health expenditure by the Indian government is less than 0.06 per cent of the total health budget (Mishra & Galhotra, 2018). The existing policies such as the National Health Policy, Integrated Child Development Scheme and National Mental Health Programme, etc. stress the need to be more comprehensive at various levels. India has adopted several national policies in different areas of child development, which include the National Policy for Children (1974), National Policy for Education (1986), POCSO Act (1982), Mental Health Act (1987), Charter for Children (2004), National Mental Health Policy (2014) etc. But none of them have serious concern over the problem of mental health and wellbeing of children and adolescents in the school setting (Shastri, 2008). Some steps are taken to improve the well-being of students by various other institutions such as the School-based campaigns started by National Institute of Mental Health and Neurosciences (NIMHANS) situated in Bangalore which aims to increase awareness about psychosocial disorders, self-awareness, and improvement in interpersonal relationships with peers and teachers (Vranda, 2015). Central Board of Secondary Education (CBSE) has made it compulsory to provide counselling services to students in every school, but even then, in most developed areas like

National Capital Region (NCR) and other metropolitan cities, less than 3 per cent of schools have counselling facilities. Schools charge heavily for counselling services and are still not guaranteed whether counselling will be done by trained counsellors (CBSE, 2008; Thacker, 2018). They do not necessarily consider all the criteria for the recruitment of counsellors. On January 7th, 2014, the National Adolescent Health Action (RKSK) was recognized by the Government of India and implemented by the state government through the National Health Mission. Under such initiative of Ministry of Human Resource Development (MHRD), recently the Government of Uttar Pradesh has started the recruitment of school counsellors in various Kendriya Vidyalaya Sangathan (a system of central government schools under the Ministry of Human Resource Development, Government of India) and other Navodaya schools (Johari, 2019). Although it has several limitations to address mental health issues, for instance, mental health is taken as taboo, and in reality; anxiety and depression are not taken as a serious concern in India (Roy *et al.*, 2019; Nebhinani & Jain, 2019). Patients with severe mental disorders are stereotypically called *Pagal* (mad) here. So the people, especially students do not hold the courage to confront their situation in front of teachers, peers or even with family members. Counsellors have the responsibility to identify such students and encourage them to share their feelings and problems. They should need continuous progression and training in their role and responsibility for school mental health promotion and special education for disabled children.

A Solution as a Holistic School-based Approach (HSBA)

Mental health is the main concern of this review paper so it broadly emphasizes the approach that needs to be focusing on students' psychological, emotional, social health and wellbeing. Schools play a large role in the holistic development of students and provide a room and scope for interventions at all levels of the schooling extent. There is a need to boost students' mental health at various levels of school. As we have already discussed the importance of all-round development of students to ensure their positive mental health, so it is necessary to collaborate and cooperate with all school stakeholders to make sure that the counselling programmes and mental health activities are successfully implemented (Low *et al.*, 2013). This is called the *Holistic Approach* which means the involvement of every aspect of school and/or people related to school incorporates accomplishing certain goals (Argyros,

2012). It is a concept that acknowledges the social, political, economic and demographic contexts within which schools operate and influence students' psychological health (Parsons *et al.,* 1996). Teaching resilience, safety, and health education, the involvement of parents and community services and working on comprehensive mental health policies are the most important contributing factors of a successful holistic approach across all years of the schooling system. This comprehensive approach is globally recognized as working holistically to promote student health and wellbeing. The Holistic school approach ensures that all aspects of the school communities contribute positively to students' health, safety, and wellbeing. Several international initiatives from the WHO, UNICEF, UNESCO, and the International Union for Health Promotion and Education (IUHPE) use different terms to describe holistic, and comprehensive approaches address to the health and well-being issues among students, school staff and the wider school community. It is not just about what happens in the curriculum, but it is about the entire school day, it is built on an assumption that learning does not only take place through the traditional curriculum but also through students' daily experience of life inside or outside of the school. It works on a theme that the good health of an individual cannot be attained just through their efforts, but health is also shaped by the surroundings within which he/she live, and work. By adopting this approach, schools can enhance the involvement of all stakeholders and increase the potential for sustainable development.

Here are some insights to initiate Holistic School-based Approach in the school system:

Require to work as a team to accomplish the same goal: The holistic school-based approach includes working together and being committed to all parts of the school. This requires teamwork among the students, school leaders, teachers and all school staff, as well as parents, and the wider community to achieve students' overall health and development (Dassanayake, Springett & Shewring, 2017). The mental health approaches should be designed to strengthen student abilities or skills using teachers as the facilitators in the schools in the following areas: promotion of positive mental health, enhancing resilience, handling academic stressors, practicing healthy lifestyles, prevention and handling sexual abuse, and bullying, developing healthy relationships, prevention of substance abuse, goal setting, prevention of suicide and developing values and life skills (Nagpal, 2017).

Development of comprehensive mental health curriculum: Schools should encompass the 'comprehensive curriculum' that can elevate the awareness among principals, teachers, managers and all students towards the factors that can promote their mental health, like, Healthy activities, Anger management, Promotion of Emotional Health, and Safety and so on. '*Happiness Curriculum*' that has been introduced by the Delhi government in over 1,000 schools between nursery to class 8. The entire curriculum is activity-based which includes yoga, meditation, exercises. It aims to stimulate a sense of self-concept, good mental health and reduce depression, anxiety among students (Staff, 2018).

Organizing programmes and campaigns to make parents and students aware of mental health: Schools must organize sequential age-appropriate programmes and campaigns to spread awareness on all dimensions of health and wellbeing. Life skills, health, and wellbeing programmes should be implemented for all students so that they become aware, accountable and empowered from all aspects of their personality and integrated with the standard of health and wellbeing. Along with this, some parenting sessions in terms of child mental health, care and resilience training and awareness are also important to under HSBA.

Appointment of Trained counsellors and special educators: Trained Counsellors and special educators should be appointed to facilitate effective guidance and counselling for students as well as their families throughout their schooling. The right counselling and guidance help them to deal with their problems and also helps them to choose their academics and career effectively. There are a few most important things to consider for children with special needs i.e. early detection and intervention of the developmental problems and disorders are necessary as part of the specialized support to these children.

Capacity building programmes for teachers: Along with this, some capacity building programmes for teachers and non-teaching staff should also be included to accommodate and equip them with the greatest skills to understand and deal with students' and their mental health concerns (Ireland, 2017).

Holistic School-based interventions programme has been increasingly recognized as an effective means of promoting the mental health of students and prevent the development of unhealthy behaviour. Increased access to mental health services and supports in schools is vital to improve the physical and psychological safety of students, as well as academic performance and problem-solving skills at schools. HSBA supports an idea that social-emotional learning, mental health, resilience, and positive relationships between students and teachers are essential to creating a harmonious school culture in which students feel confident and create an adaptive coping strategy to maintain their mental health and well-being. One of the main assumptions of HSBA is that if students feel safe and empowered to report their concerns, it is one of the most effective school safety strategies (Xaba, 2014; Diaz, 2017). Additionally, school mental health professionals can provide sustainable supports, and can help to identify and work with students with their more intense or daily needs. All programmes focused on increasing the capacity of children and adolescents produce long-lasting positive effects on the mental, social, and behavioural domains.

Conclusion

Schools should initiate various activities to ensure a complete sense of support and safety that further linked to students' physical, emotional and psychological and social health. A successful school is one that aims to promote the mental health of their students and staff and to create an environment that supports both mental health and well-being along with students' academic success. In his study, Jamtsho also supports the idea that a well-equipped programme that is developed with a motive to the acquisition of students' social, emotional competencies also has the potential to decrease the rates of behavioural disorders and emotional distress (Jamtsho, 2015).

To conclude, it is suggested that it is a shared responsibility of teachers, parents and all school communities for the overall health and wellbeing of students, so they should understand, build and maintain all parts of the school climate to make it a better and healthier environment. Additionally, it is important to have an approach as well as an evaluation system that can concern on students' overall development and progressively access their problems from time to time. High quality mental health policies and services are required to ensure their diagnosis, treatment and proper care and support. It is suggested that the schools which work with all aspects of a holistic school plan have a positive impact on students' mental health and well-being. A holistic-school approach could be an ideal way to bring about changes to policy and practice to ensure everyone is fully on board, from governors to teaching assistants.

References

Argyros, I. (2012). "Aspects of the holistic approach in teaching, presented at Modern Technologies of Teaching Foreign Languages", Selected papers from the International Scientific Conference, Ulyanovsk, Russia, vol. 1.

Bhat, R. (2012). *Mental Health Budget Analysis*, doi: 10.13140/RG.2.1.2955.8242.

Central Board of Secondary Education (CBSE) (2008). "Counselling in Schools. Circular no. 08 of 2008. www.cbse.nic.in/welcome/htm retrieved on July 27, 2009.

Collins, A. and Solomando, A.M. (2018). "The transition from child to adolescent to adult mental health services with a focus on diagnosis progression", *British Journal of Psychology Bulletin, 42*(5), 188-192.

Díaz-Vicario, A. (2017). "Practices that promote comprehensive school safety", *New Trends and Issues Proceedings on Humanities and Social Sciences.* [Online]. 01, 304-312. Available from: www.prosoc.eu.

Government of India (1982), *National Mental Health Programme for India*. New Delhi: Ministry of Health and Family Welfare. New Delhi. India.

Grover, S., Raju, V., Sharma, A., and Shah, R. (2019). "Depression in children and adolescents: A review of Indian studies", *Indian Journal of Psychological Medicine*, *41*(3), 216-27.

Hossain, M.M. and Purohit, N. (2019). "Improving child and adolescent mental health in India: Status, services, policies, and way forward", *Indian Journal of Psychiatry*, 61, 415-19.

Ireland, M.L. (2017). Increasing Teacher Capacity in Supporting Student Mental Health (Doctoral dissertation). The Organizational Improvement Plan at Western University, University of Western Ontario.

Jamtsho, S. (2015). "Implementing a Whole-School Approach to Student Wellbeing: A Study Examining the Implementation Experiences of Bhutanese and Australian Teachers in Wellbeing Leadership Roles. [Doctoral dissertation, Melbourne Graduate School of Education, The University of Melbourne].

Johri, N. (2019, Nov. 10). Navodaya Vidyalaya Samiti recruits 1,176 counsellors after incidents of suicides by students. Retrieved from https://preptube.in/news/navodaya-vidyalaya-samiti-recruits-1176-counsellors-after-incidents-of-suicides-by-students/2019/11/10/

Kessler, R.C., Berglund, P., Demler, O., Jin, R., and Merikangas, *et al.* (2005). "Lifetime prevalence and age of onset distributions of DSM-IV disorders in the national comorbidity survey replication", *Arch of Gen Psychiatry,* 62 (6), 593-602.

Keyho, K., Gujar, N.M., and Ali, A. (2019). "Prevalence of mental health status in adolescent school children of Kohima District, Nagaland", *Ann Indian Psychiatry,* 3(1), 39-42.

Lahariya, C. (2018). "Strengthen mental health services for universal health coverage in India", *Journal of Postgraduate Medicine, 64*(1), 7–9.

Low, S.K., Kok, J.K. and Lee, M.N. (2013). "A holistic approach to school-based counselling and guidance services in Malaysia", *School Psychology International. 34*(2), 190–201.

Malhotra, S., and Patra, B.N. (2014). "Prevalence of child and adolescent psychiatric disorders in India: A systematic review and meta-analysis", *Child and Adolescent Psychiatry and Mental Health, 8,* 22.

Mark, D. and Weist, M.M. (2008), Advancing School Mental Health Promotion Globally", *Advances in School Mental Health Promotion*, 1 sup1, 2-12.

Mental health: a state of well-being. (2014, August 15). Retrieved from https://www.who.int/features/factfiles/mental_health/en/.

Mental health: strengthening our response. (2018, march 30). Retrieved from https://www.who.int/news-room/fact-sheets/detail/mental-health-strengthening-our-response.

Mishra, A. and Galhotra, A. (2018). "Mental Healthcare Act 2017: Need to wait and watch", *International Journal of Applied Basic Medicine Research,* 8(2), 67-70.

Nagpal, J. (2017, April 18). *Promotion of mental health and wellbeing in schools.* Retrieved April from http://www.progressiveschool.in/promotion-of-mental-health-wellbeing-in-schools/.

Nebhinani, N. and Jain, S. (2019). "Promoting child and adolescent mental health in India*", Indian Assoc. Child Adolescent Mental Health, 15*(3), 1-8.

Patel, V., Ramasundarahettige, C., Vijayakumar, L., Thakur, J.S., Gajalakshmi, V., *et al.* (2012). "Suicide Mortality in India: A Nationality Representative Survey", *Lancet*, 379, 2343-51.

Parikh, R., Michelson, D., Sapru, M., Sahu, R., Singh, A., Cuijpers, P., and Patel, V. (2019). "Priorities and preferences for school-based mental health services in India: A multi-stakeholder study with adolescents, parents, school staff, and mental health providers", *Global Mental Health, 6*, e18.

Parsons, C., Stears, D. and Thomas, C. (1996), The Health Promoting School in Europe: conceptualising and evaluating the change", *Health Education Journal*, 55, 311–321.

Pedrelli, P. Nyer, M., Yeund, A., Zulauf, Courtesy, Wilens, T. (2015). "College students: Mental health problems and treatment consideration", *Acad. Psychiatry. 39*(5), 503-511.

Radhakrishnan, R., and Andrade, C. (2012). "Suicide: An Indian Perspective", *Indian Journal of Psychiatry, 54*(4), 304-319.

Roy, K., Shinde, S., Sarkar, B.K., *et al.* (2019). "India's response to adolescents' mental health: A policy review and stakeholder analysis", *Social Psychiatry and Psychiatric Epidemiology, 54*(4), 405-414.

Shastri, P.S. (2008). "Future perspective of planning child guidance services in India", *Indian Journal of Psychiatry*, 50, 241–243.

Solanki, N., and Rastogi, P. (2017). "Clinical profile of child and adolescent patients attending a mental hospital OPD", *IJRMS,* 5(9), 4021-4024.

Srinath, S., and Sitholey, P. (2005). "Epidemiological study of child and adolescent psychiatric disorders in urban and rural areas", In B. Shah, R. Parhee, N.

Kumar, T. Khanna, and R. Singh (Eds.). *Mental health research in India: Technical monograph on ICMR Mental Health Studies* (pp. 86–90). New Delhi: Indian Council of Medical Research.

Staff, F.P. (2018, July 12). 'Happiness curriculum' to be introduced in over 1,000 Delhi Government schools for eight lakh students between Nursery and Class 8. Retrieved from https://www.firstpost.com/india/happiness-curriculum-introduced-in-over-1000-delhi-govt-schools-for-eight-lakh-students-between-nursery-and-class-8-4726821.html

State Council of Educational Research and Training and Directorate of Education (2019). *Happiness Curriculum.* Retrieved from http://edudel.nic.in/welcome_folder/happiness/HappinessCurriculumFramework_2019.pdf.

Thacker, H. (2018, October 15). CSR: Counselling in Schools in India. Retrieved from https://thecsrjournal.in/csr-counselling-in-schools-in-india/

Thapa, A., Cohen, Guffey, and Alessandro (2013). "A Review of School Climate Research", *Review of Educational Research, 83*(3), 357-385.

Vranda, M.N. (2015). "Promotion of Mental Health and Well-Being of Adolescents in Schools: A NIMHANS Model", *Journal of Psychiatry, 18*(5), 303.

Wijaya Dassanayake, Jane Springett and Tania Shewring (2017): The impact on anxiety and depression of a whole school approach to health promotion: evidence from a Canadian comprehensive school health (CSH) initiative", *Advances in School Mental Health Promotion,* DOI:10.1080/175473 0X.2017.1333913.

World Health Organization (2001). *The World Health Report 2001. Mental health: New understanding. New hope*. Geneva, World Health Organization.

World Health Organization. (2004). *Promoting Mental Health: Concepts, emerging evidence, practice.* Geneva: World Health Organization.

Whole School Approach-Teaching Resilience, Road Safety and Drug Education. (2019). Retrieved from https://www.sdera.wa.edu.au/programs/whole-school-approach/

Xaba, M.I. (2014). "A holistic approach to safety and security at schools in South Africa", *Mediterranean Journal of Social Sciences, 5*(20), 1580-1589.

22

Aggression among Adolescents in Relation to Social Intelligence and Self-esteem

Kanchan Verma, Saroj Verma and *Purnima Awasthi*

Adolescence is the age of transition between childhood and adulthood. The beginning of adolescence is marked by puberty a flood of biological event leading to adult body size and sexual maturity. Most of the individual in this stage face developmental changes and life challenges (Zarrett & Eccles, 2006). Academic performance, relationship with family and friend, social rules etc. are some of the most challenging aspect of adolescent life and they try various ways to maintain harmony in these areas, but sometimes results are not positive due to which they show frustration, low self-esteem and aggression.

Aggression can be defined as a behaviour that is intended to harm another individual who does not wish to be harmed (Baron & Richardson, 1994). In previous studies it is found that adolescents show more aggression (Berkowitz, 1993; Reiss & Roth, 1993; Toldor, 2004; & Khan, 2006) than any other age group. Level of aggression may affect by family environment, school environment, peer group, society, gender and personal trait. With respect to gender the discrepancy could be seen in findings of various studies. Bjorkquist, Osterman and Largerspetz, (1992), Jonathan and Onukweefor (2013) conduct studies to examine the difference between male and female regarding their level of aggression and result explained that male adolescents were more aggressive than females. Level of anger and hostility were also found to be higher in boys as compared to girls (Tsorbatzoudis, Travlos & Rodafinos, 2013; Ghanizadeh, 2008) whereas some studies reported that females show more hostility and anger (Ali, Ichraf, Khaed, Liwa & Ali, 2013) and verbal aggression (Nagda, Amira, Dalia & Khalid, 2016).

The dissimilarity in level of aggression between male and female may be because of different pattern of socialization of both gender as well as their emotional and intellectual ability (e.g. self-esteem and social intelligence). Self-esteem is a subjective evaluation of his or her own worth. Self-esteem is combination of self-worth and self-respect which is developed as a result of positive and negative experiences in one's life. In respect to gender the several studies show that males have higher Self-esteem than females (Bleidom *et al.*, 2006; Agam, Tamir & Golan, 2015; Quatman & Watson, 2010; Nupur & Mahapatro, 2016). People with high self-esteem value themselves, set appropriate goals and use feedback for enhancing themselves (Wood & Hempet, 2003) whereas people with low self-esteem have tendency to critic themselves and get negative feedback for themselves and they also disturbed about their social relationship (Brown & Marshell, 2001). Low level of self-esteem is also related to aggressive behaviour (Donnellan, Trzesniewisk, Robins, Moffit & Capsi, 2005; Garofalo, Holden, Hill & Velotti, 2005). The low self-esteem weakens ties to society; and the weaker ties to society decrease conformity to social norms and increase delinquency (Hirschi, 1969). Feeling of inferiority rooted in early childhood experiences of rejection and humiliation also motivates aggression and antisocial behaviour (Horney, 1950; Adler, 1956). However there are several studies which have failed to find relationship between low Self-esteem and aggression (Bushman & Baumeister, 1998 Kirkpatrick, Waugh, Valencia & Webster, 2002; Twenge & Capmbell, 2003). Whereas a study by Baumeister, Smart and Boden (1996) reported that any link between self-esteem and aggression probably occurs at the high end of the self-esteem continuum. On the basis of literature reviewed so far, contradictory results have been observed regarding association between overall self-esteem and aggression.

Social intelligence is also a predictor of aggression (Andreon, 2006). Social intelligence is the ability to understand the feelings, thoughts and behaviour of persons in social or interpersonal situations and to act appropriately (Thorndike, 1920) Aggression is one of the opposites of social intelligence and is any form of behaviour directed towards the goal of harming or injuring another living one who is motivated to avoid such treatments. Negative correlation has been found between social intelligence and aggression in some studies (Babu, 2007; Shekarey, Ladani, Rostami, & Jamshidi, 2013). Gender differences have also been found in relation to this variable and in most studies adolescent girls were better than adolescent boys with respect to their social intelligence (Babu, 2007; Saxena, & Jain, 2013; Sembiyan & Vishvanathan, 2012) and social awareness (Sekar, 2016). Different results have been obtained in relation to the level of self-esteem and aggression among men and women. The dearth of studies examining the linkage between aggression and social intelligence was observed. Therefore, the present study attempts to assess and compare the aggression, self-esteem and social intelligence of male and female adolescents and to examine the extent of relationship of aggression with self-esteem and social intelligence.

Objectives

(1) To assess and compare various dimensions of aggression among male and female adolescents.
(2) To assess and compare various dimensions of self-esteem and social intelligence among male and female adolescents.
(3) To examine the extent of relationship of aggression with various dimensions of self-esteem and social intelligence among male and female adolescents.

Hypotheses

H1. Male adolescents would score higher on various dimension of aggression than female adolescents.

H2. Male adolescents would score higher on various dimensions of self-esteem whereas female adolescents would score higher on various dimensions of social intelligence.

H3. Aggression would be negatively correlated with self-esteem and social intelligence among male and female adolescents.

Method

Sample: The sample for the study consisted of 200 adolescents (male = 100, female = 100) of age range 12-18 years, studying in various schools of Barabanki district. Purposive sampling technique was employed for drawing the sample. All the participants belonged to middle socio-economic status. Students with any physical disability were excluded from the sample.

Tools

1. Personal Data Sheet

It contains information about the socio-demographic variables like age, gender, education, religion, socioeconomic status, parental education and occupation.

2. Aggression Questionnaire (BUSS, 1992)

It measures four aspect of aggression i.e. Physical aggression, Verbal aggression, Anger, Hostility. Scale consist 29 items. It is a five point Likert scale: 1 = extremely uncharacteristic of me, 4 = somewhat characteristic of me, 5 = extremely characteristic of me. The test retest reliability of this questionnaire is 0.97. internal consistency (Cronbach's alpha) reliability coefficient for the scale is 0.82.

3. State Self-esteem Scale (Heatherton and Polivy, 1991)

This scale consists 20 items divided in three aspect of self-esteem, i.e. performance self, Social self, Appearance self-esteem. It is a five point Likert scale where 1 indicate strongly disagree, 5 indicate strongly agree. Reliability of scale was found 0.73-0.81.

4. The Tromso Social Intelligence Scale (Silvera, Monica & Dahl, 1992)

This scale measures three dimensions of social intelligence i.e. social information processing, social awareness and social skills. It consists 21 items. Reliability (Cronbach's alpha) of the Tromso social intelligence scale is 0.72-0.86.

Procedure

Participants selected for the study were contacted personally at their respective schools. Detailed instructions given in the manual of the scales being used were given to them. Participants were allowed to take their own time to complete their questionnaires. Scoring for all the above mentioned questionnaires was done according to the method given in their manuals.

Results and Discussion

To meet the objectives of the study, gender differences on various dimensions of aggression, self-esteem and social intelligence were examined through computation of mean, SD and 't' test and results have been presented in tables 22.1, 22.2 and 22.3. Tables indicate significant gender difference regarding physical aggression (t = 2.95, p<0.01), appearance self-esteem (t = 2.88, p<.01), social information processing (t = 1.90, p<.05).

Table 22.1: Significance of the difference between mean score for males and females regarding various dimensions of aggression

Dimensions of aggression	*Male (n=100)*	*Female (n=100)*	*'t' values*
	Mean (SD)	Mean (SD)	
Physical aggression	20.82 (4.44)	19.24 (2.98)	2.95**
Verbal aggression	13.54 (3.27)	14.08 (3.27)	-1.16
Anger	18.12 (3.67)	16.55 (10.34)	1.43
Hostility	20.31 (3.81)	20.27 (3.94)	0.07

** significant at .01 level.

Comparison of mean scores of male and female participants with respect to various dimensions of aggression show significant difference on physical aggression between boys and girls. Male adolescents scored higher than female adolescents and this finding is supported by Talukdar and Deka (2014), Akhtar and Kushwaha (2015), Singh, Hassan and Wani (2017) which indicated that male adolescents show more physical aggression than females. There are some studies in support of the results which demonstrate that males are more hostile (Ahmed & Ghanizadeh, 2008; Burt, 1999) and in others female were found verbally more aggressive than males (Nagda, Amira, Dalia and Khalid, 2016). Thus, the first hypothesis of the study which assumes higher scores of males on various dimensions of aggression is partially accepted here. Females may be less aggressive due to gender role socialization as gender role discourage aggressiveness among females under certain circumstances (Hall, 1984), whereas men are expected to be tough, violent and aggressive (Cicone & Ruble,1978).

Table 22.2: Significance of the difference between mean score of males and females regarding various dimensions of Self-esteem

Dimensions of self-esteem	*Male N =100*	*Female N =100*	*'t' Value*
	Mean (SD)	*Mean (SD)*	
Performance self-esteem	24.21 (2.88)	25.11 (4.57)	-1.66
Social self-esteem	23.34 (13.92)	23.09 (2.87)	.176
Appearance self-esteem	21.48 (3.38)	20.08 (3.47)	2.88**

**significant at .01 level.

Results in Table 22.2 indicate the difference between mean scores of males and females on various dimension of self-esteem. There is no significant difference on performance self-esteem and social self-esteem between male and female adolescents. Significant difference was observed regarding appearance self-esteem ($t = 2.88, p < 0.01$) in which boys scored higher on appearance self-esteem than girls. Thus, the second hypothesis that assumes higher scores of males on various dimensions of self-esteem as compared to females is partially accepted. There are several studies in which the overall self-esteem of boys has been found higher than girls (Quatman & Watson, 2010; Agam, Tamir & Golan, 2015; Bleidon et al. 2016). Different standard of body image of both gender may be the reason of difference between males and females on appearance self-esteem as Austin et al. (2009) explained in their study that boys report dissatisfaction with their below or above average weight whereas underweight girls report greater satisfaction with their body in comparison to average weight girls.

Table 22.3: Significance of the difference between mean score for males and females regarding various dimension of social intelligence

Dimensions of social intelligence	*Male N =100*	*Female N =100*	*'t' Value*
	Mean (SD)	*Mean (SD)*	
Social information processing	24.29 (3.92)	22.25 (3.70)	2.87**
Social skill	22.25 (3.70)	24.33(19.16)	– 1.06
Social awareness	17.92 (4.39)	16.89 (3.13)	1.90*

* significant at the .05 level, ** significant at the.01 level.

Findings in Table 22.3 indicated that the male and female adolescents significantly differed regarding two dimensions of social intelligence, i.e. social information processing and social awareness. Male participants scored higher on social information processing and social awareness than their female counterparts. This finding is consistent with the results of the study by Kumar (2014) who reported that male adolescents have better social intelligence than female adolescents. The finding was not supported by Srivastav, Mathur, and Chako (2016), Sembiyan and Vishvanathan (2012), Baumgarther (2009), Babu (2007) and Sekar (2016) which indicated that females were better than males with respect to their social intelligence. Hence the third hypothesis assuming higher scores of female adolescents on social intelligence has been rejected.

Table 22.4: Coefficient of Correlation among various dimension of aggression, self-esteem and social intelligence of female adolescents

Measures	*Physical aggression*	*Verbal aggression*	*Anger*	*Hostility*	*Overall aggression*
Social intelligence	**0.00**	**-0.08**	**-0.00**	**0.02**	**-0.01**
Social information processing	**-0.05**	**-0.07**	**-0.12**	**-0.07**	**-0.14**
Social skill	0.00	-0.06	0.01	0.03	0.00
Social awareness	**0.01**	**-0.05**	**0.05**	**0.04**	**0.08**
Self-esteem	**-0.10**	**-0.10**	**-0.03**	**-0.13**	**-0.11**
Performance Self-esteem	**-0.06**	**-0.15**	**-0.09**	**-0.26****	**-0.20***
Social self-esteem	-0.08	-0.02	-0.06	0.00	0.14
Appearance self-esteem	**-0.09**	**-0.02**	**0.10**	**0.03**	**0.12**

** Significant at the 0.01 level, * significant at the 0.05 level.

As per the objective of the study about the association of aggression with Self-esteem and social intelligence correlation coefficients were computed and results have been presented in Tables 22.4 and 22.5. Results about the relationships among the aforesaid variables for females are presented in Table 22.4. Results indicated that hostility and overall aggression are negatively correlated with performance self-esteem. There are several studies providing evidence for a link between low self-esteem and aggression (Boden, Fergusson & Horwood, 2007; Donnellan, Trzensniewski, Robins, Moffitt & Caspi, 2005; Walker & Bright, 2009).

Table 22.5: Coefficient of correlation among various dimensions of aggression, self-esteem and social intelligence of male adolescents

Measures	*Physical aggression*	*Verbal aggression*	*Anger*	*Hostility*	*Aggression*
Social intelligence	**-0.08**	**-0.12**	**-0.02**	**0.02**	**-0.09**
Social information processing	-0.12	-0.05	-0.08	-0.05	-0.14
Social skill	0.02	0.07	-0.11	0.05	0.04
Social awareness	-0.04	-0.07	0.14	0.03	0.03
Self-esteem	**0.22***	**0.00**	**-0.06**	**-0.09**	**0.04**
Performance self-esteem	-0.02	0.04	-0.01	-0.09	0.04
Social self-esteem	0.23**	-0.05	-0.04	-0.06	-0.53
Appearance self-esteem	0.03	0.18	-0.09	-0.05	0.02

**significant at 0.01 level, *significant at 0.05 level.

Correlations of various dimensions of aggression with self-esteem and social intelligence among males have been presented in Table 22.5. Dimensions of social intelligence are not significantly correlated with aggression whereas social self-esteem and overall self-esteem are positively correlated with physical aggression. Different pattern of association between these two variables in male and female adolescents have been reported in several studies. Diamontopaulou et al. (2008) found that exaggerated self-evaluations of social competence were more strongly related to aggression in boys than in girls. Canning, Andrew, Murphy, Walker, Showden (2017) found that high level of social rank and high level of attractiveness predicted aggression among males whereas low level of social illusion and low level of attractiveness is found to be related with aggression among females.

Conclusion

On the basis of results it can be concluded that male and female adolescents differ with respect to physical aggression, appearance self-esteem, social awareness and social information processing (dimensions of social intelligence). Positive association of physical aggression with overall self-esteem and social self-esteem among males has been found whereas negative association of hostility and overall aggression with performance self-esteem among females have been obtained. The findings of the study may have counseling implications. Generalization of the findings is limited due to sample size. It would be better to include adolescents belonging to rural area for comparison. It may be suggested to include methods of qualitative assessment for further research.

References

Agam, R., Tamir, S., and Golan, M. (2015). Gender differences in respect to self-esteem and body image as well as response to adolescents' school based prevention programs. *Journal of Psychology and Clinical Psychiatry*, *2*(5), 00092.

Akhtar, J., and Kushwaha, A.K.S. (2015). Gender differences in aggressive behaviour of adolescents. *Research Paper*, *5*, 525-527.

Andreou, E. (2006). Social preference, perceived popularity and social intelligence: Relations to overt and relational aggression. *School Psychology International*, *27*(3), 339-351.

Austin, S.B., Haines, J., and Veugelers, P.J. (2009). Body satisfaction and body weight: Gender differences and socio-demographic determinants. *BMC Public Health*, *9*(1), 313.

Babu, M. (2007). Social Intelligence and Aggression among Senior Secondary School Students: A Comparative Sketch. *Online Submission*.

Baron, R.A., and Richardson D.R. (1994). *Human Aggression: Perspectives in Social Psychology*. Nova Iorque: Plenum Press.

Baumeister, R.F., Smart, L., and Boden, J.M. (1996). Relation of threatened egotism to violence and aggression: The dark side of high self-esteem. *Psychological Review*, *103*(1), 5.

Berkowitz, L. (1993). Pain and aggression: Some findings and implications. *Motivation and Emotion*, *17*(3), 277-293. National Research Council. (1994).

Bleidorn, W., Arslan, R.C., Denissen, J.J., Rentfrow, P.J., Gebauer, J.E., Potter, J., and Gosling, S.D. (2016). Age and gender differences in self-esteem—A cross-cultural window. *Journal of Personality and Social Psychology*, *111*(3), 396.

Boden, J.M., Fergusson, D.M., and Horwood, L.J. (2007). Self-esteem and violence: Testing links between adolescent self-esteem and later hostility and violent behaviour. *Social Psychiatry and Psychiatric Epidemiology*, *42*(11), 881-891.

Brown, J.D. and Marshall, M.A. (2001). Self-esteem and emotion: Some thoughts about feelings. *Personality and Social Psychology Bulletin*, *27*(5), 575-584.

Bushman, B.J. and Baumeister, R.F. (1998). Threatened egotism, narcissism, self-esteem, and direct and displaced aggression: Does self-love or self-hate lead to violence?. *Journal of Personality and Social Psychology*, *75*(1), 219.

Buss, A.H., and Perry, M. (1992). The aggression questionnaire. *Journal of Personality and Social Psychology*, *63*(3), 452.

Canning, A., Andrew, E., Murphy, R., Walker, J.S., and Snowden, R.J. (2017). Gender differences in the relationship between self-esteem and aggression in young people leaving care. *Violence and Gender*, *4*(2), 49-54.

Cicone, M.V. and Ruble, D.N. (1978). Beliefs about males. *Journal of Social Issues*, *34*(1), 5-16.

Diamantopoulou, S., Rydell, A.M., and Henricsson, L. (2008). Can Both Low and High Self-esteem Be Related to Aggression in Children? *Social Development*, *17*(3), 682-698.

Donnellan, M.B., Trzesniewski, K.H., Robins, R.W., Moffitt, T.E., and Caspi, A. (2005). Low self-esteem is related to aggression, antisocial behaviour, and delinquency. *Psychological Science*, *16*(4), 328-335.

Education, I. (2001). Teri Quatman, Ph.D (doctoral dissertation, Santa Clara university).

Elmasry, N.M., Fouad, A.A., Khalil, D.M. and Sherra, K.S. (2016). Physical and verbal aggression among adolescent school students in Sharkia, Egypt: Prevalence and risk factors. *Egyptian Journal of Psychiatry*, *37*(3), 166.

Garofalo, C., Holden, C.J., Zeigler Hill, V., and Velotti, P. (2016). Understanding the connection between Self-esteem and Aggression: The mediating role of emotion dysregulation. *Aggressive Behaviour*, *42*(1), 3-15.

Ghanizadeh, A. (2008). Gender difference of school anger dimensions and its prediction for suicidal behaviour in adolescents. *International Journal of Clinical and Health Psychology*, *8*(2).

Hall, J.A. (1984). Nonverbal sex differences: communication accuracy and expressive style. Baltimore, MD: Johnes Hopkin University Press.

Hirschi, T. (1969). A control theory of delinquency. *Criminology Theory: Selected Classic Readings*, 289-305.

Horney, K. (1950). The tyranny of the should. *Neurosis and Human Growth. The Struggle Towards Self Realisation*, 64-85.

Ichraf, A., Ali, B.M., Khaled, T., Liwa, M., and Ali, E. (2013). Effect of gender and type of sport on anxiety and self-esteem. *International Journal of Humanities and Social Science Invention*, *2*(3), 55-61.

Khan-szabist, F.N. (2006). Age Differences in Expression of Aggression in Men and Women. *Age*, *4*(1).

Kirkpatrick, L.A., Waugh, C.E., Valencia, A., and Webster, G.D. (2002). The functional domain specificity of self-esteem and the differential prediction of aggression. *Journal of Personality and Social Psychology*, *82*(5), 756.

Kumar, V. (2014). Gender differences among adolescents on social intelligence. *International Journal of Research*, *1*(1), 1-3.

Nupur, C., and Mahapatro, M. (2016). Gender differences in Self-esteem among young adults of Raipur, Uttar Pradesh, India. *Austin Journal of Women Health*, *5*(1), 1-4.

Onukwufor, J.N. (2013). Physical and verbal aggression among adolescent secondary school students in rivers state of Nigeria. *British Journal of Education*, *1*(2), 62-7.

Reiss, A.J. and Roth, J.A. (1994) *Understanding and Preventing Violence*. National Academy Press, Washigton, D.C.

Saxena, S., and Jain, R.K. (2013). Social intelligence of undergraduate students in relation to their gender and subject stream. *Journal of Research and Method in Education*, *1*(1), 1-4

Srivastava, M., Mathur, A., Anshu and Chacko, N. (2016). Impact of social intelligence on peer relationships among adolescents: A gender analysis, *Personality and Social Psychology*, *63*(3), 452–9

Sekar, D.J.M.A. (2016). Social intelligence and metacognition of adolescents. *North Asian International Research Journal of Social Science and Humanities*. *2*(9), 2454-9827.

Sembiyan, R., and Visvanathan, G. (2012). A study on social intelligence of college students. *International Journal of Current Research*, *4*(1), 231-232.

Shekarey, A., Ladani, H.J., Rostami, M.S., and Jamshidi, M. (2013). On the Relationship between the social intelligence and aggression: A case study of High School boy students. *International Journal of Education*, *5*(1), 94.

Singh, B., Hassan, A., and Wani, M.A. (2017). Aggression and Self-esteem among Teenagers. *Global Journal of Intellectual and Developmental Disabilities*, *3*(2)

Talukdar, R.R., Deka, R.S. (2014). A study on aggression level among adolescents. *International Journal of Social Science and Humanities Research* *2*(4): 91-94

Thorndike, E.L. (1920). Intelligence and its uses. *Harper's Magazine.140*,227-235.

Tsorbatzoudis, H., Travlos, A.K., and Rodafinos, A. (2013). Gender and age differences in self-reported aggression of high school students. *Journal of Interpersonal Violence*, *28*(8), 1709-1725.

Twenge, J.M., and Campbell, W.K. (2003). "Isn't it fun to get the respect that we're going to deserve?" Narcissism, social rejection, and aggression. *Personality and Social Psychology Bulletin*, *29*(2), 261-272.

Walker, J.S., and Bright, J.A. (2009). False inflated self-esteem and violence: A systematic review and cognitive model. *The Journal of Forensic Psychiatry and Psychology*, *20*(1), 1-32.

Wood, J.V., Heimpel, S.A., and Michela, J.L. (2003). Savoring versus dampening: self-esteem differences in regulating positive affect. *Journal of Personality and Social Psychology*, *85*(3), 566.

Zarrett, N., and Eccles, J. (2006). The passage to adulthood: Challenges of late adolescence. *New Directions for Student Leadership, 2006* (111), 13-28.

23

Child Sexual Abuse

Issues and Challenges

Sreeja Das, Rahul Varma, Tushar Singh and *Yogesh Kumar Arya*

> *Ms. S, 12 years old young girl, hailing from low socio-economic strata of a town near Varanasi, reported to the hospital, was referred for evaluation regarding to her physical illness along with complaint of school refusal for 8 months. On working with her, it was found that she was a victim of sexual abuse, admitted of being photographed, undressed. She was sexually assaulted in a classroom by a male class teacher. On refusal, the teacher would give threats of disclosing the pictures and warned not to reveal it to anyone; otherwise, he would kill her and her family. S did not reveal anything to anyone but started bunking school because of the fear of the teacher. Gradually she started staying isolated, showed disinterest in pleasurable activities. She also reported to experiencing flashbacks and extreme anxiety, loss of memory, at the time of hospital visit.*

Sexual abuse of children is a crime that our society detests in abstract but tolerate in public. This is a strong and provocative statement about a topic that is still taboo in many circles. It seems to be "too dirty", "too Freudian". Those who try to assist sexually abused children must be prepared to battle against all odds, innuendo, hostility and outright harassment. Child who is sexually abused (CSA) has a distressing effect on her/his psychological and physiological health. According to WHO (2003), CSA is "the involvement of a child in sexual activity that he or she does not fully comprehend and is unable to give informed consent to, or for which the child is not developmentally prepared, or else that violates the laws or social taboos of society". These include fondling, masturbation, sexual contact; offensive text messages/emails, displaying the genitals to a minor, penetrative intercourse, indulging in pornography, involving them into sex trafficking or any carnal act which is tormenting to a child psychologically and physiologically (WHO, 2003).

Researchers have investigated that 37 per cent children of Indian population below 18 years of age are not getting proper education, nutritious food and also not getting health care amenities. In addition to this, the sufferer is also prone to childhood maltreatment which includes sexual offense, neglect, and mistreatment but is not being discussed widely. Ministry of Women and Child Development conducted an extensive study to compute the magnitude and depth of child abuse in India (Kacker *et al.*, 2007). This study revealed that around 150 million teenage girls and 60 million boys under the age of 18 years have been forcefully exposed to sexual intercourse or for that matter any kind of carnal aggression (Kacker *et al.*, 2007). Also, studies conducted across the world have also revealed that 1 in 15 men have been sexually molested as a pre-schooler. Reid *et al.*, (2014) observed that many children have been exposed to emotional abuse and neglect by their family members, which aids as a pivotal forecaster of sexploitation for both the genders. The percentage of juveniles (Males-6.9% and Females-11.7%) population who have faced sexual exploitation is dreadful. Noemí *et al.*, (2009) has explored in Africa that there is approximately 37 per cent of occurrence rate of child sexual abuse which has been found to be highest till date followed by Europe, America and Asia which sprang up to 9.4 per cent, 1.1 per cent and 23.9 per cent respectively. Several other countries like Australia, Costa Rica, Tanzania, Israel, Sweden, United States, and Switzerland have proclaimed to have a prevalence rate of child who are sexually abused is more than 1/5th i.e., 37.8 per cent, 32.2 per cent, 31 per cent, 30.7 per cent, 28.1 per cent, 25.3 per cent and 24.2 per cent respectively with regards to female. These researchers justified that the lower rates of male cases are due to the under-reporting (Noemí *et al.*, 2009). WHO (2016) indicated that girls are subjected to sexual violence in the situation like armed conflict and refugee settings by militaries, combatants, their community members, and helping workers.

India is leading in the world with the maximum of CSA cases reported (Human Rights Watch, 2013). Childline Organization (2014) stated that minors are being exploited sexually before they reach their 10th year and have beastly abused at every 13th hour. A survey conducted by United Nations International Children Education Fund (UNICEF; Ray, 2014) in India from the period of 2005 to 2013, articulated that during the age range between 10-14 years, nearly 10 per cent girls have been brutally abused and in their age of 15-19 years the abuse rate had been escalated to 30 per cent. Ray (2014) also noted that around 42 per cent of the preteen girls in India have travelled the traumatic path of sexual violence.

Children's Vulnerability to Sexual Abuse

Concern for the victims of sexual assault has become a national priority only during recent times. The problems of child and adolescents victims have been largely unaddressed. Sexual abuse does not occur due to the traits presents in the child but rather due to the inhuman trait present in the perpetrator. Let's us try to understand why some children are more susceptible to this heinous crime and found themselves in a situation where they have felt they had to or wanted to, engage in sexual acts with an adult or older person. One of the plausible reasons is grooming.

Grooming

Grooming is the preparatory process in which the targeted child is being primed for sexual abuse. Mostly, it requires vigilant planning and it usually takes weeks, month or even year to mould the target. Grooming is about convincing a child to indulge in the sexual acts with the offender by building a relationship and emotional connection.

There are various forms which the offender uses to lure the child towards him. Some of these are the following:

- They target a victim who is deprived of affection, self-confidence and forces them in an emotional relationship by giving pretentious care to them.
- The sex offenders gain trust by becoming a dominant figure in the family by taking important decisions and by convincing the child that he is the only person who s/he can trust.
- One of the most menacing aspects of grooming is how it tries to take the child to the desolated place where he can get access to the child alone.
- Cyber grooming or cyber molestation has become a prospective opportunity for grooming as it happens without the consent of the adult's compliance.

Identifying a groomed child: One of the major steps to prevent CSA is to identify the child who is at the possible risk of grooming. A child who is being groomed behaves in such a way which disguises their internal problems. The groomed child often shows the following symptoms:

- Staying isolated, quiet, and reserved
- Does not feel comfortable is discussing about problems
- Develop mistrust in closed ones
- Noticing new clothes, accessories and expensive gadgets which was not provided to them by family
- Staying online and on phone either texting or talking for more than his/her usual time.
- The victim might develop a habit of stealing money to manage his or her expenses.
- These are the few signs which should be tracked carefully.

The Problem of Disclosure

Mostly, children do not disclose abuse directly after they have been sexually abused. The hesitancy to unveil abuse emerges from a terror of the perpetrator who has threatened by saying: "If you tell anyone I will kill you/kill your mother". The "child sexual abuse accommodation syndrome", suggested by Ronald C. Summit, has been raised by several researchers and they tried to explore the reason behind children's disclosures which are often delayed after the abuse and it becomes very difficult to get retracted.

There are innumerable reasons why the victim does not choose to disclose. The victim often feels confined and helpless as the offender continuously threatens him or her that he might cause harm to his family members or closed ones. The victim also instils the fear that nobody will believe the disclosure of abuse and s/he might become the talk of the town. Researchers have also examined that at times negative consequences are often being followed by disclosure which included: becoming the gossip, causing a crack between the family members where the offender is himself familial (Hunter, 2011; Jonzon & Lindblad, 2004; Ullman, 2007). Research reveals that as few as 8.3 per cent of children disclosed sexual abuse in formal (e.g. forensic) settings close to the occurrence of such abuse (Priebe & Svedin, 2008). Disclosure is a process rather than being a single event as it may take upto several years to respond. When the victim does disclose it is mainly to someone trustworthy to him.

In our society, disclosure is taken to be a positive thing and to encourage the same active engagement of closed ones, teachers, and friends are needed to foster such booming silence and create a conducive surrounding for the victims to speak their mind. Another major cause which was found to be the socio-economic status of the family which adds an extra layer of exposure for the offenders to assault the child sexually whilst their parents is at their work to earn their living.

Impact of Child Sexual Abuse

The immediate effects after sexual abuse are very depilating as it rifts off the self-confidence, self-esteem and a sense of powerlessness. Suicidal ideation and depression are the most commonly noticed in the victims of abuse. They constantly deal with the fear of being re-victimization which compels them to stay isolated and develop trust issues with the closed ones.

These impacts results in psychological, interpersonal, intrapersonal and behavioural abnormalities. Some of the effects are short-lived while most have a long term effects which continue till they reach adulthood. Victims of CSA are often found to have issues with self-esteem, clinical depression, panic attacks and flashbacks of the atrocious act. Few of them falls in the trap of substance abuse, eating disorder and self-harm practices. (American Academy of Child and Adolescent Psychiatry, 2004; American Academy of Paediatrics, 2006; Child Welfare Information Gateway, 2006; Elliot, 2001; Hopper, 2006).

Survivors of CSA are often found to be dealing with self-blame, self-doubt, and guilt. They often report having negative beliefs about self and surface defaming self-image. Also, the victims fail to sustain effective and significant interpersonal relationships. They lose the ability to sustain their interpersonal relationship which disturbs the home environment and are afraid to form sexual relationship with their partners which results in increased rates of separation and divorce (Mullen & Fleming, 2006). The effect of the abuse is so tormenting that it affects the formation of the personality. Subsequently, counselling intervention for the victim and his/her family turns out to be imperative. The isolation and stigmatization of CSA generate feelings of not belonging and a sense of being different. Fear of intimacy and an inability to trust can manifest in general social relationships.

The manifestation of behavioural effects often arises as social norm infringements. Victims are stated to exhibit increased rate of academic issues along with conduct problems. According to reports of Darkness to Light (2001-2005) and Rape and Sexual Abuse Centre (2002) victims are more susceptible to become expectant of a baby before becoming an adult. Self-harm, self-mutilation and suicidal ideation are associated with CSA and other self-destructive behaviour such as eating disorder, substance abuse and a range of addictive behaviours. Obsessive compulsive behaviours are seen frequently in adult survivors indulging in checking, counting and washing to ward off feelings.

The long term effects of abuse have a detrimental effect on the psychological and physical health of the victim which has been widely discussed in the literature. The physical health issue includes gastrointestinal disorders like irritable bowel syndrome, abdominal pain, gynaecological abnormalities like irregular menstrual cycle and somatization which is in regard to bodily discomforts. The psychological abnormalities which could also be seen in victims are clinical depression, anxiety attacks, flashbacks of the dreadful incidents which may lead to PTSD, inappropriate sexual behaviour, distorted cognition, addiction to alcohol/cocaine and insecurities about one's own body.

Screen the Victims of Child Sexual Abuse

Screening is the most important part in identifying child who is sexually abused and maltreated. Though it does not intend to be diagnostic but it provides a base for identifying the victims who might have serious issues. The report of his or her parents, immediate acquaintance and the victims is an essential document for further investigations and treatment. Child Behaviour Checklist 6–18 (CBCL; Achenbach & Rescorla, 2001) and the Child Sexual Behaviour Inventory (Friedrich, 1997) are the two most widely used screening tools used for the same but the tests have been found to have low reliability. Therefore, a proper combination of screening and intervention is a must for the better screening of the CSA victims.

Protection and Rehabilitation of Child

Standing against the sexual exploitation of children is a familial and social responsibility. Not only the parents but also the society as well as professional working with children (e.g. teachers, primary healthcare workers etc.) need to be informed about the issue and to be trained to be more vigilant about such issue and engage themselves in spreading awareness. It is also highly suggestive of psychotherapists to psychoeducate the victims, parents and their close ones about the abuse and its deadly consequences and take measurable steps to act effectively with the situation. Psychotherapists should also communicate to children to become more empathetic, compassionate and, the importance of consent.

Counselling and Social Support

Though it's imperative to establish a therapeutic rapport with the patient in the few initial medical assessments the victims might not feel comfortable in discussing about their abuse experiences to the practitioners at the first place. Further assessments are required to dig deep into the issue and proper diagnosis are been made. As the victims are already engrossed in fear of the accused ones it becomes very difficult for them to agree for counselling sessions. Therefore, the task of a counsellor is very challenging to engage the victims in this process. It is vital for the victims to gradually indulge them in talking about their unresolved worries and cope with the fears. Effective treatment strategies and suitable techniques like trauma-focused cognitive behaviour therapy, safe place technique, play therapy, bibliotherapy, and comfort kit are proven to be successful in handling cases of child sexual abuse. Counselling should be delivered in combination with similar services provided by schools and other community groups, who act as a co-therapist. In the initial phase, supportive therapy should be provided to victim as it becomes difficult for them to receive any sort of intervention. Mindfulness-based cognitive behavioural treatment is considered to be anoperative form of therapy for post-traumatic stress reactions which is given when the victims are normalized and ready for further intervention. Along with diagnosed psychiatric disorder, many victims have found to have comorbid conditions that also entail specific treatment.

Conclusion

Sexual abuse is a concomitant of adverse consequences and depilating effect for survivors throughout their lifetime. The victims found the offenders to be a monster who has taken away all their happiness and left within the pool of hopelessness, fear, and powerlessness. To date, CSA has been found to strongly correlated with the presence of depression, eating disorder, dissociation, alcohol and substance abuse and anxiety-related issues. The key constraint which the CSA survivors find is the delayed disclose which happens due to the unavailability of a supportive environment to access the effective services and to deal with the experiences and all its effects.

Although CSA is faced by children of both the genders, the girls are targeted more often than boys. It has been observed that the sexual exploitation depends on the socioeconomic status, children living in joint/

extended family, and multiple caregiving of children, street children, lack of recreational facilities and opportunities for families and other swarm of factors. Furthermore, law administrations must be executed to safeguard children from all kinds of exploitation and abuses. Also, NGOs and government officials should play a larger role to protect the victims from the heinous trap of the perpetrators. Additionally, counselling is imperative for the victims of child sexual abuse, their families the offenders.

References

Achenbach T.M., Rescorla L.A. (2001), *Manual for the ASEBA School-Age Forms and Profiles*. Burlington, VT: University of Vermont, Research Center for Children, Youth and Families.

American Academy of Child and Adolescent Psychiatry (2004). *Child Sexual abuse* [*Facts for Families*]. Retrieved November 2, 2006, from http://www.aacap.org/

American Academy of Paediatrics. (2006). *What is Child Sexual Abuse*? Retrieved November, 19, 2006, from http://www.medem.com/MedLB/article_detaillb.cfm?article_ID=ZZZ1LW3YA7C

Breaking the Silence. *Child sexual abuse in India*. USA, Humans Rights Watch. 2013. [Last cited on 2014 Aug 09]. Available from: http://www.hrw.org/sites/default/files/reports/india0113ForUpload.pdf.

Child Welfare Information Gateway (2007). *Recognizing Child Abuse and Neglect: Signs and Symptoms*. Retrieved November 7, 2006, from http://www.childwelfare.gov/pubs/factsheets/signs.cfm

Childline Organisation. Childline 1098 service. [Last cited on 2014 Aug 20]. Available from: http://www.childlineindia.org.in/1098/1098.htm.

Darkness to Light (2001-2005). *Statistics*. Retrieved September 22, 2006, from http://www.darkness2light.org/KnowAbout/statistics_2.asp

Elliot, M. (2001). *Why My Child? A Guide for Parents of Children who have been Sexually Abused*. London: Kidscape. Retrieved October, 25, 2004 from http://www.kidscape.org.uk

Friedrich, W.N. (1997). *Child Sexual Behaviour Inventory: Professional Manual*. Odessa, FL: Psychological Assessment Resources.

Hopper, J. (2006). *Child Abuse: Statistics, Research and Resources*. Retrieved November 29, 2006, from http://www.jimhopper.com/abstats

Hunter, S.V. (2011). "Disclosure of child sexual abuse as a life-long process: Implications for health professionals". *Australian and New Zealand Journal of Family Therapy*, *32*(2): 159-172.

Jonzon, E. and Lindblad. F. (2004). "Disclosure, reactions and social support: Findings from a sample of adult victims of child sexual abuse". *Child Maltreatment 9*(2): 190-200.

Kacker L, Mohsin N, Dixit A. (2007). *Study on Child Abuse: India 2007*. New Delhi: Ministry of Women and Child Development, Government of India.

Mullen, P.E. and Fleming, J. (2006). *Long-term Effects of Child Sexual Abuse*. [*National Child Protection Clearinghouse*.] Retrieved November 8, 2006, from http://www.aifs.gov.au/nch/issues9.html

Noemí, P., Georgina, G., Maria, F. and Juana, G.B. (2009). "The prevalence of child sexual abuse in community and student samples: A meta-analysis", *Clinical Psychology Review*, *29*(4), 328-338. doi-10.1016/j.cpr.2009.02.007.

Priebe, G. and Svedin, C.G. (2008). "Child sexual abuse is largely hidden from the adult society: An epidemiological study of adolescents' disclosures". *Child Abuse and Neglect*, *32*(12), 1095-1108.

Rape and Sexual Abuse Center (2002), *Education Statistics*. Retrieved November 29, 2006, from http://www.rasac/education/statistics.html

Ray, A. 42% of Indian girls are sexually abused before 19: Unicef. *The Times of India*. 2014 (Sep. 12). Available from: http://timesofindia.indiatimes.com/india/42-of-Indian-girls-are-sexually-abused-before-19-Unicef/articleshow/42306348.cms?

Reid, S., Reddock, R., Nickenig, T. (2014). "Breaking the silence of child sexual abuse in the Caribbean: A community-based action research intervention model". *Journal of Child Sexual Abuse*, *23*(3), 256–277

Ullman, S.E. (2007). "Relationship to perpetrator, disclosure, social reactions and PTSD symptoms in child sexual abuse survivors". *Journal of Child Sexual Abuse*, 16 (1), 19-36.

World Health Organization. Geneva: World Health Organization, *Child Sexual abuse; 2003. Child sexual abuse. Guidelines for medicolegal care for victims of sexual violence*. Available from: Whqlibdoc.who.int/publications/2004/924154628x.pdf

24

Techie to Techno-addict

Uncovering the Veiled Switch in Children

Aishwarya Jaiswal, Tushar Singh and *Yogesh Kumar Arya*

Case One: Shruti, 16, was an easygoing and extrovert girl who became a school dropout after getting addicted to social networking sites. She started spending nearly seven hours a day online, chatted with over 350 online friends, found face-to-face interactions traumatic and on being reprimanded, resorted to lying and theft to visit Internet cafes.

Case Two: Rahul, 14, was a high achiever, and excelled academically, before getting absorbed in Massively Multiplayer Online Role-Playing Games. He began to habitually outstretch more than 16 hours a day in contending with other gamers online, losing most of his social skills to his gaming addiction. Similarly, Rohit Nagpal (name changed), a Delhi boy, class topper till class XI, hasn't been able to clear class XII for the last three years after he started playing games online. In an anomalous case, two brothers aged 22 and 19, engineering and a class XII student, started to sleep intermittently, stopped studying, changing clothes, attending to phone calls or doorbell, or having a bath. They came physically and socially dysfunctional to the extent of urinating and defecating in their clothes while playing the game online.

Case Three: Riya (name changed), 14, slapped her father. The reason was that he took away her phone on which she spent hours chatting with friends who were available for online chat only. She told the counselor that without her phone she had no life.

> **Case Four:** A Bengaluru man, 26, unemployed, started to access a streaming platform to relieve himself of financial, familial and societal pressures. The binge-watching soon turned compulsive, and he started spending around 7 hours a day streaming videos which disturbed his physiological functioning and circadian rhythm. He has become the first case of reported Netflix addiction in India.

Similar cases are being reported from across the globe, giving a clear indication that getting glued to technology isn't any more limited by region or age. One of the weirdest examples is that where a 3-month-old South Korean girl starved to death after her parents went on a 12-hour playing binge.

After having read these instances, take a moment and think about the following questions:

How much time do you spend browsing the internet, using your mobile device, on Facebook, and so on? Do you lose track of time while doing so? Did you ever try cutting short your technological access? If yes, then were you able to do so? Do you think of online activities even when offline? Has any concern been raised by your family or friends regarding your technological access or gadget use? Have you suffered any physical complications or issues such as sore fingers/thumbs, eye strain, or numbness of extremities, owing to long hours of tech usage? If you have a "Yes" response to most of the statements above, then technological addiction is an issue concerning you as well. Now consider the same questions about your children or children close to you. Do the cases apply to them as well? If it's a "Yes" about the children around you, then, realize the alarming need to limit them (children) from falling prey to the heightening addiction towards technology prevalent in children. Though technology-related unhealthy behaviours and mental health issues affect people of all ages, there unpreceded high prevalence in children and adolescents has made the excessive use of technology, promotion of healthy use of the internet and digital wellness emerging concerns among mental health professionals.

Those mentioned above are just a few of the numerous instances manifesting one or the other form of the so-called "Technological Addiction" that have been reported to the Service for Healthy Use of Technology (SHUT) Clinic of the Bangalore-based psycho-neurological specialized clinic NIMHANS, the Behavioural Addiction Clinic (BAC) of the country's premier medical institute AIIMS and other psychiatric

OPDs that dealt with the technology-related psychological wellness issues and attempted to stop techno-addicts from slipping into severe psychiatric conditions. Though not classified as an official mental health condition in the mental health diagnostic manuals such as DSM-V, technology addiction is a widely acknowledged health and well-being concern globally. Since their inception, both the SHUT and the BAC weekly get around eight or more cases of addiction to gaming, social media, pornography and so on, mostly in school and college students, and in the previous few years have witnessed a two-fold rise in the number of patients visiting them. Smartphones, tablets, PDAs, laptops, music, and gaming devices have become so much of life essential in today's cyber-era that we fail to realize when our urge to use them becomes uncontrollable, or how it starts to impede the functioning of our daily lives.

Technology falls amongst the foremost boredom busters and, has become the easy way out in relieving stress, gaining social lubrication and attaining an effortless breakout from reality. Largely, it's about communication and entertainment, as the majority uses their smartphones and tablets for networking, streaming music, videos, movies and web series, and playing games. In today's information age, it has become the chief source of satisfaction of our insatiable appetite for information and the fulfillment of basic human needs for stimulation and interaction. However, it impacts our brain's pleasure systems in ways resembling alcohol and other psychoactive drugs, and thus in combination to certain altered states—emotional, psychological, social, environmental, and biological—makes us prone to technological dependence—a state where our urge to access technology doesn't remain under our control anymore. This is what marks Technological Addiction. Griffiths (1995) proposed this concept to refer to behavioural addictions, non-chemical in nature but involving strikingly enormous human-machine interaction. The nations more expressly affected include UK, USA, Italy, Korea, China, Japan, India, Taiwan, and Australia.

Internet-equipped gadgets have highly transformed our lives and have raised our dependence on technology for performing everyday routine tasks. For instance, Google Maps for locations and directions, YouTube for learning practically about anything, whether it be yoga, dance, cooking, dancing, painting, science, etc., fitness apps that monitor our health and well-being, streaming platforms such as Netflix, Amazon, etc. to stream videos on demand from anywhere, digital libraries to read books or other written materials online, smartphone apps for entertainment and social interaction such as Facebook and WhatsApp, etc., not only these but apps for almost all functional things such as water and electricity bill payments to accessing bank accounts are available. However, one more significant sphere where technology has of recent found a role is in pacifying the kids via mobile phones and tablets. An easy way out, Right? An easy way to control the kid is to hand over your smartphone to him/her. Isn't it? But those following the practice of simply handing over a smartphone or tablet as a means to pacify the kid fail to realize the repercussions that this habituation to instant gratification could follow (and, probably do follow in most cases!).

The dissonance subsisting between our natural sensitivities and the ultramodern technology has led to a slew of harmful side effects such as reduced attention spans (both short-term and long-term), online social media jealously such as Facebook jealousy that has turned life into a competition for likes and shares, polarization of democracy, impulsive outrage over dialogues and discourses, and also technological addiction —a topic of absolute concern exclusively in regard to growing children. Most people fail to realize that all online sites including social networking sites work on a business model and by utilizing sophisticated methods make all efforts to draw the user's attention and enhance the time they spend accessing the specific sites. Also, they forward all this information to advertisers who target users and attempt at maneuvering the user's behaviour to their advantage. However, most people are unaware of the depth of the issue and fail to realize the invisible problems that continual access to such sites pose for them and their growing children.

Researchers from the University of Hong Kong reported that by 2014 around 420 million people worldwide suffered from one or other forms of internet and technology addictions (Cheng & Li, 2014). Such findings make it apparent that when it comes to technological overuse and addiction, it is prevalent among individuals of all ages and youths are the most vulnerable or 'at-risk' section. The enormity of the issue for children and teens of growing ages is so much that even the Tech Giants, not to mention Apple, Google and Facebook, have been constrained to turn up with solutions that could aid in preventing the amplifying technological addiction amidst kids and adolescents. For instance, the techno giant Apple in January 2018 hinted at introducing parental control features in their products. Similarly, Google in 2015 launched YouTube Kids and in March 2017 announced to launch the Family Link-an application with certain parental control features over the child's first Google account. The social media platform Facebook in 2018 started with prioritizing "meaningful social interactions" over "relevant content". Parent control devices such as Circle with Disney, Torch that doesn't need any app installations have also been introduced.

Around 44 per cent of teens from the UK (Rideout & Robb, 2018) and 50 per cent of the teens from the US (Common Sense Media, 2016) felt addicted to their mobile devices. In the UK while 63 per cent of parents realized their teens techno-addiction, 46 per cent of them admitted that they were smartphone addicts. Close to 50 per cent of teens were found to access their mobile devices right after waking up and close to 80 per cent checked their mobiles at least once an hour. Also, screen-time was found to be amongst the three most frequent source of conflictual parent-teen relationships. It is well-demonstrated that gadget addiction adversely impacts children's cognitive and emotional development. Common Sense reports also found that as the time spent by teens on virtual interaction is at the stake of their face-to-face interaction, they have started to have a lack of focus, empathy, and find face conversations difficult. The glorification of picture-perfect lives and well-toned physiques on online platforms erode children's self-esteem and self-confidence. Screen Education's Teen Smartphone Addiction National Survey (2018) also had similar findings. The survey found that around 35 per cent of teens had more online as compared to real-time interaction with their close friends. Also, 52 per cent of teens remained silent and for long stared their smartphones during actual socialization. Children and teens who are still to attain majority are, at most times, unable to curb their technological usage and end up with technological dependence and deteriorated physical and psychological health issues. Twenge, Joiner, Rogers, and Martin (2018) found that teenagers who accessed electronic devices for more than 5 hours/day were 71 per cent more likely to undergo suicidal risk factors compared to the teens whose access was limited to just an hour. Eighth graders who spent most of their time accessing social media were found to be at 27 per cent more risk of depression than their counterparts (Twenge, 2017). As per Bankmycell reports (2019), 67 per cent of teachers found that mobile devices had a negative and distracting effect on students and, teens who spend 5 hours a day on electronic devices are 51 per cent more likely than their low use counterparts, to get under 7 hours of sleep. On the issue of who was responsible for a child's phone use, most parents (89% of all those surveyed) blamed themselves and the caregivers, while 5 per cent assigned the blame to children and 3 per cent to the device/app manufacturers. While 47 per cent of parents accepted their child's smartphone addiction, only half (50%) of them were concerned about the impact such addiction had on their child's mental health.

India is no exception to rising techno-addiction. Online media with round-the-clock and on-the-go facilities led to a 58 per cent hike, from 2016 to 2018, in the time spent by Indians in watching videos online, which is far higher than the global average for the same (Limelight Networks, 2018). The same reports revealed that while amongst western nationals' computer is the most preferred video viewing device, consumers from eastern nations (including India) preferred smartphones. A report (NDTV, 2018) indicated that AIIMS saw a two-fold rise in patients with internet addiction. Psychiatrists operating in varied specialty clinic across the nation commonly hold that two out of every 10 children who visit them suffer distress and behavioural disorganization owing to internet and gaming addiction, and are developing severe psychiatric problems. In a case report published in the *International Journal of High-Risk Behaviours and Addiction*, Sachdeva and Verma (2015) held that in spite of deep-knit family systems and parental supervision, online gaming is an evolving epidemic even in the Indian subcontinent and its access shall be restricted.

Major Techno-based Addictions

As per the Bank my cell reports, the popular drivers triggering technological addiction include—social media networks, internet pornography, information overexposure, shopping, relationship-driven content, dating apps, cybersex, gambling, etc. (Turner, 2018). The most pervasive technological addictions among youth globally, are Gadget Addiction, Internet Addiction, and Social Networking Addiction.

Gadget Addiction: Addiction to gadgets counts amongst the 21st century's major non-drug addictions. Gadgets like cell phones, smart phones, tablets, laptops, I-pads, etc. are generally accessed for communication, entertainment, movies, music, game playing, shopping, browsing educational materials, etc. Gadget addiction involves the use/ abuse of gadgets to an extent that it starts to bear negative consequences for one's health and overall quality of life. A report by Flurry, prepared by analyzing data from 5 lakh applications from over 1.3 billion mobile devices worldwide, affirmed that over a single year there was a jump of 123 per cent in the count of mobile addicts across the globe (Khalaf, 2014). Around 50 per cent of teens in the United States admitted their addiction to their mobile devices (Wallace, 2016). B2X Care Solutions in their global survey, 2014, affirmed that 83 per cent of Indians keep their smartphones close to their body, or better to say within their reach throughout the day.

The same survey reported 98 per cent of Indians to be sleeping with their smartphones kept next to them.

Internet Addiction: Internet Addiction Disorder or iDisorder or Pathological Internet Use or Problematic Internet Use or Compulsive Internet Use is an impulse control disorder where the user feels compelled to access the internet, whether it be for email, networking, gaming, shopping or pornography, to the extent that over a prolonged period their daily life functioning is hampered. For instance, they find it difficult to differentiate virtual reality from actual reality. Young (2011) held Internet-based gaming, gambling, infidelity, pornography, cyber sexual activities, information overload, and compulsive buying to be the sub-types of online addiction. The sub-type Internet Gaming Disorder is enlisted in DSM-5 (APA 2013) as a "Condition for Further Study". Internet World Stats reported the existence of 4.15 billion internet users worldwide, which constitutes nearly 54.4 per cent of the world population in 2018. A multinational meta-analysis on internet addiction showed that the global prevalence estimate of this addiction is 6 per cent (Cheng & Li, 2014). Dissatisfaction with life, pollution and traffic time are positive while the quality of life is a negative correlate of internet addiction. China and South Korea have enlisted internet and video game addiction amongst their significant public health issues. Statista Reports published in 2019 held that the number of active gamers worldwide was 2.3 billion in 2018, and this number is predicted to rise to more than 2.7 billion people in 2021. A cross-disciplinary survey conducted in the US, 2017, involving students (average age 23 years) found 10.3 per cent of them fell in the range of cybersex addiction (19% of men and 4% of women) (Giordano & Cashwell, 2017). As per Psychology Today reports (mentioned in Schuster, 2016), approximately 8 to 11 per cent of Americans suffer from a shopping addiction. The Internet and Mobile Association of India (IAMAI) reports published at the end of the financial year 2019 held that India is second in the world in terms of internet usage and 66 million out of the 451 active internet users fall in the age bracket of 5-11 years. A market research agency Kantar IMRB has predicted the number of internet users in India to reach around 627 million in 2019. The report titled "Digital India–Technology to Transform a Connection Nation' by McKinsey Global Institute (Kaka, 2019) has predicted that India will see a rise of about 40 per cent in its internet users by 2023 while those using smartphones would also double. As internet penetration is increasing, a vigilance over internet usage of children. Zimbardo, the noted Stanford psychologist in his book '*Man Disconnected*' held that online gaming is taking such a toll on adolescents and youths mental health that it could someday lead to the real Fall of Man.

Social media addiction: It involves an excessive and compelled availing of online social media, be it Facebook, Twitter, Instagram, Snapchat or any other online networking site, in a way that one's real-life and relationships are held at stake. Social networking has become the main means of communication among adolescents. The number of social media users worldwide is anticipated to reach around 2.77 billion by 2019, and that of monthly active users is estimated to be around 3.02 billion by 2021. As these estimated numbers roughly reckon a third of the entire populace of Earth, the paramountcy of online social media becomes well evident. Newport Academy cited that in the United States 24 per cent of teenagers remained almost continually online the entire day and, 76 per cent of them engaged in one or more social networking platforms (Monroe, 2017). In 2013, the count of active Facebook users in India was 63692540 million, and about 30474220 million of them fell in the age range of 18 to 24 years (Social Bakers, 2013). As per McKinsey reports, the average time spent by an Indian social media user on any social platform weekly is around 17 hours and this is more than their counterparts in China and the USA (Kaka, 2019).

Causes and Risk Factors

The explicit dynamics behind youth getting glued to technology couldn't be unfolded as the causes are many and multifarious. But, some of the most prominent causes and/or factors that further the risk of technological overuse include: the ubiquitous presence of web-equipped text-messaging, social media-enabled technology, easy accessibility of internet-based applications on computers, laptops, tablets, smartphones and watches, generation of huge personally-relevant information at unprecedented speeds, provision of an escape from reality, facilitation of stress and anxiety alleviation, provision of a sense of competence, provision of a sense of autonomy, provision of a sense of connectivity, and triggering of brain's reward center that flushes the individual being with mood-regulating neurotransmitters and hormones such as dopamine, serotonin, and adrenaline appertaining upon the level of activity. Any contingent mental or behavioural health issues such as anxiety, depression, Attention Deficit Hyperactivity Disorder (ADHD), lowered self-esteem, negative self-image and self-concept, and troubled real-life situations such as lack of familial support and poor home environment also contribute significantly.

Neurochemistry of Addiction

The sudden advent and spread of technology, in addition to being advantageous in varied regards, has also posed fresh challenges for classical addictology by making huge adolescent and pre-adolescent populations prone to technological addiction. Concerning internet addiction, Tereshchenko and Kasparov (2019) opined that each specific case of addiction results from a combination of inherited characteristics and extra-environmental factors. The inherited characteristics might include neuro-mediator and neuroreceptor activities, hormonal secretions, nervous tissue structure, bodily degradations, etc., while extra-environmental factors might count the familial backdrop, social functioning, and cultural factors.

In explaining the science behind techno-based addictions, Nir Eyal in 2014 came up with a Hooked Model. He explains that we run through four stages—trigger, action, reward and investment on accessing any online platform, and these in conjunction push an individual into the spiral of addiction. Internal trigger can be a feeling of boredom, the action that follows is the logging in on any app, the photos, comments, likes, gossip, news, emotions, laughter, etc. offered by that particular app are the rewards and all these results in repeated investments into the app or products/services/advertisements prompted and promoted by that app. Also, these activities lead to altered dopaminergic activity that in turn affects the brain's reward and punishment centers. The heightened level of neurochemical dopamine leads to increased reward recognition, motivation, excitement, goal fulfillment, reinforcement and a sense of pleasure, while low dopamine levels relate to a sense of boredom, a tendency towards procrastination, and lowered enthusiasm and self-confidence. As repeated accessing of technology-facilitated boredom-busting mediums such as smartphone apps leads to lowered dopamine secretion compared to initial exposures, also the rewards such as "likes" that earlier felt rewarding don't appear so anymore. These potentially lead to an amplified craving for reward and non-receipt of which leads to anxiety, depression and other negative consequences very similar to those suffered by alcohol addicts. A sort of "rewiring" occurs in the brain and the individual's overall homeostasis is affected.

Consequences and Risks

The detrimental payoffs that technological overuse, abuse and addiction hold for youth necessitate a need to look into and resolve the issue of unhealthy technological access. Some of the major problems associated with techno-addiction include the following:

***Somatic Problems**:* Addicts suffer from sleep disturbances, increased dopaminergic activity, and dopamine down-regulation, and lowered levels of norepinephrine (Zhang *et al.*, 2013) that make them prone to depression and low blood pressure. Cardiovascular diseases, dietary complications, obesity, increased weight on the spine, along with deficits in memory and learning skill have also been observed. All these bear a long-term impact on the addict's mental health. Vision-related problems such as strain, irritation, dryness, reduced blink rate, and blurred vision are increasingly becoming common in very young age children. Functional vision problems especially near-sightedness has raised at an enhanced frequency in Americans (The National Eye Institute, 2017). Long-term damage to the retina is posed by the blue light, or high-energy visible (HEV) light wavelengths that are commonly emitted by most digital screens these days. About 15 per cent of Americans suffer hearing difficulties due to exposure to loud sounds via earbuds (The National Institute of Deafness and Other Communication Disorders, 2017).

Neuroanatomical Changes: Technological addiction is known to alter the brain's overall volume by shrinking the gray and white matter fibers that affect emotional processing and brain functioning. Neural abnormalities such as atrophies in the dorsolateral prefrontal cortex are likely. Functional changes are apparent in the brain areas such as the prefrontal cortex associated with performing executive and higher cognitive functions like anticipation, judgment, planning, and decision-making, personality development, and social behaviour moderation. Also, cortical (e.g., temporal) regions that process memories, integrate them with sensations of taste, sound, sight and touch, and subcortical (e.g., ventral striatum) regions which form critical components of brain's reward system, and regulate reward, motivation, and decision-making processes are also affected. Dysfunctions in these regions implicated in a broad range of psychiatric disorders, from depression to drug addiction.

Mental and Emotional Health issues: Mood swings, fatigue, stress, and depression are likely. Addicts are at risk of developing Nomophobia- the irrational fear of being aloof from cellular network or phone. Negative intellectual functions such as short-term memory loss and cognitive dysfunctions such as impaired working memory become observable. Young sufferers of this addiction are at an elevated risk of suffering from attentional problems, loneliness, violent tendencies, aggression, suicidal thoughts, delinquent behaviour, and can develop disorders like Attention Deficit Hyperactivity Disorder (ADHD), Oppositional Defiant Disorder (ODD), teen depression, loneliness, and anxiety. Too much technology can also lead to dangerous conditions like psychosis and neurosis, or surfacing of narcissistic and self-absorption traits. Also, gadget-addiction leads to a common memory disorder—digital dementia.

Relationship and other issues: Technology over users suffer from intimacy issues, social phobia, and social isolation. They display attention-seeking behaviour and are more prone to cyberbullying and technology-facilitated abuse. Deteriorated academic, athletic, and social performance, school absenteeism, lowered grades, academic failure, school dropout, distraction, fatalities and worsened close relationships are probable. Their socialization pattern is also disrupted and children find themselves unable to cope with stressful situations. It has been observed that in most cases children find difficulties differentiating lived and alternate realities, and also develop a sedentary lifestyle.

Signs and Symptoms of Technological Addiction

The warning signs and symptoms, both behavioural and physical, that the guardians and care-takers shall check to prevent the surfacing of tech-addition in their children have been enlisted below.

Behavioural Symptoms: The associated behavioural symptoms incorporate the following:

- losing appeal for activities not involving technological gadgets
- being obsessed with thoughts of technological experiences
- abandoning real-life friends and happenings to focus on online activities or virtual world,
- feeling euphoric while surfing the Web,
- frequently uploading photos, images or "selfies" and making status updates on social networking sites,
- compulsively checking messages online
- feeling drowsy all through the day and falling asleep while in school
- deceiving when enquired about gadget usage
- abandoning of other social groups (clubs or sports, etc.) and withdrawing from social activities
- lengthily devoting time online despite contravening repercussions alike problems at school, lowered performance, impaired

relationships, and health botherations
- spending much of their non-school duration on the computer system or in playing video games
- experiencing frustration, anxiety, irritability and/or restlessness on being unable to have tech accessibility.

Physical Symptoms: The tech-addiction associated physical symptoms include the following:

- headache
- neck and back pain
- dry eyes and vision problems
- sleep disturbances, especially insomnia
- poor nutrition
- poor personal hygiene
- carpal tunnel syndrome .

Challenging Technological Addictions

Preventive efforts are pivotal in the early and effective curbing of technology-related adverse fallouts. Some of them include: skipping morning digital check-ins, delimitating online availability, curbing instant web search for everything, balancing activity and productivity, and nurturing pro-social identity in the real world. In case of young age children, parents could help in cubing addiction by adopting simple measures like: enforcing house rules on the duration of gadget or internet usage, installing the computer system in the living room, providing children with alternative socializing enterprises, improving parent-child relationship and family functioning, and making available familial and social support. Self-help tips for children and helpful ways that parents could utilize to reduce their child's technological dependence have been detailed further.

Self-Help Tools for Preventing Technological Addictions

In attempting to break technological addiction, firstly a realization of the habits that trigger and cause addiction is needed. It should then be followed by working upon those triggers (e.g. daily stress, academic pressure, boredom) by finding better alternatives to them. Self-awareness is the best way to overcome gadget addiction. Those with excessive technological abuse shall take control of their digital lives with the aid of better tools and habits. Tim Elmore (2014) suggested some self-help ways for students to adopt a balanced approach towards smartphone usage. They are: (1) Make daily times when your cell phone is switched off; (2) Try to experience solitude or aim for in-person conversations whenever possible; (3) Try to strike a balance between screen time and face-to-face interaction time; (4) Keep technology fast each month; (5) While sleeping, try to place the cellular device at least 15 feet away from you; (6) Divide the day into time zones, where there are separate blocks for organic and genuine interaction apart from the time to be spent on technological access.

Conclusion

Bringing to a close, technology has an undeniable role in our lives today. It provides a platform for learning, knowledge expansion, creativity and expression, metacognition, communication, and socialization. Notwithstanding this, its overuse holds associated physical, mental and social costs. This necessitates the bearing of a healthy and balanced approach towards technology use. Though the lack of standardized diagnostic criteria makes us unable to discern the true prevalence of technological addiction, it demonstrably leads to multifarious disadvantageous consequences and correlates highly with comorbid psychiatric disorders. Hence, the time is ripe for the proliferation of public awareness on the issue of growing technological addiction among youth and, a multidisciplinary and collaborative approach is required on the part of educational, social, mental health and government agencies to come up with a comprehensive solution towards managing technological addiction in youth.

References

American Psychiatric Association (2013). *Diagnostic and Statistical Manual of Mental Disorders* (DSM-5®). American Psychiatric Pub.

Cheng, C. and Li, A.Y. (2014). "Internet addiction prevalence and quality of (real) life: a meta-analysis of 31 nations across seven world regions". *Cyberpsychology, Behaviour and Social networking*, *17*(12), 755–760. https://doi.org/10.1089/cyber.2014.0317

Common Sense Media (2016). New Report Finds Teens Feel Addicted to Their Phones, Causing Tension at Home. Commonsensemedia.Org.

Elmore, T. (2014, August 26). Curing Students of Nomophobia. HuffPost. https://

www.huffpost.com/entry/curing-students-of-nomoph_b_5710427

Eyal, N. (2014). *Hooked: How to build habit-forming products*. Penguin.

Giordano, A.L. and Cashwell, C.S. (2017). "Cybersex addiction among college students: A prevalence study". *Sexual Addiction and Compulsivity*, *24*(1-2), 47-57.

Griffiths, M.D. (1995). *Adolescent Gambling*. London: Routledge.

Internet Growth Statistics 1995 to 2019—the Global Village Online. (2019). Internetworldstats.Com. https://www.internetworldstats.com/emarketing.htm

Kaka, N. (2019). Digital India: Technology to transform a connected nation.

Khalaf, S. (2014). *The Rise of the Mobile Addict*. Flurry blog.

Limelight Networks. (2018). THE STATE OF ONLINE VIDEO 2018. https://www.limelight.com/resources/white-paper/state-of-online-video-2018/

Monroe, J. (2017, March 27). Looking for "Likes": Teens and Social Media. Newport Academy. https://www.newportacademy.com/resources/mental-health/teens-social-media-addiction/

National Eye Institute (2017). Myopia: A close look at efforts to turn back a growing problem. https://www.nei.nih.gov/about/news-and-events/news/myopia-close-look-efforts-turn-back-growing-problem

NDTV. (2018, October 9). At AIIMS, Internet Addiction Patients Have Doubled In Last 2 Years. NDTV.Com. https://www.ndtv.com/india-news/visitors-at-aiims-facility-for-internet-addiction-has-doubled-in-2-years-1929505

Rideout, V. and Robb, M.B. (2018). *Social Media, Social Life: Teens reveal their experiences*. San Francisco, CA: Common Sense Media.

Sachdeva, A. and Verma, R. (2015). "Internet gaming addiction: A technological hazard". *International Journal of High Risk Behaviours and Addiction*, *4*(4).

Schuster, D. (2016, August 11). Online shopping has created a whole new breed of addicts. *New York Post*; New York Post. https://nypost.com/2016/08/11/online-shopping-has-created-a-whole-new-breed-of addicts/#:~:text=Psychology%20Today%20reported%20that%20an,lives%20in%20the%20Bay%20Area.

Screen Education (2018). Teen Smartphone Addiction National Survey. https://www.screeneducation.org/uploads/1/1/6/6/116602217/teen_smartphone_addiction_national_survey_2018_report_6.21.18_upload_version_1.2.pdf

Social Bakers (2013) Facebook-statistics in India. http://www.socialbakers.com/facebook-statistics/india

Tereshchenko, S., Kasparov, E. (2019). Neurobiological Risk Factors for the Development of Internet Addiction in Adolescents. Behav Sci (Basel). *9*(6):62. Published 2019 Jun 14. doi:10.3390/bs9060062

The National Institute of Deafness and Other Communication Disorders, (2017). U.S. adults aged 20 to 69 years show signs of noise-induced hearing loss. (2017, February 7). https://www.nidcd.nih.gov/news/2017/us-adults-aged-20-69-years-show-signs-noise-induced-hearing-loss

Turner, A. (2018, June 4). Smartphone Addiction and Cell Phone Usage Statistics in 2019. BankMyCell. https://www.bankmycell.com/blog/smartphone-addiction/

Twenge, J.M. (2017). IGen: Why today's super-connected kids are growing up less rebellious, more tolerant, less happy--and completely unprepared for adulthood--and what that means for the rest of us. Simon and Schuster.

Twenge, J.M., Joiner, T.E., Rogers, M.L. and Martin, G.N. (2018). "Increases in depressive symptoms, suicide-related outcomes and suicide rates among US adolescents after 2010 and links to increased new media screen time". *Clinical Psychological Science*, *6*(1), 3-17.

Wallace, K. (2016). Half of teens think they're addicted to their smartphones. CNN, Turner Broadcasting.

Young, K. (2011). *Internet Addiction A Handbook and Guide to Evaluation and Treatment.*

Zhang, H.X., Jiang, W.Q., Lin, Z.G., Du, Y.S. and Vance, A. (2013). "Comparison of psychological symptoms and serum levels of neurotransmitters in Shanghai adolescents with and without internet addiction disorder: a case-control study". *PloS One*, *8*(5), e63089.

25

Increasing Strength in Children

The Role of Counselor in School Setting

Aradhana Shukla

Introduction

The role of guidance and counseling in school setting can not be denied. It plays a leading role in the harmonious development and future progress of the child. Counseling is based on the fact that it is a transformative process of helping/assisting people to learn those issues which are learnt in and out of the schools and are necessary for personality development. It is the job of a counselor to guide and suggest the device to the needy ones and help to develop them in all walks of life. In this paper an attempt has been made to describe the role and need of the counselor in school setting.

Guidance and counseling are two streams but two sides of a coin. Guidance refers to help the students to provide them overall development (Lei Yeugn, 2014; Gysbers & Handerson, 1994; Yuen, 2006), while counselling suggests the optimum solution of any problem with operational process and significance of the suggestion. Guidance is vast but counselling is problem foucused. Akinade (2012) has defined guidance and counseling as, "a process of helping an individual become fully aware of his/her self and the ways in which he is responding to the influences of his her environment. It further assists him to establish some personal meaning for this behaviour and to develop and classify a set of goals and values for future behaviour."

Guidance and counseling are considered as a major educational devices that can change the child's mind from negative direction (planted by peers or any body else) to positive ones. This changing of the mind and persisting it till a long time needs a well-trained, skill handed and acceptable conservationist who can take this big responsibility on his/ her shoulders and can solve the matter. That is why the school counselor is regarded as a role model by the students. It is the duty and ethics of a counselor to listen the child carefully, be empathetic, be unconditional and offer guidance and counseling to the needy one. Egbo (2013) has stated that "the total development of a child can only take place in an environment conducive for teaching and learning." Truly speaking, all educational services promoting teaching and learning in schools are designed by curriculum planners and policy makes so, it can be said that guidance and counseling services in schools shall develop, assess and improve educational programmes, enhance teaching and inculcate the competence of teaches and reduce thc unhealthy relationship of children.

In accordance with Oviogbodu (2015) counseling is involved more in more dependent on personalized feelings like emotions and feelings, value, attitudes and it is dependent on client-counselor relationship and trust (Geshinde, 1991).

In this way it can said that counseling is a definite and structural permissive relationship which allows the client to gain and understanding to himself to a degree which enables him to take positive steps in the light of his new orientations. It needs to be pointed out that counseling interview is a person to person relation in which one individual with problem and needs turns to another person for assistance. Counseling aims to:

- provide self-knowledge and awareness
- develop a sense of self-acceptance
- develop social harmony
- provide realization of students potentials
- develop children to solve their problem by own self
- help in school curriculum construction and development
- help in reciprocity building between teacher and taught and
- help the students use outer and additional sources of development.

Although counseling movement in India was appearing in the beginning of psychology in India (Rao, 1991), formal counseling age is not so old. Truly speaking, the relative significance of counseling and its emergence can be termed as vocational guidance in early 1938 (Arulmani, 2007). Short courses on vocational guidance were found available in India since early 1958 (Fuster, 1963; Joneja, 2006), but the emergence of post graduate diploma in guidance and counseling originated recently. Everyday a large group of passed out graduates appears and most of them get them placed in various settings like, educational institutions, HIV/AIDS clinics, psychiatric clinics, psychiatric hospitals, family counseling centres, corporate sectors, family courts, rehabilitation centres, de-addiction centres and so many more (Janardhan & Rayan, 2015).

Counseling is needed to encourage the child for better development and effective teaching.

In 1981 the Lark branch of the Institute of Guidance Counseling presented the job list for a counselor:

1. The counselor counsels individually/in group to the students who are in need or can do better after counseling. He administers psychological prescribed tests or situational measures as per requirements and provides educational and vocational guidance to them.
2. Not only the counselor provides educational or vocational guidance but also helps the needy students to understand and solve their personal, social and emotional problems.
3. The counselor advices the study techniques and suggests to modify the study habits of the students and the teachers of the school are also be benefited by the counselor because they are also suggested to improve their teaching strategies.
4. The counselor does the complete care of the school. Although he is appointed for students counseling yet he takes care of the whole school and helps as per requirement and need.
5. The counselor, not only co-ordinates a school system of pastoral care, but also he enjoys the freedom and flexibility in the organization of counseling activities in accordance with the need of the school.

On the basis of these notions the counselor works in the schools with full zeal and courage and proves him a necessary assets.

Ethics of the counselor: The counselor should do following jobs. They must be followed as per circumstances.

Not to cross the limit: The counselor should always keep it in that mind the every person although a client has his own dignity and privacy so, the way to be more personal and near must be avoided by the counselor. It is the will and wish of the client to expand his limitation for counselor for better counseling.

Not to impose the problem: The counselor should always treat the client as a normal person and counsel him that the problem which he/she (client) is facing are the commonalties of life. Although the counselor thinks and knows the complexity of the problem and he has to make a path to get rid of from them yet it should not be imposed on the client.

Open the doors for the client: It is the job of a counselor to provide all facilities and possibilities to the client following which and adopting any one of them, he can get rid of from the problem. It is not the duty and ethics of a counselor to focus on any possibility specially and force the client to follow.

Complete and detailed record keeping: Counseling is a systematic process which cannot be shaped without proper and complete setup. Therefore, the counselor should always prepare complete record of the client and all necessary information must be kept. On the basis of these complete records the counselor can facilitate the client about the problem later on also and can get help also. Valid and reliable information like, educational, personal, training and grassroots of related problems must be kept in counselors records.

Skillfulness in counseling session: A counselor should be well-trained, skilled and completely well-organized prior to start counseling session. Organization of testing/counseling session, testing devices, testing session and follow-up sessions are the key jobs and duties that a counselor must know and will be well skilled and equipped too. These devices and they should be properly followed by him.

Emotional care and support: It is the first and foremost duty of the counselor to be attentive, supportive and empathetic towards the client. Providing physical care, gestural empathy and care, emotional support, understanding the potentials and ascertaining the client under psychological underpinnings are the important and essential features of the behaviour of a counselor.

Understanding the students: Counseling is not only limited in counseling centres but it is also provides in schools. Students, due to their age, career and other circumstances need counseling more than the other segments of society. During the period of adolescents, which is also termed as, "brain storming period" need regular counseling. So, it comes under the ethics of counselor to watch, guide and counsel the students to maintain their mental health and better future.

Delivery required system: It is also the duty of a counselor to deliver required system to the client like, counseling, consultancy, referral, appraisal, and guidance, placement and collaboration, and referred.

In addition to achieve the best results for the student, the school counselor regularly assesses their progress to determine its impact, inform improvement should in students after school counseling, design and delivery and last prediction, assessment and intervene.

The career of a counselor is very tough. It is not the bed of roses. The counselor faces a lot of challenges and problems in daily course of life. In India the status of a counselor is very pathetic. As psychology is not so popular as it should be. Therefore, the counselor are also not regarded according to their place, role and significance. They do a lot of work and share the curriculum in the school and get a very few time to counsel the students. Moreover, the students do not share the entire problem to the counselor, therefore as a results, counselor finds himself unable to study the children. Also, it is observed that the students sometimes take the suggestions from the other non-psychological resources and this blocks the normal course of counseling. Moreover, it is also noticed that though the counselor must be cognizant about the needs of the students but the neither the school nor the student and his family provide them the pertinent information records so, the counseling process disturbs and it does not bond the mutual relation between the school and the student. Orodho (2013, 2014) and Heyden (2011) stated that teacher's subject matter knowledge, teaching capacity are also the leading factors for the school test development of the child on one side and unnecessary exhibition of the superiority and disturbance of the teachers create a block in the normal course of work for the counselor which is other side of the coin. It is the duty of the teachers to apply their own strategies to the students to increase not only the academic achievement but also to give them better ways to lead a smooth and positive life and use positive coping skills (Goodstein, Nolan and Pfeiffer, 2006). Also, it will help the school counselor.

Problem, Difficulties, Issues and challenges faced by the counselor: In regard to the problems faced by the counselors so many studies have taken place. Bain (2012) studied contemporary issues of school counselors in America and noted that the school counselors face so many challenges related to job description, mental health issue, family and communities, student success, leadership and issues in technology and many more. It disturbs them and blocks the roots of counseling.

Pereira and Rekha (2017) have placed counselor under two types, novice counselor and beginning counselors. Novice counselors are trainee counselors and growing to be therapist. They have many challenges like being self-critical in practice and having troubling reactions to clients (Hell, Sullivan, Knox and Ronnesteaeb, 2007). They experience stress, (Kumary & Baper, 2008; Skovholt & Ronnesteed, 2003) anxiety and counter-transference management (Anasta Siou, 2006). They easily react with negative and undesirable responses because they do not know the seriousness of the session (De Stefano, D'iuso, Blake Fitzpatrick

Drapeau and Chamodraka, 2007). Also, novice counselors face many more difficulties during the sessions (Duggal & Rao, 2016; Skovholt, 2003). Beginning counselor are somewhat superior than novice counselor but they are not well-skilled. In addition, beginning counselor feel more problems as compared to other counselors (Pereira & Rekha, 2017). (Nystul (2003) has identified some common problems of beginning counselors like; focusing on the first issue in a session, overlooking physical or medical issues, wanting to rescue clients from their unhappiness, having like perfectionist, holding unrealistic expectations, getting carried away with the latest technique, getting lost in the counseling process, using inappropriate phrases, having an excessive and uncontrolled desire to help the client, having as excessive need to be liked or favoured, having difficulty in differently between normal and abnormal, being uncertain about self-disclosure and being uncertain about confidentiality. Due to their new experience, they feel nervousness and uncomfortable during sessions and reluctant in job responsibilities (Coreej, 2005; Theriault, Gazzola and Richardson, 2009; Busacca & Wester, 2006). Anagbogu, Nwokolo, Anyamene and Umezylike (2013) studied professional challenges faced by primary school counselors in Nigeria and found that lack of counseling clinic, lack of computers for data storage, unavailability of internet facilities, lack of equipment like tape recorder and other relevant psychological measures, low counselor-client ratio and lack of dedicated time for counseling in the school time table were found as the topmost challenges. Arowolo (2013) noted that secondary school counselor in Nigeria have faced problems like, wrong ideas and misconceptions of school head and other staff, lack of infrastructure, shortage of funds to run the process of counseling smoothly and lack of exposure. Further, Agarwal (2015) stated that psychologists face several challenges like, poor salaries, lack of job opportunity and licensing, lack of awareness in society about psychological issues and many more. Very recently Pereira and Rekha (2017) studied the problems and conditions of counselors in India and they noted that counselors use to face many problems like lack of awareness of counseling among people, inadequate job assignments and salaries, absence of professional border to regulate counseling, lack of network of counselor and mental health professionals for seeking supervision and consultation.

However, the most common and prevalent problems faced by the counselor are as follows:

- Lack of significance of counseling and awareness in people as a result, very few people visit their clinics, even that they need it.

- Psychological disorders and behavioural deformities are considered as very normal so people do not take it seriously. As a results, psychologist and mental health care professional are treated second grade as compared with medical professionals.
- In this time almost all people think and consider psychology near to their door so they think the psychological consultancy as a wastage of time and money. Also, many people think impertinent that they can do their own counseling and do not know the discrepancy between "suggestion" and "counseling". This overspreading tendency of people has made the counselor on the crossroad.
- Financial crisis and meagre salary has created a sense of financial uncertainty in counselors.
- Temporary and/or part time appointment in the schools also creates problem for counselors. Normally the schools appoint the counselors only for one session (maximum 10 months) which makes them economically deprived with insecure future.
- Absence of professional bodies to regulate the functions of counseling properly has also laid its impact on the counselors. They feel alone and helpless.
- Less cooperation from the organizational authorities also creates problem in the field of counseling. They depute them so many other school assignments so that their basic aim of counseling hampers. In addition, the officials do not pay attention on the basic requirements like personal chamber, psychological tools etc. Therefore, proper counseling does not take place. So, there is need of fully equipped infrastructure and support to the counselor.
- Lack of network of counselor and mental health professionals for cooperation and understanding is also an important factor. They seek the cooperation and support from the professional bodies but in vain.
- During counseling, the counselor faces some challenges and dilemma like, will he/she work with the client, under which direction the counseling should be taken place, level and type of interruption, level, frequency and type of enthusiasm, revision of past trauma and traumatic experiences, curiosity of the counselor about the client, confrontation, and time and effort to reach up to the conclusion. These are the main challenges that a counselor faces during the process of counseling and they influence his

ability of counseling. The counselors should keep them in mind and take it in their cognizance while performing daily counseling.

Ways of developing good counseling: There are some ways following which foster the new ways of counseling. It is a message for the counselor. In case, they use, they can make their future better:

- Enhancement of micro skills
- Constant learning
- Improvement in effectiveness
- True understanding of the client
- Empathetic
- Flexible
- Continuous search for new ways of counseling
- Problem-focused nature
- Skillfullness in questioning
- Confrontation
- Good understanding and sensitivity
- Believe the fact, "Every two are not same"
- Making distinction between goals and values
- Avoiding arguments
- Optimistic and supportive.

It is the time bound need and present day learned that a good counselor should develop these attributes in them. They will help them to meet with the needs, demands and expectations of client and establish their role and performance in the world of psychology.

References

Agrawal, G. (2015). "Psychology in India: A career with uncertain opportunities", *Online Journal of Multidisciplinary Research*, *1*(2), 1-7, www.ojmer.in

Akinade, E.A. (2012). *Modern Behaviour Modification, Principles and Practices*, Ibadan: Bright Way Publishers.

Arowolo, D.O. (2013). "Counsellors' perception of problems facing guidance and counselling services in Nigerian schools", *Journal of Education and Practice*, *4*(24). 115-118. http://iiste.org.

Anagbogu, Nwokolo, Anyamene and Umezylike (2013). "Professional challenges to counseling practice in primary schools in Ananbrastate, Nigeria: The way forward", *International Journal of Psychology and Counseling*, 5 (s), 97-103, www.AcademicJournal.org

Arulmani, G. (2007). "Counselling psychology in India: At the confluence of two traditions", *Applied Psychology: An International Review, 56*(1), 69-82.

Bain, S. (2012). "School counselor: A review of contemporary issues", *Research in Higher Education Journal, 18*, 1-7. http://www.Aabri.com.

Busacca, L.A. and Wester, K.L. (2006). "Career concerns of master's level community and school counselor trainees", *The Career Development Quarterly, 55*(12), 179-190.

Cole, Kothari. (2005). *Research Methodology: Methods and Techniques.* Inyata: KWTS Publishers.

Corey, G. (2005). *Theory and Practice of Counselling and Psychotherapy* (6th ed.) Belmont. CA: Thomson Brooks/Cole.

De Stefano, J., D'iuso, N., Blake, E., Fitzpatrick, M., Drapeau, M. and Chamodraka. M. (2007). "Trainees' experiences of impasses in counselling and the impact of group supervision on their resolution: A Pilot study", *Counselling and Psychotherapy Research, 7*(1), 42-47, doi: 10. 1080/14733140601140378

Duggal, C. and Rao, M. (2016). "Challenges Experienced by Novice Counsellors", In S. Sriram (ed.), *Counselling in India,* Singapore: Springer.

Egbo, A.C. (2013). *Development of Guidance and Counselling.* Enugu: Joe Best Publishers.

Fuster, M.J. (1963). "Psychological counselling in India", *Indian Journal of Psychiatry, 5*(1), 39-47. http:/www.indianjpsychiatry.org.

Goodstein, L.D., Nolan, T.M., and Pfeiffer, J.W. (2006). *Applied Strategic Planning: An Introduction. Applied Strategic Planning: A Comprehensive Guide.*

Gysbers, N.C., and Henderson, P. (1994). *Developing and managing your school guidance programme.* Alexandria, V.A.: American Counselling Association.

Heyden, S.M. (2011). *Counseling Children and Adolescents.* Belmont, CA: Brooks.

Hill, C.E., Sullivan, C., Knox, S. and Schlosser, L.Z. (2007). *Becoming Psychotherapists: Experiences of Novice Trainees in a Beginning Graduate Class.* Marquette University e-Publications@Marquette. 1-27, http:// epublications, Marquette.edu.

Janardhan, S. and Rajan, P. (2015). "Closing the credibility gap: Credentialing for counselling professionals in India", *International Journal of Psychosocial Research* (special Issue). 73-77.

Joneja, G.K. (2006). "A follow-up study of trained guidance counsellors", *Journal of the Indian Academy of Applied Psychology*, (32)*3*, 153-170, http:/medind. nic.in.

Kumary, A. and Baker, M. (2008). "Stresses reported by UK trainee counselling psychologists", *Counselling Psychology Quarterly, 2*(1): 19-28, doi: 10. 1080/09515070801895626

Nystul, M.S. (2003). *Introduction to Counselling: An Art and Science Perspective* (2nd ed.) Boston: Allyn & Bacon.

Orodho, A.J. (2013). *Techniques of Writing Proposals and Research Reports in Education and Social Science Research Methods*, Maseno, Kenya: Kanezja Publishers.

Orodho, A.J. (2014). "Policies on free primary and secondary education in East Africa: Are Kenya and Tanzania on course to attain Education for All (EFA) Goals by 2015?", International Organization of Scientific Research (IOSR) *Journal of Humanities and Social Sciences (IOSR-JHSS) 19*(I), 11-20.

Oviogbodu, C.O. (2015). Perceived impact of guidance and counseling in the development of Niger Delta Region. Paper present at Niger Delta University conference with the theme: education and sustainable development in the Niger Delta region of Nigeria. Held at the University Entrepreneur Centre new site Niger Delta University, Wilberforce Island, Amasoma, Bayalsa State Nigeria from 9th-12th August.

Pereira, M. and Rekha, S. (2017). "Problem, difficulties and challenges faced by counsellors", *The International Journal of Indian Psychology*, *4*(3), 65-72.

Rao, N.S. (1991). *Counselling and Guidance* (2nd ed.). New Delhi: Tata McGraw.

Skovholt, T.M. and Ronnestad, M.H. (2003). "Struggles of the novice counselor and therapist", *Journal of Career Development*, *30*(1), 45-58.

Theriault, A., Gazzola, N. and Richardson, B. (2009). "Feelings of incompetence in novice therapists: Consequence, coping, and corrective", *Canadian Journal of Counselling*. 43(2). 105-119. www.mentalhealthacademy.com

Yuen, M. (2002). "Exploring Hong Kong Chinese guidance teachers' positive beliefs: A focus group study", *International Journal for the Advancement of Counselling, 24*, 169–182.

Index